Alzheimer Disease and Other Dementias

Editor

JOHN E. MORLEY

CLINICS IN GERIATRIC MEDICINE

www.geriatric.theclinics.com

November 2018 • Volume 34 • Number 4

ELSEVIER

1600 John F. Kennedy Boulevard • Suite 1800 • Philadelphia, Pennsylvania, 19103-2899

http://www.theclinics.com

CLINICS IN GERIATRIC MEDICINE Volume 34, Number 4
November 2018 ISSN 0749–0690, ISBN-13: 978-0-323-64149-4

Editor: Jessica McCool
Developmental Editor: Laura Fisher

Clinics in Geriatric Medicine (ISSN 0749-0690) is published quarterly by Elsevier Inc., 360 Park Avenue South, New York, NY 10010-1710. Months of issue are February, May, August, and November. Business and Editorial Offices: 1600 John F. Kennedy Blvd., Suite 1800, Philadelphia, PA 191023-2899. Periodicals postage paid at New York, NY, and additional mailing offices. Subscription prices are $278.00 per year (US individuals), $602.00 per year (US institutions), $100.00 per year (US student/resident), $320.00 per year (Canadian individuals), $763.00 per year (Canadian institutions), $195.00 per year (Canadian student/resident), $402.00 per year (international individuals), $763.00 per year (international institutions), and $195.00 per year (international student/resident). Foreign air speed delivery is included in all *Clinics* subscription prices. All prices are subject to change without notice. POSTMASTER: Send address changes to *Clinics in Geriatric Medicine*, Elsevier Health Sciences Division, Subscription Customer Service, 3251 Riverport Lane, Maryland Heights, MO 63043. **Telephone: 1-800-654-2452 (U.S. and Canada); 314-447-8871 (outside U.S. and Canada). Fax: 314-447-8029. E-mail:** journalscustomerservice-usa@elsevier.com **(for print support) or** journalsonlinesupport-usa@elsevier.com **(for online support).**

Reprints. For copies of 100 or more, of articles in this publication, please contact the Commercial Reprints Department, Elsevier Inc., 360 Park Avenue South, New York, New York 10010-1710. Tel.: 212-633-3874; Fax: 212-633-3820, E-mail: reprints@elsevier.com.

Clinics in Geriatric Medicine is covered in *MEDLINE/PubMed (Index Medicus), EMBASE/Excerpta Medica, Current Contents/Clinical Medicine (CC/CM),* and the *Cumulative Index to Nursing & Allied Health Literature.*

Contributors

EDITOR

JOHN E. MORLEY, MB, BCh
Dammert Professor of Gerontology, Director, Division of Geriatric Medicine, Saint Louis University School of Medicine, St Louis, Missouri, USA

AUTHORS

ROULA AL-DAHHAK, MD
Assistant Professor, Department of Neurology, Saint Louis University, St Louis, Missouri, USA

HIDENORI ARAI, MD, PhD
Director, National Center for Geriatrics and Gerontology, Obu, Aichi, Japan

BIRONG DONG, MD, PhD
Professor, The Center of Gerontology and Geriatrics, West China Hospital, Sichuan University, Chengdu, China

SUSAN A. FARR, PhD
Professor, Division of Geriatric Medicine, Saint Louis University School of Medicine, Research and Development Service, VA Medical Center, St Louis, Missouri, USA

GEORGE T. GROSSBERG, MD
Professor of Neurology, Department of Psychiatry and Behavioral Neuroscience, Saint Louis University, St Louis, Missouri, USA

RITA KHOURY, MD
Department of Psychiatry and Behavioral Neuroscience, Saint Louis University, St Louis, Missouri, USA

KOICHI KOZAKI, MD, PhD
Professor, Department of Geriatric Medicine, Kyorin University School of Medicine, Mitaka, Tokyo, Japan

SANDRA MARIA LIMA RIBEIRO, PhD
School of Public Health and School of Arts, Sciences and Humanities, University of São Paulo, São Paulo, Brazil

MILTA O. LITTLE, DO, CMD
Division of Geriatric Medicine, Associate Professor, Department of Internal Medicine, Saint Louis University Health Center, St Louis, Missouri, USA

JOHN E. MORLEY, MB, BCh
Dammert Professor of Gerontology, Director, Division of Geriatric Medicine, Saint Louis University School of Medicine, St Louis, Missouri, USA

SHIRLEY STEFFANY MUÑOZ FERNÁNDEZ, MSc
Department of Nutrition, School of Public Health, University of São Paulo, São Paulo, Brazil

ANDREW D. NGUYEN, PhD
Assistant Professor, Division of Geriatric Medicine, Saint Louis University School of Medicine, St Louis, Missouri, USA

MARTIN ORRELL, PhD, FRCPsych
Division of Psychiatry and Applied Psychology, Faculty of Medicine and Health Sciences, Research Fellow, Institute of Mental Health, University of Nottingham, Jubilee Campus, University of Nottingham Innovation Park, Nottingham, United Kingdom

RONALD C. PETERSEN, MD, PhD
Professor of Neurology, College of Medicine, Mayo Clinic, Rochester, Minnesota, USA

ERUM QAZI, MD
Department of Psychiatry and Behavioral Neuroscience, Saint Louis University, St Louis, Missouri, USA

HARLEEN RAI, MSc
Division of Psychiatry and Applied Psychology, Institute of Mental Health, School of Medicine, University of Nottingham, Jubilee Campus, Nottingham, United Kingdom

ANGELA M. SANFORD, MD
Assistant Professor of Internal Medicine, Division of Geriatrics, Saint Louis University School of Medicine, St Louis, Missouri, USA

SHOSUKE SATAKE, MD, PhD
Chief, Section of Frailty Prevention, Department of Frailty Research, Center for Gerontology and Social Science, Department of Geriatric Medicine, National Center for Geriatrics and Gerontology, Obu, Aichi, Japan

ERIC G. TANGALOS, MD
Professor of Medicine, College of Medicine, Mayo Clinic, Rochester, Minnesota, USA

LADISLAV VOLICER, MD, PhD, FGSA, FAAN
University of South Florida, Tampa, Florida, USA

ZIQI WANG, MD, PhD
Department of Neurology, Chengdu Fifth People's Hospital, Chengdu, China

LAUREN YATES, BSc, PhD
Division of Psychiatry and Applied Psychology, Director, Head, Institute of Mental Health, School of Medicine, University of Nottingham, Jubilee Campus, University of Nottingham Innovation Park, Nottingham, United Kingdom

Contents

CLINICS IN GERIATRIC MEDICINE

SERIES OF RELATED INTEREST

Neurologic Clinics
Medical Clinics
Primary Care: Clinics in Office Practice

THE CLINICS ARE AVAILABLE ONLINE!
Access your subscription at:
www.theclinics.com

Preface

Patient-Centered Care and Cognitive Dysfunction

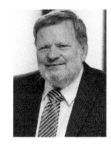

John E. Morley, MB, BCh
Editor

Cognitive dysfunction is one of the most common conditions to plague older persons.[1] Approximately 20% of persons over 70 years of age have dementia and another 20% have mild cognitive impairment. Physicians are not very good at recognizing older persons with cognitive impairment. This results in the patients following medical instructions poorly (eg, taking medicines improperly, inability to use inhalers or to measure glucose levels accurately). In addition, cognitively impaired older persons tend to continue to drive when it is dangerous and often continue to manage their own financial affairs. In addition, early recognition of cognitive dysfunction allows patients to develop advance directives to express their desires. Early recognition of cognitive impairment allows treatment of reversible causes of cognitive impairment, such as removing ear wax, treating sleep apnea and depression, and avoiding anticholinergic drugs. Finally, there is increasing evidence that a Mediterranean diet with extra virgin olive oil, exercise, socialization, mental stimulation, and early management of cardiovascular risk factors can slow the rate at which cognitive dysfunction develops.[2]

This issue of the *Clinics in Geriatric Medicine* provides a detailed overview of the causes of cognitive impairment and dementia. It stresses the need for appropriate screening for cognitive impairment and provides rapid screening tests that can be used in the office of the primary care physician. Further available behavioral approaches can be as successful as medicines at improving cognitive function in persons with dementia.[3]

This *Clinics in Geriatric Medicine* issue also delves into the rapidly developing scientific knowledge concerning Alzheimer disease and other dementias.[4] It stresses that much of the confusion associated with developing drugs to treat Alzheimer disease is the failure to recognize that amyloid-beta at physiologic levels is a memory enhancer, and it is only at pathologic levels that it is amnestic.

Clin Geriatr Med 34 (2018) ix–x
https://doi.org/10.1016/j.cger.2018.08.013
0749-0690/18/© 2018 Published by Elsevier Inc.

Overall, those reading this issue should recognize the importance of patient-centered medicine in developing an individualized management plan for persons with cognitive impairment.[5]

John E. Morley, MB, BCh
Division of Geriatric Medicine
Saint Louis University School of Medicine
1402 South Grand Boulevard, Room M238
St. Louis, MO 63104, USA

E-mail address:
john.morley@health.slu.edu

REFERENCES

1. Morley JE, Morris JC, Berg-Weger M, et al. Brain health: the importance of recognizing cognitive impairment: an IAGG consensus conference. J Am Med Dir Assoc 2015;16(9):731–9.
2. Ngandu T, Lehtisalo J, Solomon A, et al. A 2 year multidomain intervention of diet, exercise, cognitive training, and vascular risk monitoring versus control to prevent cognitive decline in at-risk elderly people (FINGER): a randomised controlled trial. Lancet 2015;385(9984):2255–63.
3. Morley JE, Berg-Weger M, Lundy J. Editorial: nonpharmacological treatment of cognitive impairment. J Nutr Health Aging 2018;22(6):632–3.
4. Morley JE. New horizons in the management of Alzheimer disease. J Am Med Dir Assoc 2015;16(1):105.
5. Morley JE, Vellas B. Patient-centered (P4) medicine and the older person. J Am Med Dir Assoc 2017;18(6):455–9.

An Overview of Cognitive Impairment

John E. Morley, MB,BCh

KEYWORDS

- Cognition • Aging • Dementia • Frailty • Olive oil • Exercise

KEY POINTS

- Increase in processing time is a key component of aging-associated memory disturbances.
- Oxidative damage due to mitochondrial dysfunction is a key to brain aging.
- The Rapid Cognitive Screen can screen for mild cognitive impairment and dementia in less than 3 minutes.
- Case finding for cognitive difficulties is essential for health professionals to allow them to recognize when patients may not be able to follow instructions.
- Hearing deficits, including ear wax, are a major cause of cognitive deficits.

Time robs of us of all, even memory

—*Virgil in Eclogues IX*

In 700 BC, Salon noted that intelligence declines from the mid-50s. This article gives a brief overview of cognition and the aging process.

COGNITIVE AGING

The first study documenting a decline in memory between the ages of 20 and 70 years was conducted by Willoughby[1] in 1929. He did a digital substitution test and found that there was a peak in memory at 22 from childhood and a slow decline toward old age.[1] Following the original study by Birren[2] in 1956 showing that there is an increase in processing time, numerous studies have demonstrated that longer processing time is the key to the memory disturbances associated with aging.[3]

Fluid intelligence is the ability to learn and use new information and use it to problem solve. These are the memories that are generally affected by aging. In cross-sectional aging, memory ability peaks by 25 and then slowly deteriorates at a rate of approximately 0.5% per year.[4] The exception is verbal memory, which peaks at

Disclosure: The author has nothing to disclose.
Division of Geriatric Medicine, Saint Louis University School of Medicine, 1402 South Grand Boulevard, M238, St Louis, MO 63104, USA
E-mail address: john.morley@health.slu.edu

approximately age 45 and remains stable for much of the lifespan. In longitudinal studies, most memories peak somewhat later, with the exception of perceptual speed, which peaks at 25 and shows the most rapid decline. Spatial navigation tasks, inductive reasoning, and spatial orientation peak in the late 40s and decline slowly thereafter. Numeric ability also peaks in the late 40s but has a more rapid decline.

With the exception of spatial ability, women tend to perform better than men on most standardized tests when corrected for education.[5] In longitudinal studies, women decline more slowly than men in verbal ability, language fluidity, and episodic memory. Similarly, the decline in the Mini-Mental State Examination (MMSE) with aging is less in women.

Overall, these changes do not prevent older persons from functioning as they age. For certain professions in which processing speed may be especially important, for example, pilots, fire-fighters, air traffic controllers, and surgeons, regular cognitive testing may be particularly important[6] Although it may appear ageist, it is important that in professions in which in-depth knowledge and reasoning are important for their practice, for example, judges and physicians, regular cognitive testing in those older than 70 would appear not unreasonable. It is important to recognize it is ability, not age, that determines the ability to continue practicing one's profession.[7] Most industrial psychology studies have suggested that optimum performance occurs between 35 and 55 years of age.

THE AGING BRAIN

Cellular senescence of neurons and microglia are central to brain aging.[8] These changes include exhaustion of neural stem cells, increased cellular apoptosis, aggregation of proteins, mitochondrial dysfunction with increased reactive oxygen species and oxidative damage to protein and lipids, and accumulation of DNA damage.[9] Early in the aging process there is an increase in intraneuronal calcium due to an increase in calcium entry into cells and a decline in mechanisms removing calcium from the brain.[10] Calcium plays a key role in memory and also prevents cell death of neurons.

These molecular changes lead to changes in the anatomic structure of the brain. There is a reduction in the number of neurons and a decrease in brain volume of approximately 5% per decade after the age of 40 years.[11]

The brain is responsible for one-fifth of the body's energy consumption.[12] Central to this is the need for energy to be supplied through the anaerobic oxidation of glucose. Brain aging is associated with a decrease in glucose uptake. This is due to a decrease in neuronal glucose transporters: GLUT-3 and GLUT-4.[13] The decline in glucose transport into the brain is associated with a decline in cognitive function. Most of the energy (ATP) within the cell is produced by mitochondria, where glucose is oxidized to carbon dioxide. With aging there is a decrease in the functionality of the oxidative phosphorylation (OXPHOS) system in mitochondria leading to decreased ATP production.[14,15] Damage to the OXPHOS system also leads to increased reactive oxygen species and oxidative damage to the mitochondria and neurons as a whole. Damage to mitochondrial DNA with aging leads to impaired mitochondrial fission, mitochondrial bioenergetics, and mitophagy.[5] This results in accumulation of defective mitochondria. Finally, alterations in microglia with aging result in increase in inflammation and inflammatory cytokines. Inflammatory cytokines can directly decrease memory.[16]

Fig. 1 summarizes the factors that occur with brain aging.

Screening for Memory Problems

The utility of screening and case finding for cognitive impairment is controversial.[17,18] This is based in part on the lack of evidence that these screenings would benefit the person screened. There are a number of reasons why case finding should provide

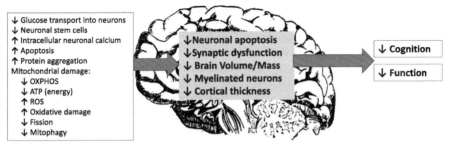

Fig. 1. Factors affecting brain aging. ↑, increase; ↓, decrease; ROS, reactive oxygen species.

benefit. The major one is that health professionals provide their patients with complex information and instructions that are unlikely to be understood or carried out if the person is cognitively impaired. Other reasons include the following:

- There are a number of treatable causes of cognitive function, for example, medications, depression, hearing deficits, hypothyroidism, vitamin B12 deficiency, normal-pressure hydrocephalus, atrial fibrillation, and sleep apnea.[19] Not looking for cognitive impairment would delay treatment of these conditions.
- Advance directives should be executed while the person is at an optimum level to understand the choices.[20]
- There is increasing evidence that lifestyle changes and early treatment of cardiovascular risk factors may lead to a delay in cognitive decline.[21]
- Drugs for the treatment of Alzheimer disease work only in the mild to moderate stages.[22]
- There are a number of interventions that are important for both the person with dementia and the public health of the community; for example, removal of guns from house, no longer driving, home safety, a "safe return" bracelet, and protection against fraud.[19]
- Cognitive stimulation therapy works in moderate, but not late dementia.[23–25]

Many screening tests exist for dementia. Although the MMSE has been extensively used, it is a poor test to detect mild cognitive impairment (MCI).[26] Both the Montreal Cognitive Assessment and the St. Louis University Mental Status test (SLUMS) can identify MCI with reasonable sensitivity and specificity. These 3 tests all take longer than 6 minutes to complete.[27–29]

Three rapid tests for dementia that are suitable for a primary care health professional's office have been validated. These are the MiniCog,[30] the Rapid Cognitive Screen (RCS),[31] and the Ascertain Dementia 8-item questionnaire.[32] The Rapid Cognitive Screen also identifies MCI. All 3 tests can be completed within 3 minutes. Only the SLUMS and RCS are not copyrighted and thus can be guaranteed to be cost free.

Our experience with the Perry County Demonstration Project suggests that the RCS can be incorporated into the physician's practice and/or as part of the Medicare Wellness Visit.[33] In screening or case finding in more than 8000 persons in the Missouri area, we have found that approximately 40% of the persons older than 65 screen positive for MCI or dementia. Twenty percent of persons with diabetes mellitus between 50 and 65 years of age have cognitive impairment.[34]

Mild Cognitive Impairment

MCI results in an intermediate stage of cognitive impairment between those with memory changes normally seen with aging and those who have clear dementia.[35] Persons with

MCI have a mild decline in memory and other thought processes.[36] They do not have functional decline. Testing must take into account educational attainment. In general, it can be divided into amnestic and nonamnestic types. The nonamnestic type involves language difficulties, lack of attention, or navigational skills. The amnestic type is a pure inability to use short-term memory. The prevalence of MCI is between 10% and 20%.[37]

It has been suggested that approximately 50% will progress to dementia in 5 years and 20% to 30% of persons with MCI will revert to normal.[38] A recent study of 357 participants at Saint Louis University demonstrated that with careful assessment for reversible causes, including hearing and visual deficits, 47% had returned to normal 7.5 years later.[39] Hearing deficits lead to early reversible cognitive difficulties and, in the long term, dementia.[40–42]

Cognitive frailty is a form of MCI associated with the physical phenotype of frailty.[43,44] Frailty can be diagnosed by the Fried Frailty criteria[45] or by the simple FRAIL test.[46] Persons with cognitive frailty have a high propensity for falling, which can lead to traumatic encephalopathy that can accelerate the progress to dementia.[47] This is often associated with the presence of white matter hyperintensities in the brain.[48] Persons with cognitive frailty are at increased risk to develop early functional impairment.[49]

Dementia

There are more than 100 causes of dementia. The majority are never considered by most physicians. In the postmortem study by the Seattle-based Adult Changes in Thought study, it was found that 45% had Alzheimer disease, 33% had vascular-based lesions, and 10% had Lewy body dementia. From 2000 to 2012, dementia decreased from 11.6% to 8.6% in the United States.[50] This is most probably because of the increase in treatment of cardiovascular risk factors in middle-aged persons leading to a decrease in vascular dementia.[51]

Other causes of dementia are as follows:

- Primary age-related tauopathy leads to neurofibrillary tangles alone and may occur in up to 5% of persons
- Pick disease (frontotemporal dementia) includes apathy, social problems, loss of meaning of words, and nonfluent aphasia
- Hippocampal sclerosis of dementia is the most common dementia in persons older than 100 years
- Dementia of diabetes, which appears to be a mixture of an abnormal metabolism and vascular disease
- Prion diseases, for example, Creutzfeldt-Jakob disease, Kuru, bovine spongiform encephalopathy
- CADASIL (cerebral autosomal-dominant arteriopathy with subcortical infarcts and leukoencephalopathy)
- Fragile X syndrome associated with essential tremor
- Progressive supranuclear palsy is associated with problems with vertical gaze
- Corticobasal deterioration, in which one may have problems using a limb and the limb may move without the persons recognizing that their brain did it: "alien limb"
- Chronic traumatic encephalopathy: a condition in which severe or repeated trauma leads to memory problems
- Cerebral vasculitis, such as systemic lupus erythematosus
- Multiple sclerosis, an autoimmune-mediated disorder producing demyelination
- Hypoxic encephalopathy due to diseases such as chronic obstructive pulmonary disease, atrial fibrillation, and congestive heart failure
- Toxic encephalopathy due to diseases such as liver failure and kidney failure

Overall, this limited list of causes of dementia reminds us that we must be very careful in labeling diseases as Alzheimer disease. We are developing more diagnostic techniques, which is moving the diagnosis and management of dementia into a highly specialized area. It therefore increases the importance of early recognition of cognitive problems and the development of specific treatments for each cause.

Art and Dementia

A number of artists have continued to paint as they developed Alzheimer disease. Of these, Carolus Horn's painting of the Venice bridge clearly delineates the changes with Alzheimer disease. His changes show a marked change in visuospatial perspective and an increase in bright colors. William Utermohlen also showed a shift to bright colors early in his Alzheimer disease, although late in the disease he returned to dark colors and a loss of facial features. Of interest was Wilhelm de Kooning, an abstract expressionist, whose paintings became much simpler with age, which one art critic described as "Haiku-like." This change was applauded by many art critics but most probably represented a loss of visuospatial perspective.

Gretton and Ffytche[52] studied a number of artists who were known to develop dementia. Artists with Alzheimer disease were characterized by having visuospatial problems and a color shift. Artists with frontotemporal dementia showed preservation of themes and their paintings became more realistic. Persons with Lewy body dementia were found to have simple bizarre content.

PREVENTION OF COGNITIVE DECLINE

Epidemiologic studies suggest that a Mediterranean diet and exercise both are associated with protection against cognitive decline and dementia.[53,54] The PREDIMED study supported the use of extra virgin olive oil and the Mediterranean diet as preventive of dementia.[55] Animal studies in the SAMP8 mouse show a positive effect of extra virgin olive oil on memory and oxidative brain damage.[56]

For exercise, the data are less clear, although the 2013 Cochrane Analysis concluded that "exercise programs can have a significant impact in improving ability to perform Activities of Daily Living and possibly in improving cognition in people with dementia, although some caution is advised in interpreting these findings." Physically active videogames (exergames) appear to improve cognition.[57]

The FINGER study, using a combination of a Mediterranean diet, exercise, socialization, computer games, and treatment of cardiovascular risk factors, slowed cognitive decline in older persons.[58] Exercise alone has failed to protect against cognitive decline in cognitively intact older persons.

Animal studies lend support to the possible effects of fish oils,[59] polyphenols,[60] and curcumin[61] on memory. Souvenaid, a nutritional supplement containing uridine monophosphate, doahexanoic acid, eicosapentaenoic acid, choline, and phospholipids, has shown minor effects in early cognitive dysfunction but not in those with well-established cognitive dysfunction.[62] Although omega-3 polyunsaturated fatty acids improve memory in mice, the human studies have given disappointing outcomes.[63,64]

SUMMARY

It seems prudent to suggest the following approach to cognitive impairment in older persons:

- All older persons should have a yearly cognitive assessment, for example, the RCS, as part of the Annual Medicare Wellness visit.

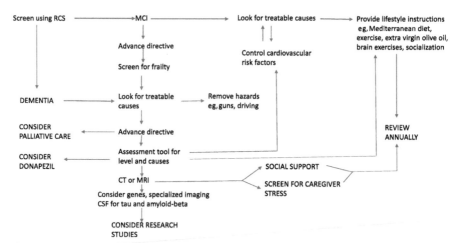

Fig. 2. Precision approach to dementia. CSF, cerebrospinal fluid; CT, computed tomography.

- A computer-assisted management algorithm using the principles of precision medicine should be developed to help health care professionals manage cognitive dysfunction (**Fig. 2**).
- Lifestyle modification sheets for patients with cognitive dysfunction should be developed; for example, Mediterranean diet, extra virgin olive oil, fruits rich in polyphenols, physical exercise, brain exercises from computer to sudoku and crossword puzzles, and socialization.
- Check for caregiver stress in the primary caregiver and provide support when required.
- Provide cognitive stimulation programs in the community.

REFERENCES

1. Willoughby RR. Incidental learning. J Educ Psychol 1929;20:671–82.
2. Birren JE. The significance of age changes in speed of perception and psychomotor response. In: Anderson TE, editor. Psychological aspect of aging. Washington, DC: American Psychological Association; 1956. p. 97–104.
3. Salthouse TA. The processing-speed theory of adult age differences in cognition. Psychol Rev 1996;103:403–28.
4. Salthouse TA. Selective review of cognitive aging. J Int Neuropsychol Soc 2010; 16:754–60.
5. McCarrey AC, An Y, Kitner-Triolo MH, et al. Sex differences in cognitive trajectories in clinically normal older adults. Psychol Aging 2016;31:166–75.
6. Dellinger EP, Pellegrini C, Gallagher TH. The aging physician and the medical profession: a review. JAMA Surg 2017;152:967–71.
7. Kaups KL. Competence not age determines ability to practice: ethical considerations about sensorimotor agility, dexterity, and cognitive capacity. AMA J Ethics 2016;18:1017–24.
8. Raz N, Daugherty AM. Pathways to brain aging and their modifiers: free-radical-induced energetic and neural decline in senescence (FRIENDS) model–a mini-review. Gerontology 2017. https://doi.org/10.1159/000479508.
9. Boccardi V, Comanducci C, Baroni M, et al. Of energy and entropy: the ineluctable impact of aging in old age dementia. Int J Mol Sci 2017;18:2672.

10. Chandran R, Kumar M, Kesavan L, et al. Cellular calcium signaling in the aging brain. J Chem Neuroanat 2017. https://doi.org/10.1016/j.jchemneu.2017.17.006.
11. Skullerud K. Variations in the size of the human brain. Influence of age, sex, body length, body mass index, alcoholism, Alzheimer changes, and cerebral atherosclerosis. Acta Neurol Scand Suppl 1985;102:1–94.
12. Grimm A, Eckert A. Brain aging and neurodegeneration: from a mitochondrial point of view. J Neurochem 2017;143:418–31.
13. Mooradian AD, Morin AM, Cipp LJ, et al. Glucose transport is reduced in the blood-brain barrier of aged rats. Brain Res 1991;14:145–9.
14. Yin F, Sancheti H, Patil I, et al. Energy metabolism and inflammation in brain aging and Alzheimer's disease. Free Radic Biol Med 2016;100:108–22.
15. Tonnies E, Trushina E. Oxidative stress, synaptic dysfunction, and Alzheimer's disease. J Alzheimers Dis 2017;57:1105–21.
16. Banks WA, Farr SA, La Scola ME, et al. Intravenous human interleukin-1 alpha impairs memory processing in mice: dependence on blood-brain barrier transport into posterior division of the septum. J Pharmacol Exp Ther 2001;299:536–41.
17. Lin JS, O'Connor E, Rossom RC, et al. Screening for cognitive impairment in older adults: a systematic review for the U.S. Preventive Services Task Force. Ann Intern Med 2013;159:601–12.
18. Morley JE, Morris JC, Berg-Weger M, et al. Brain health: the importance of recognizing cognitive impairment: an IAGG consensus conference. J Am Med Dir Assoc 2015;16:731–9.
19. Morley JE. Editorial: can we improve care for patients with dementia? J Nutr Health Aging 2011;15:523–5.
20. Abele P, Morley JE. Advance directives: the key to a good death? J Am Med Dir Assoc 2016;17:279–83.
21. Morley JE. Mild cognitive impairment—a treatable condition. J Am Med Dir Assoc 2014;15:1–5.
22. Birks J, Harvey RJ. Donepezil for dementia due to Alzheimer's disease. Cochrane Database Syst Rev 2018;(6):CD001190.
23. Woods B, Aguirre E, Spector AE, et al. Cognitive stimulation to improve cognitive functioning in people with dementia. Cochrane Database Syst Rev 2012;(2):CD005562.
24. Berg-Weger M, Tebb S, Henderson-Kalb J, et al. Cognitive stimulation therapy: a tool for your practice with persons with dementia? J Am Med Dir Assoc 2015;16:795–6.
25. Morley JE, Cruz-Oliver DM. Cognitive stimulation therapy. J Am Med Dir Assoc 2014;15:689–91.
26. Trivedi D. Cochrane review summary: Mini-Mental State Examination (MMSE) for the detection of dementia in clinically unevaluated people aged 65 and over in community and primary care populations. Prim Health Care Res Dev 2017;18:527–8.
27. Tariq SH, Tumosa N, Chibnall JT, et al. Comparison of the Saint Louis University mental status examination and the mini-mental state examination for detecting dementia and mild neurocognitive disorder—a pilot study. Am J Geriatr Psychiatry 2006;14:900–10.
28. Cummings-Vaughn LA, Chavakula NN, Malmstrom TK, et al. Veterans Affairs Saint Louis University mental status examination compared with the Montreal Cognitive Assessment and the Short Test of Mental Status. J Am Geriatr Soc 2014;62:1341–6.

29. Shaik MA, Chan QL, Xu J, et al. Risk factors of cognitive impairment and brief cognitive tests to predict cognitive performance determined by a formal neuro-psychological evaluation of primary health care patients. J Am Med Dir Assoc 2016;17:343–7.

30. Borson S, Scanlan JM, Watanabe J, et al. Simplifying detection of cognitive impairment: comparison of the Mini-Cog and Mini-Mental State Examination in a multiethnic sample. J Am Geriatr Soc 2005;53:871–4.

31. Malmstrom TK, Voss VB, Cruz-Oliver DM, et al. The Rapid Cognitive Screen (RCS): a point-of-care screening for dementia and mild cognitive impairment. J Nutr Health Aging 2015;19:741–4.

32. Dong Y, Pang WS, Lim LB, et al. The informant AD8 is superior to participant AD8 in detecting cognitive impairment in a memory clinic setting. J Alzheimers Dis 2013;35:159–68.

33. Morley JE, Abele P. The Medicare Annual Wellness visit in nursing homes. J A Med Dir Assoc 2016;17:567–9.

34. Liccini A, Malmstrom TK, Morley JE. Metformin use and cognitive dysfunction among patients with diabetes mellitus. J Am Med Dir Assoc 2016;17:1063–5.

35. Petersen RC. Clinical practice. Mild cognitive impairment. N Engl J Med 2011; 364:2227–34.

36. Gauthier S, Reisberg B, Zaudig M, et al. International Psychogeriatric Association Expert Conference on mild cognitive impairment. Mild cognitive impairment. Lancet 2006;367:1262–70.

37. Petersen RC, Roberts RO, Knopman DS, et al. Prevalence of mild cognitive impairment is higher in men. The Mayo Clinic Study of Aging. Neurology 2010; 75:889–97.

38. Larrieu S, Letenneur L, Orgogozo JM, et al. Incidence and outcome of mild cognitive impairment in a population-based prospective cohort. Neurology 2002;59: 1594–9.

39. Cruz-Oliver DM, Malstrom TK, Roegner M, et al. Cognitive deficit reversal as shown by changes in the Veterans Affairs Saint Louis University Mental Status (SLUMS) examination scores 7.5 years later. J Am Med Dir Assoc 2014;15: 687.e5-10.

40. Huh M. The relationships between cognitive function and hearing loss among the elderly. J Phys Ther Sci 2018;30:174–6.

41. Thompson RS, Auduong P, Miller AT, et al. Hearing loss as a risk factor for dementia: systematic review. Laryngoscope Investig Otolaryngol 2017;2:69–79.

42. Loughrey DG, Kelly ME, Kelley GA, et al. Association of age-related hearing loss with cognitive function, cognitive impairment, and dementia: a systematic review and meta-analysis. JAMA Otolaryngol Head Neck Surg 2017. https://doi.org/10.1001/jamaoto.2017.2513.

43. Malmstrom TK, Morley JE. The frail brain. J Am Med Dir Assoc 2013;14:453–5.

44. Canevelli M, Cesari M. Cognitive frailty: what is still missing? J Nutr Health Aging 2015;19:273–5.

45. Shimada H, Makizako H, Lee S, et al. Impact of cognitive frailty on daily activities in older persons. J Nutr Health Aging 2016;20:729–35.

46. Malmstrom TK, Miller DK, Morley JE. A comparison of four frailty models. J Am Geriatr Soc 2014;62:721–6.

47. Merchant RA, Chen MZ, Tan LWL, et al. Singapore Healthy Older People Everyday (HOPE) study: prevalence of frailty and associated factors in older adults. J Am Med Dir Assoc 2017;18:734.e9-e14.

48. Morley JE. White matter lesions (laukoaraiosis): a major cause of falls. J Am Med Dir Assoc 2015;16:441–3.
49. Roppolo M, Mulasso A, Rabaglietti E. Cognitive frailty in Italian community-dwelling older adults: prevalence rate and its association with disability. J Nutr Health Aging 2017;21:631–6.
50. Langa KM, Larson EB, Crimmins EM, et al. A comparison of the prevalence of dementia in the United States in 2000 and 2012. JAMA Intern Med 2017;177:51–8.
51. Reamy BV, Williams PM, Kuckel DP. Prevention of cardiovascular disease. Prim Care 2018;45:25–44.
52. Gretton C, Ffytche DH. Art and the brain: a view from dementia. Int J Geriatr Psychiatry 2014;29:111–26.
53. Petersson SD, Philippou E. Mediterranean diet, cognitive function, and dementia: a systematic review of the evidence. Adv Nutr 2016;7:889–904.
54. Martinez-Lapiscina EH, Clavero P, Toledo E, et al. Virgin olive oil supplementation and long-term cognition: the PREDIMED-NAVARRA randomized, trial. J Nutr Health Aging 2013;17:544–52.
55. Strohle A, Schmidt DK, Schultz F, et al. Drug and exercise treatment of Alzheimer disease and mild cognitive impairment: a systematic review and meta-analysis of effects on cognition in randomized controlled trials. Am J Geriatr Psychiatry 2015; 23:1234–49.
56. Farr SA, Price TO, Dominguez LJ, et al. Extra virgin olive oil improves learning and memory in SAMP8 mice. J Alzheimers Dis 2012;28:81–92.
57. Bamidis PD, Fissler P, Papageorgiou SG, et al. Gains in cognition through combined cognitive and physical training: the role of training dosage and severity of neurocognitive disorder. Front Aging Neurosci 2015;7:152.
58. Ngandu T, Lehtisalo J, Solomon A, et al. A 2 year multidomain intervention of diet, exercise, cognitive training, and vascular risk monitoring versus control to prevent cognitive decline in at-risk elderly people (FINGER): a randomised controlled trial. Lancet 2015;385:2255–63.
59. Petursdottir AL, Farr SA, Morley JE, et al. Effect of dietary n-3 polyunsaturated fatty acid composition, learning ability, and memory of senescence-accelerated mouse. J Gerontol A Biol Sci Med Sci 2008;63:1153–60.
60. Farr SA, Niehoff ML, Ceddia M, et al. Effect of botanical extracts containing carnosic acid or rosmarinic acid on learning and memory in SAMP8 mice. Physiol Behav 2016;165:328–38.
61. Goozee KG, Shah TM, Sohrabi HR, et al. Examining the potential clinical value of curcumin in the prevention and diagnosis of Alzheimer's disease. Br J Nutr 2016; 115:449–65.
62. Kamphius PJ, Verhey FR, Olde Rikkert MG, et al. Efficacy of a medical food on cognition in Alzheimer's disease: results from secondary analyses of a randomized, controlled trial. J Nutr Health Aging 2011;15:720–4.
63. Moon SY, de Souto Barreto P, Chupin M, et al. Association between red blood cells omega-3 polyunsaturated fatty acids and white matter hyperintensities: the MAPT study. J Nutr Health Aging 2018;22:174–9.
64. Canhada S, Castro K, Perry IS, et al. Omega-3 fatty acids' supplementation in Alzheimer's disease: a systematic review. Nutr Neurosci 2017;3:1–10.

Screening for Cognitive Impairment in Geriatrics

Ziqi Wang, MD, PhD[a], Birong Dong, MD, PhD[b],*

KEYWORDS

- Cognitive impairment • Screening • Geriatrics • Dementia
- Early detection of disease • Assessment • Neuropsychology

KEY POINTS

- The Mini-Mental State Examination is still the most commonly used in screening dementia, the Mini-Cog and the Addenbrooke Cognitive Examination–Revised (ACE-R) also showed excellence in screening dementia.
- For mild cognitive impairment, the Montreal Cognitive Assessment and ACE-R had better performance than the other dementia screening tests.
- Using neuropsychological batteries that include main cognitive domains (learning and memory, language, executive function, complex attention, and social cognition) may predict preclinical disease, such as Alzheimer disease.
- It is better to choose instruments for screening cognitive impairment in geriatrics by considering the settings, stages, conditions, and specific people.
- Practitioners also need to consider goals and harm for use of the different cognitive tests.

INTRODUCTION

Dementia corresponds to the major neurocognitive disorder (major NCD),[1] an acquired decline in 1 or more cognitive domains severe enough to affect social or occupational functioning.[2] In the world, there were approximately 47 million people living with dementia in 2015, which will increase to triple that by 2050.[3] The 2015 worldwide cost of dementia was estimated to be US $818 billion, and the figure will cross US $1 trillion by 2018.[4] Mild cognitive impairment (MCI), also categorized as mild neurocognitive disorder (mild NCD),[1] differs from dementia in that it preserves independence in daily life[1]; however, it may be useful for predicting dementia. Cumulative dementia incidence was 14.9% in older adults with MCI by follow-up of 2 years.[5] Both the major NCD and mild NCD can be caused by many diseases, such as Alzheimer disease (AD), vascular, Lewy bodies, Parkinson disease, frontotemporal, traumatic brain injury,

Disclosure: The authors have nothing to disclose.
[a] Department of Neurology, Chengdu Fifth People's Hospital, No. 33 Mashi Street, Chengdu, Sichuan, China 611130; [b] The Center of Gerontology and Geriatrics, West China Hospital, Sichuan University, No. 37 Guoxue Lane, Chengdu, Sichuan, China 610041
* Corresponding author.
E-mail address: birongdong@163.com

Clin Geriatr Med 34 (2018) 515–536
https://doi.org/10.1016/j.cger.2018.06.004
0749-0690/18/© 2018 Elsevier Inc. All rights reserved.

human immunodeficiency virus infection, substance/medication-induced, Huntington disease, prion disease, and so on.[1] Cognitive impairment is identified at an early stage in the disease process and may allow patients and their families to receive earlier care, which may lead to improved prognosis and decreased morbidity.[6] A wide range of instruments has been developed to aid the clinician in this process.

SCREENING TOOLS

For there are a wide range of tools developed to assess cognitive function.[7] An appropriate choice depends both on the time available and the purpose of assessment. The Mini-Mental State Examination (MMSE) was the most widely used cognitive screening tool. However, in practice, there is a need for a briefer test than the MMSE that retains reasonable sensitivity and specificity.[7] For secondary and tertiary care where cognitive screening routinely forms part of the differential diagnostic process, comprehensive cognitive screening measures, such as the Addenbrooke Cognitive Examination–Revised (ACE-R)[8] and DemTect[9] are more useful.[10]

Very Brief Cognitive Tests

Clock-drawing test
There are many scoring systems of the clock-drawing test (CDT),[11] the most common score in screening AD is total score 1 to 10[12] and 0 to 5/1 to 6.[13] The CDT was 67% to 97.9% sensitivity and 69% to 94.2% specificity in screening cognitive impairment[14]; however, there are multiple scoring methods for interpreting the CDT (each with varying degrees of complexity) and no consensus on the best method.[14]

Mini-Cog
The Mini-Cog includes the CDT adding a 3-item word recall test.[15] Administration time for the Mini-Cog is 2 minutes. It has moderate to high sensitivity (76%–99%[15,16]) and moderate to great specificity (85.3%–96.0%[15,17]) to classify dementia from cognitive normal and is not influenced by education or language.[15] As with excellent screening characteristics and spending less time, the Mini-Cog could be considered to be used as a screening tool among communities to help to diagnose dementia early.[17]

Memory impairment screen
The memory impairment screen (MIS) is a brief 4-item delayed free and cued recall memory impairment test.[18]

   With a cut-point of 4, the sensitivity of MIS in screening dementia ranged from 43% to 86% and specificity ranged from 93% to 97%.[14]

Verbal fluency tests
Verbal fluency tests (VFTs) can be category (assesses language ability) or letter fluency tests (assesses executive functioning) that measure the ability to name as many items in a category (eg, animals, fruits, first names) or starting with a specific letter in 1 minute.[14] VFTs have a wide range of sensitivity (37.0%–89.5%) and specificity (43%–97%), with likely unacceptably low sensitivity (37.0%–89.5%) for lower thresholds (12 or 13) and low specificity (43%–94%) for higher cut-points (14 or 15).[14]

Short test of mental status
The short test of mental status (STMS) can be used for patients in inpatient and outpatient settings in approximately 5 minutes, and it contains items that test orientation, attention, immediate recall, arithmetic, abstraction, construction, information, and delayed recall.[19,20] The sensitivity of the test in identifying dementia is 86.4% to 95.5%, with a specificity of 87.9% to 93.5% at a score of 29 or less.[19,20]

Brief Cognitive Tests

Mini-mental state examination
The MMSE is a 30-point cognitive test that includes 11 items[21] and takes approximately 8 minutes to complete.[22] A cutoff of 23 versus 24 (23/24) was recommended in persons with at least 8 years of education.[21] Scores of 21 to 24, 10 to 20, and 9 or less indicate mild, moderate, and severe cognitive impairment, respectively.[23] It estimates that the sensitivity and specificity were 88.3% and of 86.2%, respectively.[6] The MMSE with best value for ruling out a diagnosis of dementia in community and primary care had a negative predictive value of 98.5% and 95.7%, respectively.[24] It also has a ceiling; individuals with MCI may score in the "normal" range of 25 to 30 points, particularly if they have high educational attainment. **Table 1** lists some common tools for screening cognitive impairment in geriatrics.

Montreal cognitive assessment
The Montreal cognitive assessment (MoCA) is a 30-point test administered in 10 minutes and was developed as an instrument to screen persons who present with mild cognitive complaints.[25] Using a cutoff of 26, the MoCA assesses several domains of cognition (ie, memory, visuospatial abilities, executive functions, naming, attention, language, abstraction, delayed recall, and orientation) with excellent sensitivity in recognizing MCI and AD (90% vs 100%, respectively). The MoCA also shown a high specificity in identifying 87% of healthy controls.[25] MoCA is better than the MMSE in the detection of MCI among patients older than 60.[26]

Abbreviated mental test
The abbreviated mental test (AMT) is a 10-item assessment that is commonly used in hospitals. The total scores are 10. A score of ≤7 suggests cognitive impairment.[23] AMT has a sensitivity ranging from 42.0% to 92.3% and a high specificity ranging from 93.0% to 95.4% at the cut-point of 7/8.[14] A 4-item version is taken in less than 1 minute and is used in emergency departments or acute assessment units.[27] Failure on any of the 4 items (age, date of birth, place, and year) implies cognitive impairment.[23]

Free and cued selective reminding test
Free and cued selective reminding test (FCSRT) is a verbal episodic memory test used to identify individuals with encoding specificity impairment, such as AD.[28] The FCSRT has a sensitivity of 86% to 100% and specificity of 73.0% to 87.2% at a cut-point of 25.[14]

7-minute screen
The 7-minute screen (7MS) is a combination of 4 individual tests (the Benton Temporal Orientation Test, Enhanced Cued Recall test, the CDT, and the animal VFT) representing 4 cognitive areas typically compromised in AD.[29] Sensitivity is 100% and specificity ranges from 95.1% to 100%.[14]

Six-item cognitive impairment test
The 6-item cognitive impairment test (6CIT)[30] is designed to screen dementia and cognitive impairment. It includes 1 memory, 2 calculations, and 3 orientation questions. A higher score (maximum 28) represents more significant cognitive impairment. To screen dementia in primary care, the 6CIT gives a sensitivity and specificity of 78.6% and 100% (cutoff 7/8), which is better than the MMSE.[31]

Table 1
Screening cognitive tools for cognitive impairment

Instruments	Total Score	Sensitivity, %	Specificity, %	Cut-Points	Components of Tests
Very brief (<5 min)					
CDT	10	67–97.9	69–94.2	<7	Visuospatial and executive function
Mini-Cog	5	76–99	85.3–96	≤3	Memory, visuospatial, and executive function
MIS	8	43–86	93–97	≤4	Memory
VFT	NA	37–89.5	43–97	12/13 or 14/15	Memory and language
STMS	38	86.4–95.5	87.9–93.5	31~27 (age-related)	Orientation, memory, attention, and executive function
Brief (6–10 min)					
MMSE	30	88.3	86.2	23/24 or 24/25	Orientation, memory, language, attention, and visuospatial
MoCA	30	90–100	87	26	Orientation, memory, language, attention, and executive function
AMT	10	42–92.3	93–95.4	7/8	Orientation, memory, and attention
FCSRT	48	86–100	73–87.2	25	Memory
7MS	28	100	95.1–100	0	Orientation, memory, language, visuospatial and executive function
6CIT	28	78.6	100	7/8	Orientation, memory, and calculations
TICS	41	74–88	86–97	30/31	Orientation, memory, attention, calculation, and executive function
SLUMS	30	92–100	76–100	23.5 (<high school), 25.5 (≥high school)	Memory, language, attention, calculation, visuospatial, and executive function

GPCOG	15	85	86	10/11	Orientation, memory, language, visuospatial, executive function, and other daily living functions
DemTect	18	100	92	≤12	Memory, language, and executive function
Self-administered (<20 min)					
IQCODE-26/16	26–130/16–80	75–83	65–90	3.3	Orientation, memory, language, and other daily living functions
AD8	8	74–85	86	≥2	Orientation, memory, language, and executive function
Neuropsychological batteries (>20 min)					
ACE-R	100	84–94	89–100	82 or 88	Orientation, memory, language, attention, visuospatial, and executive function
CAMCOG	106	92	96	<80	Orientation, language, memory, attention, praxis, calculation, abstract thinking, perception

Abbreviations: 6CIT, 6-item cognitive impairment test; 7MS, 7-minute screen; ACE-R, Addenbrooke cognitive examination revise; AD8, 8-item informant interview; AMT, abbreviated mental test; CAMCOG, Cambridge cognitive examination; CDT, clock-drawing test; FCSRT, free and cued selective reminding test; GPCOG, general practitioner assessment of cognition; IQCODE, informant questionnaire on cognitive decline in the elderly; MIS, memory impairment screen; MMSE, Mini-Mental State Examination; MoCA, Montreal cognitive assessment; SLUMS, Saint Louis University mental status examination; STMS, short test of mental status; TICS, telephone interview for cognitive status; VFT, verbal fluency test.

Telephone interview for cognitive status

The telephone interview for cognitive status (TICS) is an 11-item tool that can be administered by phone or in person, does not require vision, and therefore can be used in visually impaired individuals.[32] The face-to-face administration of TICS is a reliable and valid alternative in persons who cannot be evaluated by MMSE.[33] The sensitivity ranges from 74% to 88% and specificity from 86% to 87%.[14]

The Saint Louis University mental status examination

The Saint Louis University mental status examination (SLUMS)[34] is a 30-point screening questionnaire that tests for orientation, memory, attention, and executive functions. It takes approximately 7 minutes to complete. The optimal cutoff scores for SLUMS for mild NCD with less than a high school education and high school or higher education were 23.5 and 25.5, respectively.[34] The sensitivities are 92% and 95%, respectively, and the specificities are 81% and 76%, respectively.[34] The cutoff scores for SLUMS for dementia were 19.5 and 21.5 for less than high school education and high school or higher education, respectively.[34] The sensitivities are 100% and 98%, respectively, and the specificities are 98% and 100%, respectively.[34]

General practitioner assessment of cognition

The general practitioner assessment of cognition (GPCOG) was specifically designed for use in primary care and consists of cognitive test items and historical questions asked of an informant. Patient interviews take less than 4 minutes to administer and informant interviews less than 2 minutes.[35] It has a sensitivity of 85%, a specificity of 86%, a misclassification rate of 14%, and positive predictive value of 71.4%.[35]

DemTect

The DemTect is easy to administer and takes 8 to 10 minutes to complete.[9] Its subtests include a word list, a number transcoding task, a semantic verbal fluency task, digit span reverse, and delayed recall of the word list.[9] Its transformed total score (maximum 18) is independent of age and education. The DemTect helps in deciding whether cognitive performance is adequate for age (13–18 points), or whether MCI (9–12 points) with sensitivity of 80% and specificity of 92%, or dementia (8 points or below) should be suspected with sensitivity of 100% and specificity of 92%.[9]

Self-Administered Instruments

Informant questionnaire on cognitive decline in the elderly

The full informant questionnaire on cognitive decline in the elderly (IQCODE) is a 26-item questionnaire that asks an informant (ie, caregiver, family, close friend) about changes in an older adult's everyday cognitive function with the aims to assess cognitive decline independent of premorbid ability.[36] The IQCODE has a sensitivity of 79% to 83% and specificity from 65% to 90% for a cut-point of approximately 3.3.[14] There is also a 16-item short form IQCODE[37] with a sensitivity of 75% to 81% for dementia and specificity from 68% to 80% for a cut-point of approximately 3.3.[14] Both the short and the full IQCODEs are the most well-studied in a primary care–relevant population.[38]

Eight-item informant interview

The 8-item informant interview (AD8) differentiates between clinical dementia rating (CDR) 0 (nondemented) and CDR 0.5 (very mildly impaired conditions) and queries memory, orientation, judgment, and function.[39] Its sensitivity is 74%, and specificity is 86%.[39] When AD8 is used to screen mild to severe dementia, the sensitivity is 85%.[39]

Neuropsychological Batteries

Addenbrooke cognitive examination–revised

The Addenbrooke cognitive examination–revised (ACE-R) includes 5 subdomain scores (orientation/attention, memory, verbal fluency, language, and visuo-spatial). When cutoffs are defined as 88 for evaluating dementia, the sensitivity is 94% and specificity 89%. Although the cutoffs are defined as 82, the sensitivity is 84% and specificity 100%. The ACE-R is recommended in both modest (such as primary care or general hospital settings) and high prevalence settings (such as memory clinics).[40]

Cambridge cognitive examination

The Cambridge cognitive examination (CAMCOG) is a brief neuropsychological battery with 8 major subscales (orientation, language, memory, attention, praxis, calculation, abstract thinking, perception) designed to assess the range of cognitive functions required for a diagnosis of dementia, and to detect mild degrees of cognitive impairment.[41] The total CAMCOG score is up to 106, with a cutoff of less than 80 being typical to diagnose cognitive impairment and there is no ceiling effect[41] (92% sensitivity and 96% specificity[42]). It is estimated to take 30 minutes to complete.

Screening tools used in different cognitive domains

According to the *Diagnostic and Statistical Manual of Mental Disorders, Fifth Edition* (DSM-V), 6 key domains of cognitive function are defined, and each of these has subdomains[1] (**Table 2**).

Learning and memory There are a number of components to memory. Following DSM-V,[1] memory is categorized to recent memory (relating to assessing the process of encoding new information), semantic (memory for facts), autobiographical long-term memory (memory for personal events or people), and implicit learning (procedural unconscious learning of skills). There are 3 subdomains of recent memory: free recall, cued recall, and recognition memory.[1] Some simple questions and special tests, such as California Verbal Learning Test (CVLT),[43] Cued Selective Reminding Test (CSRT),[44] Rey-Osterrieth Complex Figure (ROCF) Test,[45] Delayed Word Recall Test (DWR),[46] Visual Reproduction Subtest of the Wechsler Memory Scale,[47] can be used to evaluate memory.

Language The submains of a language disturbance include expressive (naming, word finding, fluency), grammar and syntax, and receptive language.[1] For detecting a receptive dysphasia, the patient is asked to obey first 1-stage, and then more complex instructions (eg, point to the window, then the ceiling, and then the door).[7] Expressive dysphasia is identified by asking the patient to name objects or pictures (eg, the Boston Naming Test[48]), or count animals or letters in 1 minute.[1,7] The grammar and syntax errors, which can be observed during naming and fluency tests, are compared with norms to assess frequency of errors and compare with normal slips of the tongue.[1] This may include semantic errors (the insertion of incorrect, but related words), such as saying "dog" instead of "cat," or "conductive aphasia," which causes particular impairment with the repetition of phrases (eg, "no ifs, ands or buts") in the MMSE.[49]

Executive function Executive function includes components such as planning, decision-making, working memory, responding to feedback/error correction, overriding habits/inhibition, and mental flexibility.[1] Many techniques are available to the clinician to assess executive functions. They include the Trail Making Test, Part B

Table 2
Neurocognitive domains and tests

Key Domains	Subdomains		Definition	Simple Questions Tests	Special Tests
Learning and memory	Immediate memory span		Ability to repeat a list of words or digits, also as working memory		California Verbal Learning Test, Cued Selective Reminding Test, Rey-Osterrieth Complex Figure Test, Delayed Word Recall Test, Visual Reproduction Subtest of the Wechsler Memory Scale
	Recent memory	Free recall	Assesses the process of encoding new information	The person is asked to recall as many word diagrams, or elements of a story as possible	
		Cued recall		Examiner aids recall by providing semantic cues such as "List all the food items on the list" or "Name all of the children from the story"	
		Recognition memory		Examiner asks about specific items, eg, "Was 'apple' on the list?" or "Did you see this diagram or figure?"	
	Semantic		Memory for facts		
	Autobiographical long-term memory		Memory for personal events or people		
	Implicit learning		Procedural unconscious learning of skills		

Domain	Subdomain	Description	Identification of objects or pictures	Test
Language	Expressive language — Naming, Word finding, Fluency, Grammar and syntax	Omission or incorrect use of articles, prepositions, auxiliary verbs	Animals count or letter count in 1 min; Errors observed during naming and fluency tests are compared with norms to assess frequency of errors and compare with normal slips of the tongue (eg, saying "dog" instead of "cat")	The Boston Naming Test
	Receptive language	Performance of actions/activities according to verbal command	Comprehension (word definition and object-pointing tasks involving animate and inanimate stimuli, such as point to the window, then the ceiling, and then the door)	
Executive function	Planning		Ability to find the exit to a maze; interpret a sequential picture or object arrangement	The Trail Making Test, Part B, Stroop Interference Test, Self-Ordering Test, Porteus Mazes, Alpha Span Test, Digit Span Backward
	Decision-making	Performance of tasks that assess process of deciding in the face of competing alternatives	Simulated gambling	
	Working memory	Ability to hold information for brief period and to manipulate	Adding up a list of numbers or repeating a series of numbers or words backward	
	Responding to feedback/ error correction	Ability to benefit from feedback to infer the rules for solving a problem		
	Overriding habits/Inhibition	Ability to choose a more complex and effortful solution to be correct	Looking away from the direction indicated by an arrow; naming the color of a word's font rather than naming the word	
	Mental/cognitive flexibility	Ability to shift between 2 concepts, tasks, or response rules	From number to letter, from verbal to key-press response, from adding numbers to ordering numbers, from ordering objects by size to ordering by color	

(continued on next page)

Table 2
(continued)

Key Domains	Subdomains	Definition	Simple Questions Tests	Special Tests
Perceptual-motor function	Visual perception		Line bisection tasks, motor-free perceptual tasks (including facial recognition), and decision of whether a figure can be "real" or not based on dimensionality	Clock-drawing test, the Rey Complex Figure, the Wechsler Memory Scale
	Visuo-constructional reasoning		Drawing, copying, and block assembly	
	Perceptual-motor coordination		Inserting blocks into a form board without visual cues; rapidly inserting pegs into a slotted board	
	Praxis		Wave goodbye; "Show me how you would use a hammer"	
	Gnosis		Recognition of faces and colors	
Complex attention	Sustained attention	Maintenance of attention over time	Pressing a button every time a tone is heard, and over a period of time	Digit Span Forward, Trail Making Test, Part A, and Cued Reaction Time
	Divided attention	Attending to 2 tasks within the same time period	Rapidly tapping while learning a story being read	
	Selective attention	Maintenance of attention despite competing stimuli and/or distractors	Hearing numbers and letters read and asked to count only letters	
	Processing speed		Time to put together a design of blocks; time to match symbols with numbers; speed in responding, such as counting speed or serial 2 speed	
Social cognition	Recognition of emotions		Identification of emotion in images of faces representing a variety of both positive and negative emotions	
	Theory of mind	Ability to consider another person's mental state (thoughts, desires, intentions) or experience	Story cards with questions to elicit information about the mental state of the individuals portrayed, "Where will the girl look for the lot bag?"	

(TMT-B),[50] Stroop Interference Test,[51] Self-Ordering Test,[52] Porteus Mazes,[53] Alpha Span Test,[54] and Digit Span Backward.[47]

Perceptual-motor function Perceptual-motor impairment is that dysfunction in visual perception, visuo-constructional reasoning, perceptual-motor coordination, praxis, and gnosis.[1] Visuospatial disturbances tend to be more severe when the nondominant hemisphere is involved.[7] They are common in both dementia and delirium with rarely "nonorganic" cognitive disorders.[7] The usual method of detecting such a deficit is to ask the patient to draw, copy (eg, copying the CDT, Rey Complex Figure,[45] the Wechsler Memory Scale[55]), and block assembly.[1] More complex and 3-dimensional objects also may be used. Visual perception can be tested by line bisection tasks, motor-free perceptual tasks (including facial recognition), and decision of whether a figure can be "real" or not based on dimensionality.[1] Perceptual-motor coordination can be tested like rapidly inserting pegs into a slotted board.[1] Wave goodbye can be used to test praxis, and recognition of faces and colors tested gnosis.[1]

Complex attention The submain of complex attention includes sustained attention, divided attention, selective attention, and processing speed.[1] The sustained attention is maintenance of attention over time, which can be tested as "pressing a button every time a tone is heard, and over a period of time."[26] The divided attention is attending to 2 tasks within the same time period, for example, rapidly tapping while learning a story being read.[1] Selective attention is defined as maintenance of attention despite competing stimuli and/or distractors, and can be tested by hearing numbers and letters read and asked to count only letters.[13] Processing speed can be quantified on any task by timing it.[1] Some scales also can test attention, such as Digit Span Forward,[47] Trail Making Test, Part A (TMT-A),[50] and Cued Reaction Time.[56]

Social cognition Social cognition contains recognition of emotions, theory of mind, and insight.[1] Recognition of emotions can be tested by identification of emotion in images of faces representing a variety of both positive and negative emotions.[1] Theory of mind is an ability to consider another person's mental state (eg, thoughts, desires, and intentions) or experience.[1] The theory of mind can be tested by story cards with questions to elicit information about the mental state of the individuals portrayed, for instance, "Where will the girl look for the lost bag?"[1]

SCREENING INSTRUMENTS USED IN DIFFERENT SETTINGS

Brief instruments to screen for cognitive impairment in primary care can adequately detect dementia,[6] and are tools that take 10 minutes or less to administer. The MIS, GPCOG, and Mini-Cog may be most suited in primary care,[57,58] CDT, MMSE, MoCA, SLUMS, and AMT may be most suited to specialty care (**Table 3**).[14,57] In addition to brief tests, more extensive screening and diagnostic instruments are available for use in secondary care (eg, memory clinic, mixed specialist hospital) or other settings, although their longer administration time (10–45 minutes) renders them infeasible for use in primary care. Those major tools include ACE-R, CAMCOG, MoCA, 7MS,[59] and AMT.[60] However, for acute hospital care services, there are no instruments that have high sensitivity and specificity and further work is required.[49]

SCREENING TOOLS USED IN DIFFERENT STAGES
Preclinical Stage

Although there were insufficient data to make any recommendations regarding cognitive screening of asymptomatic individuals,[61] episodic memory deficits may serve as

Table 3
Screening tools in different settings

Settings	Tools
Primary care	Most suited: *MIS, GPCOG, Mini-Cog*; Suited: CAMCOG, CDT, MMSE, MoCA
Specialist services: Memory clinic, mixed specialist hospital, community psychiatry services, neurology	CAMCOG, MoCA, 7MS, AMT, ACE-R, DemTect

Abbreviations: 7MS, 7-minute screen; ACE-R, Addenbrooke cognitive examination revise; AMT, abbreviated mental test; CAMCOG, Cambridge cognitive examination; CDT, clock-drawing test; GPCOG, general practitioner assessment of cognition; MIS, memory impairment screen; MMSE, Mini-Mental State Examination; MoCA, Montreal cognitive assessment.

preclinical cognitive markers for AD that can be detected by memory special tests, such as the CVLT,[62,63] although annual decline in the executive function/working memory domain is relative to persons without AD neuropathology.[63] Neuropsychological batteries, which usually include main cognitive domains (memory, executive function, language, spatial ability, attention, and general intelligence) (**Table 4**), may predict preclinical AD.[64]

Mild Cognitive Impairment

Following the famous Petersen criteria,[65] MCI is a clinical condition of persons involving impaired memory but functioning well and not meeting clinical criteria for dementia. Except for the Petersen criteria (or "in the spirit" of the Petersen criteria), other major criteria included the international working definition by Winblad and colleagues,[66] and suboptimal performance on cognitive testing (eg, between 1–2 SDs below norm, CDR score of 0.5) without evidence of functional limitations.[14] It is necessary to evaluate and clinically monitor individuals with MCI due to their increased risk for developing dementia.[61] The MMSE[21] is the most commonly used in clinical practice[67]; however, its ability to distinguish MCI sufferers from healthy elderly adults has not been established.[10] The sensitivity and specificity of the MMSE to diagnose MCI

Table 4
Screening tools in different stages

Cognitive Impairment Degrees	Tools
Preclinical stage	Suited: Neuropsychological batteries include main cognitive domains (memory, executive function, language, spatial ability, attention and general intelligence)
MCI	Most suited: *MoCA, ACE-R*; Suited: MMSE, SLUM, DemTect
Dementia	Most suited: *MMSE, Mini-Cog, ACE-R*; Suited: CDT, VFT, IQCODE, MIS, AMT, FCSRT, 7MS, TICS

Abbreviations: 7MS, 7-minute screen; ACE-R, Addenbrooke cognitive examination revise; AMT, abbreviated mental test; CDT, clock-drawing test; FCSRT, free and cued selective reminding test; IQCODE, informant questionnaire on cognitive decline in the elderly; MIS, memory impairment screen; MMSE, Mini-Mental State Examination; MoCA, the Montreal cognitive assessment; SLUMS, Saint Louis University mental status examination; TICS, telephone interview for cognitive status; VFT, verbal fluency test.

also varied (18.1% −85.7% vs 48.0%–100%[24]). With sensitivity of 92% to 95% and specificity of 76% to 81%, the SLUMS is possibly better at detecting mild NCD that the MMSE failed to detect.[34] Compared with the MMSE, the MoCA was better in detecting MCI among patients older than 60[26] and was likely to be the best alternative for MCI.[68] Both MoCA[25] and ACE-R[8] have high sensitivity (90% vs 84%) and excellent specificity (87% vs 100%) for screening MCI; however, both of them failed to discriminate between minimally educated patients with MCI and age and education matched healthy controls.[10] DemTect screened MCI with sensitivities of 80%.[9] ACE-R[8] and the DemTect[9] have been validated for use within a range of non-AD dementias in conjunction with MCI, more useful in secondary and tertiary care than community or primary care.[10]

Dementia

DSM-III or DSM-IV or National Institute of Neurologic and Communicative Disorders and Stroke and the Alzheimer's Disease and Related Disorders Association (NINCDS-ADRDA) criteria are the most common for diagnosing dementia.[14] The MMSE is the most widely used brief screening tool for dementia[69] and should be considered as cognitive screening instruments in elderly patients for the detection of dementia in individuals with suspected cognitive impairment.[61] The MMSE demonstrated a moderate specificity (71%) and sensitivity (86%) with a poor positive predictive value (34%) and excellent negative predictive value (97%) when the base rate of disease was 14%. Other most commonly evaluated screening instruments included (most to least common): CDT, verbal/category fluency tests, short or full IQCODE, MIS, Mini-Cog, AMT, FCSRT, 7MS, and TICS.[14] The Mini-Cog test and the ACE-R were likely to be the best alternative screening tests for dementia.[68]

SCREENING TOOLS USED IN DIFFERENT CONDITIONS
Alzheimer Disease

AD is the major type of dementia and one of the great health care challenges of the twenty-first century.[70] The typical presentation of AD is memory impairment and executive dysfunction interfering with daily life activities.[70] Highly selective tests (eg, GPCOG, MIS, Mini-Cog, and CDT) (**Table 5**) have been validated as screening tests

Table 5	
Screening tools in different cognitive impairment condition	
Cognitive Impairment Condition	**Tools**
Alzheimer disease	Suited: MIS, GPCOG, Mini-Cog, CDT, LM-II + AVLT + TMT-B/TMT-A
Frontal lobe dementia	Suited: FAB, EXIT-25
Vascular	Suited: TMT + DS, IBCST, MoCA, MMSE, CAMCOG, ACE-R
Parkinson disease dementia	Most suited: *PD-CRS*; Suited: MoCA, SCOPA-COG, ACE-R

Abbreviations: ACE-R, Addenbrooke cognitive examination revise; AVLT, Rey auditory verbal learning test; CAMCOG, Cambridge cognitive examination; CDT, clock-drawing test; DS, digit span; EXIT-25, executive interview; FAB, frontal assessment battery; GPCOG, general practitioner assessment of cognition; IBCST, informant-based cognitive screening tests; LM-II, logical memory story A delayed recall; MIS, memory impairment screen; MMSE, Mini-Mental State Examination; MoCA, Montreal cognitive assessment; PD-CRS, Parkinson disease cognitive rating scale; SCOPA-COG, scales for outcomes of Parkinson disease–cognition; TMT-A, Trail Making Test, part A; TMT-B, Trail Making Test, part B.

for patients with moderate AD.[60] Although designed to detect AD, they may be less able to detect other forms of dementia; patients with dementia of Lewy bodies may have poor score on the CDT.[60] Episodic memory impairment in MCI was defined as scores < −1 SD below normative references on 2 measures (Logical memory story A delayed recall [LM-II], Rey auditory verbal learning test [AVLT]), which can predict AD with 75.9% accuracy.[71] Although the cutoffs were less than −1.5 SD and −2.0 SD on one memory test, the accuracy in predicting AD was 66.6% and 76.5%, respectively.[71] TMT-B/TMT-A ratio can improve predictive accuracy.[71]

Frontotemporal

Some instruments are focused on detecting impairments in executive function which are important for diagnosing a range of dementia types, such as frontotemporal dementia (FTD).[72] The Frontal Assessment Battery (FAB) is estimated to take approximately 10 minutes to complete.[73] Subjects are allocated a score between 0 and 18, with lower scores indicating more severe impairment.[74] It is effective at differentiating patients with frontal lobe impairment from healthy controls.[74] The Executive Interview (EXIT-25) is a 25-item screening tool of executive function that is estimated to take 10 minutes to complete, with higher scores representing greater impairment.[75] The FAB and the EXIT-25 have similar diagnostic efficiency for distinguishing FTD from AD.[72]

Vascular

Vascular diseases, such as cerebral small vessel disease (SVD) and post-stroke dementia (PSD), are a common cause of cognitive impairment and vascular dementia. The cognitive deficit of SVD differs from that in AD, with greater executive/attentional dysfunction and relatively intact episodic memory. The best brief executive assessment is using the combination of TMT and digit span, which can offer good sensitivity and specificity for identifying subjects with ischemic leukoaraiosis (sensitivity 88%, specificity 88%).[76] For diagnosis of PSD, MoCA at thresholds less than 22/30 offers short assessment time with sensitivity 0.84 and specificity 0.78 for diagnosis of dementia and multidomain cognitive impairment in stroke.[77] Informant-Based Cognitive Screening Tests (IBCST) has a summary sensitivity 0.81 and summary specificity 0.83 for diagnosis of dementia and multidomain cognitive impairment in stroke.[78] Other screening tools for diagnosis of PSD include ACE-R (thresholds <88/100) with sensitivity 0.96 and specificity 0.70, MMSE (thresholds <27/30) with sensitivity 0.71 and specificity 0.85, and Rotterdam-CAMCOG (thresholds <33/49) with sensitivity 0.57 and specificity 0.92.[77]

Parkinson Disease

Cognitive impairment in Parkinson disease (PD) includes fronto-subcortical (attention and executive function) and cortical (prefrontal tasks, visuospatial skills, and memory) dysfunction.[79] The CDT may be used to discriminate PD from dementia with Lewy bodies (68% overall classification).[80] The MoCA may be well-suited to screen for cognitive impairment in PD.[81] The Scales for Outcomes of Parkinson's disease–cognition (SCOPA-COG) is a 10-item, reliable, specific, and valid instrument that is sensitive to identifying cognitive deficits in PD.[82] The maximum score of SCOPA-COG is 43 and the test-retest reliability of the total score was 0.78.[82] ACE-R has a cut-off less than 89 with a sensitivity of 69% and specificity of 84% in detecting MCI in PD.[83] Parkinson's Disease Cognitive Rating Scale (PD-CRS) was designed to cover both the fronto-subcortical and cortical dysfunction of cognitive defects associated with PD.[79] The PD-CRS has an excellent sensitivity (94%) and specificity (94%) to diagnose PD dementia.[79]

SCREENING TOOLS USED IN SPECIAL PEOPLE
Hearing or Visually Disabled Patients

Poor hearing and visual function increase in prevalence with age, as do a decline in cognitive function.[84,85] However, cognitive screening tools mostly rely on items being correctly heard or seen. Confounding of cognitive tests with hearing or visual loss results in false-positive identification of cognitive impairment, overestimation of the severity of cognitive impairment, and reduced test specificity.[86] MMSE and MoCA are the frequently adapted tests in individuals with hearing or vision impairment (**Table 6**).[86] Adaptations for hearing impairment involved deleting (eg, MoCA-H) or creating written versions (eg, written version of the MMSE) for hearing-dependent items.[86] Adaptations for vision impairment involved deleting vision-dependent items (eg, "MMSE-blind" and MoCA-Blind) or spoken versions of visual tasks (eg, the vision-independent MMSE).[86] The Digit Symbol Substitution Test (DSST) is also used to test cognitive function in adults 60 years and older with hearing or vision impairment.[84,85] Verbal Clock Test (VCT) is used to test individuals with vision impairment.[87] But, no study reported the validity and specificity of these tests in relation to detection of dementia in people with hearing or vision impairment.

Illiterate and Low-Educated Older Adults

Illiteracy and low educational background are common in older low-income and middle-income country populations, especially in rural areas. Most older adults with dementia also live in those areas.[4] Because literacy level can affect the results of screening of dementia among illiterate people,[88] there are many challenges in cognitive function assessed by the most of the popular neuropsychological tools.[89] Special attention should be paid to evaluation of functional scales and activity of daily living scales (ADLs) compatible with the culture of each society.[90] Instead of schematic pictures, illustrative cards with real can use for delayed recall assessment.[90] Proverbs and metaphors compatible with ethnicity can be used to assess abstract thinking. Questions about traditions, religious rituals, and historical events can be used to

Table 6
Screening tools in special people

Special People	Tools
Hearing- disabled patients	Suited: MMSE, MoCA; Maybe suited: MMSE-blind, MoCA-blind, the vision-independent MMSE
Visually disabled patients	Suited: MMSE, MoCA; Maybe more suited: DSST, VCT
Illiterate and low-educated older adults	Suited: ADLs, Illustrative cars, proverbs, metaphors, traditions, religious rituals and historical events, naming months of the year forward and backward
Intellectual disabilities	Suited: DRS, DMSE, M-SRT, DLSQ, DSQIID, CCIID, WGB, SIB

Abbreviations: ADLs, activities of daily living scale; CCIID, cognitive computerized test battery for individual's with intellectual disabilities; DLSQ, daily living skills questionnaire; DMSE, Down syndrome mental status examination; DRS, Dementia Rating Scale; DSQIID, dementia screening questionnaire for individuals with intellectual disabilities; DSST, digit symbol substitution test; MMSE, Mini-Mental State Examination; MoCA, Montreal cognitive assessment; M-SRT, the modified version of the selective re- minding test; SIB, severe impairment battery; VCT, verbal clock test; WGB, working groups battery.

evaluate general information and praxis. Asking about how to cook a special dish, especially among women, can be useful to evaluate planning. For attention, concentration, and working memory, naming months of the year forward and backward can be useful.[90]

People with Intellectual Disabilities

Individuals with intellectual disabilities (ID), such as Down syndrome, often experience onset of aging characteristics earlier than in the general population.[91] Instruments used for ID usually are cataloged to direct cognitive test, informant reports, and test batteries.[92] For direct cognitive tests, various tools test memory, overall cognitive functioning, and mental status. However, many tests (eg, MMSE,[93] PCFT,[94] and CAM-COF[95]) have floor effects when participants have several IDs. The Dementia Rating Scale (DRS[96]) and the Down's Syndrome Mental Status Examination (DMSE[97]) may have good clinical utility and be suitable for dementia diagnostics in ID.[92] The modified version of the Selective Reminding Test (M-SRT[98]) could detect and pick up cognitive changes between 1 and 3 years before dementia diagnosis.[99] Informant reports assess noncognitive concepts, such as ADLs and functioning.[92] Informant reports have an effective way of aiding in dementia diagnostics and are exceedingly suitable for individuals who have severe ID.[92] The Daily Living Skills Questionnaire (DLSQ[100]) was shown to be effective in early detection, showing cognitive changes 3 to 4 years before diagnosis of dementia.[92] The Dementia Screening Questionnaire for Individuals with Intellectual Disabilities (DSQIID[101]) is informative but needs to consider the influence of other demographic factors on dementia status.[92] Because the Activities of Daily Living Questionnaire[102] is better explained by disability level and comorbidity than dementia status, it would not be an effective tool for diagnosing dementia in ID.[92] Test batteries, such as the Cognitive Computerized Test Battery for Individuals with Intellectual Disabilities (CCIID[103]), Working Groups Battery (WGB),[104] Severe Impairment Battery (SIB[105]), which includes both direct cognitive tests and informant reports, were effective in ID dementia diagnosis.[92] However, for the Boston Naming Task (BNT[48]), which is most affected by aging, it is advised to remove the BNT from the battery.[92] It is noteworthy that all the participants in these tools application were not based on older adults and lack of longitudinal studies. Clinicians must be careful when using these instruments to make a decision regarding dementia diagnosis. When the ID is more severe, a shorter instrument may be better to complete.[92]

THE HARM FOR EARLY SCREENING FOR COGNITIVE IMPAIRMENT

Although cognitive impairment screening is important and common, there is as yet no evidence that when given early enough the natural history can be changed.[106] Because every screening instrument has false-positives or false-negatives, screening for cognitive impairment may have direct or indirect harms from the diagnostic inaccuracy of screening.[14] Furthermore, there are many adverse effects, such as adverse effects from workup for false-positives, adverse effects from labeling or treating someone with dementia without diagnostic testing, or adverse effects from missed or delayed diagnosis (false-negatives).[14]

SUMMARY

Although many tools for screening for cognitive impairment in geriatrics are available, few are widely used, and many have limited evidence regarding their performance. Despite its limitations, the MMSE is still the most commonly used in screening dementia; the Mini-Cog and ACE-R also showed excellence in screening for dementia. In

MCI, the MoCA and ACE-R had better performance than the other dementia screening tests. Although there were insufficient data to make any recommendations regarding cognitive screening in the preclinical stage, but by using neuropsychological batteries which main cognitive domains may predict preclinical, such as AD. We highlighted it is better to choose instruments for screening cognitive impairment in geriatrics by considering the settings, stages, conditions, and specific people. Practitioners also need to consider goals and harm for use of the different cognitive tests. A stepped approach may be appropriate with the use in specialist settings of a short instrument followed by a longer one (eg, neuropsychological batteries).

REFERENCES

1. American Psychiatric Association. Diagnostic and statistical manual of mental disorders (DSM-V). Arlington (VA): American Psychiatric Association; 2013.
2. American Psychiatric Association. Diagnostic and statistical manual of mental disorders (DSM-IV). Washington, DC: American Psychiatric Association; 1994.
3. Livingston G, Sommerlad A, Orgeta V, et al. Dementia prevention, intervention, and care. Lancet 2017;390(10113):2673–734.
4. Wimo A, Guerchet M, Ali GC, et al. The worldwide costs of dementia 2015 and comparisons with 2010. Alzheimers Dement 2017;13(1):1–7.
5. Petersen RC, Lopez O, Armstrong MJ, et al. Practice guideline update summary: mild cognitive impairment: report of the guideline development, dissemination, and implementation subcommittee of the American Academy of Neurology. Neurology 2018;90(3):126–35.
6. Lin JS, O'Connor E, Rossom RC, et al. Screening for cognitive impairment in older adults: a systematic review for the U.S. Preventive Services Task Force. Ann Intern Med 2013;159(9):601–12.
7. Woodford HJ, George J. Cognitive assessment in the elderly: a review of clinical methods. QJM 2007;100(8):469–84.
8. Mioshi E, Dawson K, Mitchell J, et al. The Addenbrooke's Cognitive Examination Revised (ACE-R): a brief cognitive test battery for dementia screening. Int J Geriatr Psychiatry 2006;21(11):1078–85.
9. Kalbe E, Kessler J, Calabrese P, et al. DemTect: a new, sensitive cognitive screening test to support the diagnosis of mild cognitive impairment and early dementia. Int J Geriatr Psychiatry 2004;19(2):136–43.
10. Lonie JA, Tierney KM, Ebmeier KP. Screening for mild cognitive impairment: a systematic review. Int J Geriatr Psychiatry 2009;24(9):902–15.
11. Agrell B, Dehlin O. The clock-drawing test. Age Ageing 1998;27(3):399–403.
12. Sunderland T, Hill JL, Mellow AM, et al. Clock drawing in Alzheimer's disease. J Am Geriatr Soc 1989;37(8):725–9.
13. Shulman KI, Shedletsky R, Silver IL. The challenge of time: clock-drawing and cognitive function in the elderly. Int J Geriatr Psychiatry 1986;1(2):135–40.
14. Lin JS, O'Connor E, Rossom RC, et al. Screening for cognitive impairment in older adults: an evidence update for the US Preventive Services Task Force. Rockville (MD): Agency for Healthcare Research and Quality; 2013.
15. Borson S, Scanlan J, Brush M, et al. The Mini-Cog: a cognitive 'vital signs' measure for dementia screening in multi-lingual elderly. Int J Geriatr Psychiatry 2000;15(11):1021–7.
16. Borson S, Scanlan JM, Chen P, et al. The Mini-Cog as a screen for dementia: validation in a population-based sample. J Am Geriatr Soc 2003;51(10):1451–4.

17. Yang L, Yan J, Jin X, et al. Screening for dementia in older adults: comparison of mini-mental state examination, mini-cog, clock drawing test, and AD8. PLoS One 2016;11(12):e0168949.

18. Buschke H, Kuslansky G, Katz M, et al. Screening for dementia with the memory impairment screen. Neurology 1999;52(2):231–8.

19. Kokmen E, Naessens JM, Offord KP. A short test of mental status: description and preliminary results. Mayo Clin Proc 1987;62:281–8.

20. Kokmen E, Smith GE, Petersen RC, et al. The short test of mental status: correlations with standardized psychometric testing. Arch Neurol 1991;48(7):725–8.

21. Folstein MF, Folstein SE, McHugh PR. "Mini-mental state": a practical method for grading the cognitive state of patients for the clinician. J Psychiatr Res 1975; 12(3):189–98.

22. Swain DG, O'Brien AG, Nightingale PG. Cognitive assessment in elderly patients admitted to hospital: the relationship between the abbreviated mental test and the mini-mental state examination. Clin Rehabil 1999;13(6):503–8.

23. Young J, Meagher D, Maclullich A. Cognitive assessment of older people. BMJ 2011;343:d5042.

24. Mitchell AJ. A meta-analysis of the accuracy of the mini-mental state examination in the detection of dementia and mild cognitive impairment. J Psychiatr Res 2009;43(4):411–31.

25. Nasreddine ZS, Phillips NA, Bédirian V, et al. The Montreal Cognitive Assessment, MoCA: a brief screening tool for mild cognitive impairment. J Am Geriatr Soc 2005;53(4):695–9.

26. Ciesielska N, Sokolowski R, Mazur E, et al. Is the Montreal Cognitive Assessment (MoCA) test better suited than the Mini-Mental State Examination (MMSE) in mild cognitive impairment (MCI) detection among people aged over 60? Meta-analysis. Psychiatr Pol 2016;50(5):1039–52.

27. Schofield I, Stott DJ, Tolson D, et al. Screening for cognitive impairment in older people attending accident and emergency using the 4-item Abbreviated Mental Test. Eur J Emerg Med 2010;17(6):340–2.

28. Ivnik RJ, Smith GE, Lucas JA, et al. Free and cued selective reminding test: MOANS norms. J Clin Exp Neuropsychol 1997;19(5):676–91.

29. Solomon PR, Hirschoff A, Kelly B, et al. A 7 minute neurocognitive screening battery highly sensitive to Alzheimer's disease. Arch Neurol 1998;55(3):349–55.

30. Katzman R, Brown T, Fuld P, et al. Validation of a short Orientation-Memory-Concentration Test of cognitive impairment. Am J Psychiatry 1983;140(6):734–9.

31. Brooke P, Bullock R. Validation of a 6 item cognitive impairment test with a view to primary care usage. Int J Geriatr Psychiatry 1999;14(11):936–40.

32. Brandt J, Spencer M, Folstein M. The telephone interview for cognitive status. Neuropsychiatry Neuropsychol Behav Neurol 1988;1(2):111–7.

33. Ferrucci L, Del Lungo I, Guralnik J, et al. Is the telephone interview for cognitive status a valid alternative in persons who cannot be evaluated by the Mini Mental State Examination? Aging Clin Exp Res 1998;10(4):332–8.

34. Tariq SH, Tumosa N, Chibnall JT, et al. Comparison of the Saint Louis University mental status examination and the mini-mental state examination for detecting dementia and mild neurocognitive disorder—a pilot study. Am J Geriatr Psychiatry 2006;14(11):900–10.

35. Brodaty H, Pond D, Kemp NM, et al. The GPCOG: a new screening test for dementia designed for general practice. J Am Geriatr Soc 2002;50(3):530–4.

36. Jorm A, Jacomb P. The Informant Questionnaire on Cognitive Decline in the Elderly (IQCODE): socio-demographic correlates, reliability, validity and some norms. Psychol Med 1989;19(4):1015–22.
37. Jorm A. A short form of the informant questionnaire on cognitive decline in the elderly (IQCODE): development and cross-validation. Psychol Med 1994;24(1): 145–53.
38. Pfeiffer E. A short portable mental status questionnaire for the assessment of organic brain deficit in elderly patients. J Am Geriatr Soc 1975;23(10): 433–41.
39. Galvin J, Roe C, Powlishta K, et al. The AD8. A brief informant interview to detect dementia. Neurology 2005;65(4):559–64.
40. Larner AJ, Mitchell AJ. A meta-analysis of the accuracy of the Addenbrooke's Cognitive Examination (ACE) and the Addenbrooke's Cognitive Examination-Revised (ACE-R) in the detection of dementia. Int Psychogeriatr 2014;26(4): 555–63.
41. Huppert FA, Brayne C, Gill C, et al. CAMCOG—a concise neuropsychological test to assist dementia diagnosis: socio-demographic determinants in an elderly population sample. Br J Clin Psychol 1995;34(4):529–41.
42. Roth M, Tym E, Mountjoy C, et al. CAMDEX. A standardised instrument for the diagnosis of mental disorder in the elderly with special reference to the early detection of dementia. Br J Psychiatry 1986;149(6):698–709.
43. Delis DC, Kramer JH, Kaplan E, et al. CVLT: California verbal learning test-adult version: manual. San Antonio (TX): Psychological Corporation; 1987.
44. Grober E, Buschke H. Genuine memory deficits in dementia. Dev Neuropsychol 1987;3(1):13–36.
45. Rey A. L'examen psychologique dans les cas d'encéphalopathie traumatique. Arch de Psychologie 1941;28:286–340.
46. Knopman DS, Ryberg S. A verbal memory test with high predictive accuracy for dementia of the Alzheimer type. Arch Neurol 1989;46(2):141–5.
47. Wechsler D. The Wechsler adult intelligence scale– revised. New York: The Psychological Corporation; 1988.
48. Kaplan E, Goodglass H, Weintraub S. Boston naming test. Philadelphia: Lea & Febiger; 1983.
49. Velayudhan L, Ryu S-H, Raczek M, et al. Review of brief cognitive tests for patients with suspected dementia. Int Psychogeriatr 2014;26(8):1247–62.
50. Reitan RM. Validity of the trail making test as an indicator of organic brain damage. Percept Mot Skills 1958;8(3):271–6.
51. Stroop JR. Studies of interference in serial verbal reactions. J Exp Psychol 1935; 18(6):643.
52. Petrides M, Milner B. Deficits on subject-ordered tasks after frontal-and temporal-lobe lesions in man. Neuropsychologia 1982;20(3):249–62.
53. Porteus SD. The Maze test and clinical psychology. Palo Alto (CA): Pacific Books; 1959.
54. Craik FI, Klix F, Hagendorf H. A functional account of age differences in memory. Amsterdam: North-Holland; 1986.
55. Wechsler D. A standardized memory scale for clinical use. J Psychol 1945; 19(1):87–95.
56. Baker EL, Letz R, Fidler A. A computer-administered neurobehavioral evaluation system for occupational and environmental epidemiology. Rationale, methodology, and pilot study results. J Occup Med 1985;27(3):206–12.

57. Cordell CB, Borson S, Boustani M, et al. Alzheimer's Association recommendations for operationalizing the detection of cognitive impairment during the Medicare Annual Wellness Visit in a primary care setting. Alzheimers Dement 2013; 9(2):141–50.

58. Brodaty H, Low L-F, Gibson L, et al. What is the best dementia screening instrument for general practitioners to use? Am J Geriatr Psychiatry 2006;14(5): 391–400.

59. Appels BA, Scherder E. The diagnostic accuracy of dementia-screening instruments with an administration time of 10 to 45 minutes for use in secondary care: a systematic review. Am J Alzheimers Dis Other Demen 2010;25(4):301–16.

60. Brown J. The use and misuse of short cognitive tests in the diagnosis of dementia. J Neurol Neurosurg Psychiatry 2015;86(6):680–5.

61. Petersen RC, Stevens JC, Ganguli M, et al. Practice parameter: early detection of dementia: mild cognitive impairment (an evidence-based review) report of the Quality Standards Subcommittee of the American Academy of Neurology. Neurology 2001;56(9):1133–42.

62. Bondi MW, Monsch AU, Galasko D, et al. Preclinical cognitive markers of dementia of the Alzheimer type. Neuropsychology 1994;8(3):374.

63. Mortamais M, Ash JA, Harrison J, et al. Detecting cognitive changes in preclinical Alzheimer's disease: a review of its feasibility. Alzheimers Dement 2017; 13(4):468–92.

64. Albert MS, Moss MB, Tanzi R, et al. Preclinical prediction of AD using neuropsychological tests. J Int Neuropsychol Soc 2001;7(5):631–9.

65. Petersen RC, Smith GE, Waring SC, et al. Mild cognitive impairment: clinical characterization and outcome. Arch Neurol 1999;56(3):303–8.

66. Winblad B, Palmer K, Kivipelto M, et al. Mild cognitive impairment-beyond controversies, towards a consensus: report of the International Working Group on Mild Cognitive Impairment. J Intern Med 2004;256:240–6.

67. Shulman KI, Herrmann N, Brodaty H, et al. IPA survey of brief cognitive screening instruments. Int Psychogeriatr 2006;18(2):281–94.

68. Tsoi KK, Chan JY, Hirai HW, et al. Cognitive tests to detect dementia: a systematic review and meta-analysis. JAMA Intern Med 2015;175(9):1450–8.

69. Boustani M, Peterson B, Hanson L, et al. Screening for dementia in primary care: a summary of the evidence for the US Preventive Services Task Force. Ann Intern Med 2003;138(11):927–37.

70. Scheltens P, Blennow K, Breteler MM, et al. Alzheimer's disease. Lancet 2016; 388(10043):505–17.

71. Callahan BL, Ramirez J, Berezuk C, et al. Predicting Alzheimer's disease development: a comparison of cognitive criteria and associated neuroimaging biomarkers. Alzheimers Res Ther 2015;7(1):68.

72. Bentvelzen A, Aerts L, Seeher K, et al. A comprehensive review of the quality and feasibility of dementia assessment measures: the dementia outcomes measurement suite. J Am Med Dir Assoc 2017;18(10):826–37.

73. Dubois B, Slachevsky A, Litvan I, et al. The FAB: a frontal assessment battery at bedside. Neurology 2000;55(11):1621–6.

74. Wildgruber D, Kischka U, Faßbender K, et al. The frontal lobe score: part II: evaluation of its clinical validity. Clin Rehabil 2000;14(3):272–8.

75. Royall DR, Mahurin RK, Gray KF. Bedside assessment of executive cognitive impairment: the executive interview. J Am Geriatr Soc 1992;40(12):1221–6.

76. O'sullivan M, Morris R, Markus H. Brief cognitive assessment for patients with cerebral small vessel disease. J Neurol Neurosurg Psychiatry 2005;76(8): 1140–5.

77. Lees R, Selvarajah J, Fenton C, et al. Test accuracy of cognitive screening tests for diagnosis of dementia and multidomain cognitive impairment in stroke. Stroke 2014;45(10):3008–18.

78. McGovern A, Pendlebury ST, Mishra NK, et al. Test accuracy of informant-based cognitive screening tests for diagnosis of dementia and multidomain cognitive impairment in stroke. Stroke 2016;47(2):329–35.

79. Pagonabarraga J, Kulisevsky J, Llebaria G, et al. Parkinson's disease-cognitive rating scale: a new cognitive scale specific for Parkinson's disease. Mov Disord 2008;23(7):998–1005.

80. Cahn-Weiner DA, Williams K, Grace J, et al. Discrimination of dementia with Lewy bodies from Alzheimer disease and Parkinson disease using the clock drawing test. Cogn Behav Neurol 2003;16(2):85–92.

81. Dalrymple-Alford J, MacAskill M, Nakas C, et al. The MoCA well-suited screen for cognitive impairment in Parkinson disease. Neurology 2010;75(19):1717–25.

82. Marinus J, Visser M, Verwey N, et al. Assessment of cognition in Parkinson's disease. Neurology 2003;61(9):1222–8.

83. McColgan P, Evans JR, Breen DP, et al. Addenbrooke's cognitive examination-revised for mild cognitive impairment in Parkinson's disease. Mov Disord 2012; 27(9):1173–7.

84. Lin FR, Yaffe K, Xia J, et al. Hearing loss and cognitive decline in older adults. JAMA Intern Med 2013;173(4):293–9.

85. Chen SP, Bhattacharya J, Pershing S. Association of vision loss with cognition in older adults. JAMA Ophthalmol 2017;135(9):963–70.

86. Pye A, Charalambous AP, Leroi I, et al. Screening tools for the identification of dementia for adults with age-related acquired hearing or vision impairment: a scoping review. Int Psychogeriatr 2017;29(11):1771–84.

87. Cercy SP. The verbal clock test: preliminary validation of a brief, vision-and mo-tor-free measure of executive function in a clinical sample. Clin Neuropsychol 2012;26(8):1312–41.

88. Avila R, Moscoso MAA, Ribeiz S, et al. Influence of education and depressive symptoms on cognitive function in the elderly. Int Psychogeriatr 2009;21(3): 560–7.

89. Paddick S-M, Gray WK, McGuire J, et al. Cognitive screening tools for identifi-cation of dementia in illiterate and low-educated older adults, a systematic re-view and meta-analysis. Int Psychogeriatr 2017;29(6):897–929.

90. Noroozian M, Shakiba A, Iran-Nejad S. The impact of illiteracy on the assess-ment of cognition and dementia: a critical issue in the developing countries. Int Psychogeriatr 2014;26(12):2051–60.

91. Lin J-D, Wu C-L, Lin P-Y, et al. Early onset ageing and service preparation in people with intellectual disabilities: institutional managers' perspective. Res Dev Disabil 2011;32(1):188–93.

92. Elliott-King J, Shaw S, Bandelow S, et al. A critical literature review of the effec-tiveness of various instruments in the diagnosis of dementia in adults with intel-lectual disabilities. Alzheimers Dement (Amst) 2016;4:126–48.

93. Deb S, Braganza J. Comparison of rating scales for the diagnosis of dementia in adults with Down's syndrome. J Intellect Disabil Res 1999;43(5):400–7.

94. Nihira K, Leland H, Lambert NM. Adaptive behavior scale, residential and com-munity. 2nd edition. Austin (TX): Pro-ed; 1993.

95. Hon J, Huppert FA, Holland AJ, et al. Neuropsychological assessment of older adults with Down's syndrome: an epidemiological study using the Cambridge Cognitive Examination (CAMCOG). Br J Clin Psychol 1999;38(2):155–65.

96. Mattis S. Dementia rating scale (DRS). Odessa (FL): Psychological Assessment Resources.; 1988.

97. Haxby JV. Neuropsychological evaluation of adults with Down's syndrome: patterns of selective impairment in non-demented old adults. J Intellect Disabil Res 1989;33(3):193–210.

98. Hill A, Wisniewski K, Devenny-Phatate D, et al. Cognitive functioning of older people with Down syndrome. Paper presented at the 8th International Congress of the International Association for Scientific Study of Mental Deficiency. Dublin, Ireland, August 21-25,1988.

99. Krinsky-McHale S, Devenny D, Silverman W. Changes in explicit memory associated with early dementia in adults with Down's syndrome. J Intellect Disabil Res 2002;46(3):198–208.

100. National Institute of Aging. The daily living skills questionnaire. Bethesda (MD): National Institute of Aging, Laboratory of Neurosciences; 1989.

101. Deb S, Hare M, Prior L, et al. Dementia screening questionnaire for individuals with intellectual disabilities. Br J Psychiatry 2007;190(5):440–4.

102. Mahoney FI, Barthel DW. Functional evaluation: The barthel index. Md State Med J 1965;14:61–5.

103. Wardt VVD, Bandelow S, Hogervorst E. Development of the Cognitive Computerized Test Battery for Individuals with Intellectual Disabilities (CCIID) for the Classification of Athletes with Intellectual Disabilities. New York: Nova Science Publishers; 2011.

104. Burt DB, Aylward EH. Test battery for the diagnosis of dementia in individuals with intellectual disability. J Intellect Disabil Res 2000;44(2):175–80.

105. Saxton J, McGonigle K, Swihart A, et al. The severe impairment battery. London: Thames Valley Test Company; 1993.

106. Fox C, Lafortune L, Boustani M, et al. The pros and cons of early diagnosis in dementia. Br J Gen Pract 2013;63(612):e510–2.

Reversible Dementias

Milta O. Little, DO

KEYWORDS

- Cognitive impairment • Dementia • Reversible

KEY POINTS

- Not all dementia is Alzheimer disease and many dementing illnesses are reversible to some extent.
- Every memory or cognitive complaint should be accompanied by a thorough evaluation for a potentially reversible cause.
- The DEMENTIAS mnemonic can help to guide practitioners in the evaluation, diagnosis, and management of dementing illnesses.

INTRODUCTION

Cognitive impairment has become a major worldwide public safety issue because the prevalence seems to be increasing globally. In addition to global health policy to address risk factors for dementia, interprofessional health education is needed to better appreciate the many different types of dementing illnesses that present in the various clinical settings. There are many metabolic, cardiovascular, and metabolic risk factors that, when ameliorated, can help to prevent cognitive decline and dementia.[1–3] The appropriate management of dementia begins with the understanding that not all dementing illnesses are Alzheimer disease and many dementing illness can be reversed to some extent. Therefore, the first step in the evaluation of mild or major neurocognitive disorder is to rule out one or more of the potential reversible dementias.

A reversible dementia is caused by a readily treatable and potentially curable underlying disease. **Fig. 1** is a mnemonic that can help practitioners to easily recall the most common reversible dementias. The prevalence of reversible dementias is difficult to estimate because many go undetected, but it is thought to range from 5% to 40%, with a decreasing likelihood of full reversibility with advancing age.[4–6] One person may have multiple reversible and irreversible causes of memory loss and functional impairment, so it is important to be thorough in the evaluation stage of disease management. This is also why the treatment of a reversible dementia may not result in the full reversal of cognitive damage that has already

Disclosure Statement: No relevant financial disclosures.
Division of Geriatric Medicine, Department of Internal Medicine, Saint Louis University Health Center, 1402 South Grand Boulevard Room M238, St Louis, MO 63104, USA
E-mail address: Milta.little@health.slu.edu

Clin Geriatr Med 34 (2018) 537–562
https://doi.org/10.1016/j.cger.2018.07.001
0749-0690/18/© 2018 Elsevier Inc. All rights reserved.
geriatric.theclinics.com

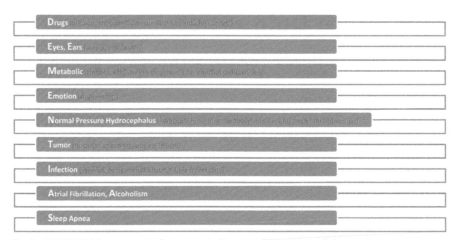

Fig. 1. DEMENTIAS mnemonic for potentially reversible causes of dementia.

taken place. Patients and caregivers need to be made aware of this possibility to set realistic expectations. In some cases, the best outcome is a stall in disease pathology and clinical progression.

Many of the treatable causes of dementia can be excluded clinically with a good history and physical examination that includes a comprehensive geriatric assessment without further investigation; however, most people who present with cognitive impairment should at least have basic laboratory work and imaging.[7,8]

DRUGS

A growing body of evidence shows that medication use, particularly in the setting of polypharmacy, can negatively impact cognition. Older adults are particular sensitive to medications because of physiologic changes that occur with aging that affect pharmacodynamics and pharmacokinetics (**Table 1**).

Table 1
Age-related changes pertinent to geropharmacology

Parameter	Age-Related Changes	Clinical Effect
Tissue sensitivity	Alteration in receptor number and affinity	Patients may be more or less sensitive to a drug
Absorption	Gastric motility and blood flow (decrease) Gastric pH (increase)	Insignificant, unless there are other underlying gastrointestinal diseases
Distribution	Total body water and lean body mass (decrease → V_d decrease) Total body fat (increase → V_d increase)	Water-soluble drugs → higher plasma concentration Fat soluble drugs → longer half-life
Metabolism	Reductions of hepatic blood flow and decline in phase I drug metabolism	Decreased clearance of drugs metabolized by liver; first-pass metabolism also affected
Excretion	Renal blood flow reduced and average clearance declines	Longer half-life and/or higher serum concentrations

Abbreviation: V_d, volume of distribution.
Adapted from Cepeda OA, Morley JE. Polypharmacy, is this another disease? In: Pathy MS, Sinclair A, Morley JE, editors. Principles and practice of geriatric medicine. 4th edition. London: John Wiley & Sons; 2006. p. 217; with permission.

Pharmacodynamics deals with the body's responsiveness or sensitivity to a particular substance at a given concentration. Although pharmacodynamics is less extensively studied than pharmacokinetics, we know that the sensitivity to drugs may increase (as with sedatives[9,10] and narcotics[11,12]) or decrease with age (drugs mediated by beta-adrenergic receptors[13]). The response of older persons to any given medication is also extremely variable, so understanding the common side effects and minimizing the use of drugs are essential. Any patient complaint, in particular one related to memory or cognition, should prompt an investigation into a possible medication reaction. Even seemingly unlikely medications may be the cause and cessation of these drugs could lead to improved symptoms.[14]

Pharmacokinetics is related to how a drug moves through the body and the resultant action the drug has in the body over time. It is affected by 4 factors: absorption, distribution, biotransformation (metabolism), and excretion. Medications undergo either hepatic or renal metabolism to be cleared from the body and toxicity is more likely in the presence of organ dysfunction. Liver size may decrease with age and decreases in blood flow of 25% to 47% have been reported in persons between the ages of 25 and 90.[15] Drugs that are metabolized by the liver depend on hepatic blood flow and, if hepatic blood flow is decreased, systemic bioavailability is increased, putting patients at risk for adverse effects, including cognitive impairment. Unfortunately, there are no systematic ways to determine hepatic blood flow in the clinical setting. What can be analyzed is phase I metabolism through the cytochrome P450 system, which is most affected by aging. Substrates are medications metabolized by particular P450 enzymes. Inhibitors impair the ability of specific P450 enzymes to metabolize their target substrates, thus increasing blood levels and likely the toxicity of the substrate medications. Conversely, inducers increase the production of particular P450 enzymes, leading to increased metabolism (decreased effectiveness) of the substrates of that P450 enzyme.[16] **Table 2** lists the 5 most common cytochrome P450 enzymes with which clinicians need to be familiar. This table allows prescribers to enter the medications from a patient's medication list into the appropriate column to determine potential drug toxicity leading to cognitive impairment.

Renal metabolism can be easily estimated clinically using a formula, such as the Cockgroft-Gault, and should be calculated at every medication review or when a new medication is initiated.

Many of the medications that cause dementia do so by acting as anticholinergic agents,[17] which are commonly used for upper respiratory infections, atopic conditions,

Table 2
Practical tool to identify drugs that interact with common cytochrome P450 enzymes resulting in higher risk of side effects

Cytochrome P450 Enzymes	Substrates	Inhibitors	Substrate Side Effects	Inducer	Substrate Therapeutic Effects
1A2					
2C9					
2C19					
2D9					
3A4					
Metabolized by liver but enzyme unknown					
Not metabolized by liver					

nausea, and urinary incontinence. Acetylcholine is a critical neurotransmitter that acts in the central nervous system on nicotinic and muscarinic receptors for awareness, short-term memory, and long-term learning. The activity of acetylcholine decreases with age, which places older adults at a greater risk for cognitive decline.[18] Anticholinergic agents impair nicotinic and muscarinic receptors, blocking the ability for acetylcholine to act on these receptors. Prospective studies have shown that older adults taking anticholinergic medications for an extended period of time perform worse on cognitive testing and have statistically and clinically significantly more cognitive impairment than those not on anticholinergic medications.[17,19–27] In addition, anticholinergic agents may worsen memory and cognitive function in people with preclinical or mild Alzheimer disease and should be avoided if possible in these patients.[17,28] Caution should be taken when prescribing any agent with a high anticholinergic burden to an aging adult and the use of selective, peripherally acting agents is preferred.[8,17,18,26] In addition, medications that depress the central nervous system (particularly benzodiazepines) have been associated with a statistically significant increase in the incidence of dementia[18,25,29–31] and should be used sparingly and started at the lowest doses in older adults (**Table 3**). The cumulative effects of anticholinergic and psychotropic medications over time seem to be important in the risk of developing significant cognitive impairment.[28,32–34] Several tools exist that help a prescriber to determine which medications may have greater risks of causing adverse cognitive effects, including the American Geriatrics Society BEERS criteria[35] and the European START/STOPP criteria.[36] **Table 4** is from the 2015 Update BEERS criteria and lists the most common medications with high anticholinergic burden. Note must be made that this set of criteria is based on medications that are available in the United States; therefore, some of these medications may not be applicable to prescribers in other countries. Section D of the START/STOPP criteria lists, with rationale, medications that may affect the central nervous system. The Anticholinergic Burden Scale and Anticholinergic Risk Scale have been developed to assess the impact of these medications on patients. Higher Anticholinergic Burden Scale and Anticholinergic Risk Scale scores have been associated with worse cognitive function.[37,38] These tools may be useful to prescribers and pharmacists when deprescribing.

There is a large body of evidence demonstrating that deprescribing can be done safely[39–41] and improves clinical outcomes, including cognitive and psychomotor function.[25,42–44]

EYES AND EARS

Hearing impairment is the most common sensory deficit affecting people across the lifespan and is a major global health issue, with more than 350 million people affected by disabling hearing loss worldwide and it is estimated that by 2025 more than 900 million people will be affected.[45–47] About one-third of people between 60 and 70 years of age experience hearing loss and more than 80% of those more than age 85 years are affected.[48] Hearing loss leads to sensory deprivation, social isolation, depression, increased health care costs, and increased cognitive load.[45,46,48,49] Visual impairment increases with age and is caused by a variety of conditions, including age-related macular degeneration, glaucoma, and cataracts. Vision loss also leads to social isolation and can lead to visual hallucinations, called Charles Bonnet syndrome, which may be mistaken for psychiatric illness.[50] Both hearing loss and vision loss have been associated with changes in brain structure and an increased risk of dementia and cognitive decline, but it is unclear if this association is causal.[45,48,51–66] The combination of vision and hearing loss may lead to more significant and rapid functional and

Table 3
BEERS criteria for drugs to avoid in cognitive impairment

Disease or Syndrome	Drug(s)	Rationale	Recommendation	Quality of Evidence	Strength of Recommendation
Dementia or cognitive impairment	Anticholinergics	Avoid because of adverse central nervous system effects	Avoid	Moderate	Strong
	Benzodiazepines H2 receptor antagonists Nonbenzodiazepine, benzodiazepine receptor agonist hypnotics Antipsychotics, chronic and as-needed use	Avoid antipsychotics for behavioral problems of dementia or delirium unless nonpharmacologic options (eg, behavioral interventions) have failed or are not possible and the older adult is threatening substantial harm to self or others Antipsychotics are associated with greater risk of cerebrovascular accident (stroke) and mortality in persons with dementia			

From American Geriatrics Society BEERS Criteria Update Expert Panel. American Geriatrics Society 2015 updated BEERS criteria for potentially inappropriate medication use in older adults. J Am Geriatr Soc 2015;63(11):2238; with permission.

Table 4
Drugs with strong anticholinergic properties

Antihistamines	Antiparkinsonian agents	Skeletal muscle relaxants
Brompheniramine	Benztropine	Cyclobenzaprine
Carbinoxamine	Trihexyphenidyl	Orphenadrine
Chlorpheniramine		
Clemastine		
Cyproheptadine		
Dexbrompheniramine		
Dexchlorpheniramine		
Dimenhydrinate		
Diphenhydramine (oral)		
Doxylamine		
Hydroxyzine		
Meclizine		
Triprolidine		
Antidepressants	Antipsychotics	Antiarrhythmic
Amitriptyline	Chlorpromazine	Disopyramide
Amoxapine	Clozapine	
Clomipramine	Loxapine	
Desipramine	Olanzapine	
Doxepin (>6 mg)	Perphenazine	
Imipramine	Thioridazine	
Nortriptyline	Trifluoperazine	
Paroxetine		
Protriptyline		
Trimipramine		
Antimuscarinics (urinary incontinence)	Antispasmodics	Antiemetic
Darifenacin	Atropine (excludes ophthalmic)	Prochlorperazine
Fesoterodine	Belladonna	Promethazine
Flavoxate	alkaloids	
Oxybutynin	Clidinium-chlordiazep oxide	
Solifenacin	Dicyclomine	
Tolterodine	Homatropine (excludes ophthalmic)	
Trospium	Hyoscyamine Propantheline	
	Scopolamine (excludes ophthalmic)	

From American Geriatrics Society BEERS Criteria Update Expert Panel. American Geriatrics Society 2015 updated BEERS criteria for potentially inappropriate medication use in older adults. J Am Geriatr Soc 2015;63(11):2243; with permission.

cognitive decline.[50,67] It is possible that these sensory impairments are modifiable risk factors for dementia or that they share a common neurodegenerative pathway as dementia.[45,49,68] The identification of hearing or vision loss should prompt an evaluation for early cognitive impairment and complaints of cognitive issues should prompt an evaluation of hearing and vision. The correction of vision and hearing impairment may help to prevent dementia, stabilize cognitive decline, and improve global functioning but further research into this area is needed.[45–49,51,68] There is evidence that treatment of cerumen impaction (a major cause of conductive hearing impairment in older adults and long-term care residents) can improve cognitive scores.[69,70] A pilot trial was conducted to test the feasibility of a randomized trial to assess the impact of treating hearing loss on cognition and recruitment for the full trial is currently underway.[71] Assessment of every patient with cognitive impairment should include questions regarding visual and hearing function and loss,[72] as well as a full neurologic, ophthalmologic, and otoscopic examination. Cerumen removal and referrals to appropriate interprofessional specialists should happen early in the disease process to maximize the potential benefits of sensory correction.

EPILEPSY

Subclinical seizure activity (subtle or clinically unrecognized) has been described in case reports and cases series to be a contributing factor to cognitive decline in people with Alzheimer pathology.[73] Adequate treatment of epileptiform activity has been associated with stabilization of decline and maintenance of independent function.[74] Clinicians should maintain a high index of suspicion for undiagnosed seizure activity in early-onset dementia and in people exhibiting a rapid decline in cognition. Diagnosis is made by serial or extended electroencephalographic monitoring in the ambulatory setting, which may be difficult to obtain. More research into this area is needed.

METABOLIC
Thyroid Disease and Cognition: Recognition and Management

Thyroid hormones exert important physiologic effects on cognition and behavior, especially during neural development. Abnormal thyroid function tests, in particular, elevated thyroid-stimulating hormone and decreased triiodothyronine and thyroxine levels, have been correlated with cortical ischemia, vascular dementia, and cognitive decline.[75–79] However, this evidence is mixed[77,78,80,81] and there is little evidence for hypothyroidism as a sole cause of dementia or for treatment with thyroid hormone replacement to reverse cognitive impairment.[79,82] The same can be said for hyperthyroidism, with higher thyroxine levels associated with increased risk of Alzheimer disease brain pathology,[77,79,83] but little evidence for improved cognition with treatment of such abnormalities. Although more evidence is needed to confirm the relationship of thyroid disease with dementia and the impact of treatment, it is still recommended to test thyroid function in the workup of cognitive impairment[8] because thyroid disease can lead to other issues that impact functional trajectories in dementia, such as depression, weight loss, or cardiac arrhythmias.

Vitamin Deficiencies

Vitamin B_{12} and folate are critical for normal neural function and severe deficiency is associated with anemia and cognitive decline.[8,82] The most common cause of vitamin B_{12} deficiency in older adults is malabsorption and decreased oral intake. B_{12} and folate deficiency are also associated with alcohol abuse (discussed elsewhere in this article). Folate deficiency, even in the absence of anemia, may lead to high homocysteine levels, which is associated with vascular disease and Alzheimer pathology.[84,85] Unfortunately, metaanalyses have not found a statistically significant benefit of repletion of vitamin B_{12} or folate on cognition or mood.[84,86] Niacin (vitamin B_6) deficiency is also associated with dementia that is fully reversible once replenished; however, it is very unusual to see cases of pellagra in developed countries, where food is fortified with niacin,[82] and there is no evidence for the benefit of adding a niacin supplement regimen for people with cognitive impairment with or without anemia.[87]

Disorders of Sodium and Water Metabolism

Sodium abnormalities are unique electrolyte disturbances because it is not a simple matter of having an excess or insufficient supply of sodium. Sodium and water metabolism involves a complex interplay between the vascular, neural, and renal systems. Older adults experience physiologic changes that predispose them to the syndrome of inappropriate antidiuretic hormone and are also more likely to have comorbid conditions and drugs that further worsen the syndrome of inappropriate antidiuretic hormone. People are more likely to experience confusion and encephalopathy related to sudden and dramatic changes in sodium levels; however, chronic hyponatremia and hypernatremia have also been associated with cognitive decline.[82,88] The treatment of sodium abnormalities begins with a thorough investigation into the underlying cause, starting with an assessment of plasma osmolality and fluid status. Any potentially offending medications should be discontinued or have the dosages reduced. Correction with saline versus water intake versus water restriction versus diuresis depends on the underlying cause. Salt tablets should not be used for the correction of hyponatremia.

Parathyroid and Calcium Metabolism

Hyperparathyroidism leading to hypercalcemia and hypoparathyroidism leading to hypocalcemia have both been associated with cognitive decline and dementia. Correction of the parathyroid abnormalities with parathyroid resection (hyperparathyroid) or calcitriol (hypoparathyroid) has been associated with improved mentation.[82,89]

A Word on Diabetes

A full article in this special edition focuses on dementia associated with diabetes mellitus. It is important for providers to understand that people with diabetes have a very high risk of developing cognitive impairment[90] and dementia in diabetes seems to be a unique condition with a combination of vascular disease, hippocampal volume loss, brain volume loss, and amyloid deposition. Both hypoglycemia and hyperglycemia have been associated with cognitive changes and decline.[82,91] Careful management of diabetes to avoid frequent episodes of either low or high blood sugars is imperative to avoid more rapid cognitive decline.

EMOTION

It is well-established that there is a strong association between depression and dementia. Older adults with depression may present primarily with apathy and difficulties with concentration, which may be mistaken for memory decline. This has traditionally been referred to as pseudodementia and the associated cognitive dysfunction was thought to be completely reversible. This relationship seems to be far more complicated. Early and late-life depression have been shown to be risk factors for developing dementia and depression is often a comorbid condition in all stages of dementia.[92–97] However, an exact causal link either way has not yet been established and evidence on this topic is mixed.[92] It is unlikely that there is 1 set chain of events but rather a complex relationship between the presence of risk factors for both depression and dementia and the fact that the presence of either condition leads to further neural changes and diminished cognitive reserve that predispose to progressive mood and cognitive decline.[92,98,99] This relationship has been described as the web of causation or the multiple pathways model.[100,101] Regardless of causality, every comprehensive evaluation of dementia should include a screen for depression, because treatment may help to improve quality of life, decrease institutionalization, and, in some cases, improve cognitive function.[99,102] Recent animal studies have shown that the treatment of depression with the serotonin reuptake inhibitor citalopram improved memory, cognition, and beta-amyloid deposition.[103,104] Human studies showing similar results are emerging,[105,106] but there have also been negative trials[107,108] so further studies are needed to confirm the benefit of treatment with antidepressants for the prevention or treatment of cognitive impairment.[109] Depression is often minimized or more subtle in older adults, so it is imperative to use validated tools to regularly screen people for depression over time. In mild cognitive impairment, one may use the Geriatric Depression Scale or Patient Health Questionnaire-9 (**Fig. 2**). These screening tests may not be accurate in people exhibiting moderate cognitive impairment, when one can use the Saint Louis University AM SAD tool (**Fig. 3**)[110] or the Hamilton Depression Rating Scale, or in those with advanced cognitive impairment, when it is recommended to use a caregiver assessment scale such as the Cornell Scale for Depression in Dementia (**Fig. 4**).[99,111,112]

Over the last 2 wk, how often have you been bothered by any of the following problems? (Use "✔" to indicate your answer)	Not at all	Several days	More than half the days	Nearly every day
1. Little interest or pleasure in doing things	0	1	2	3
2. Feeling down, depressed, or hopeless	0	1	2	3
3. Trouble falling or staying asleep, or sleeping too much	0	1	2	3
4. Feeling tired or having little energy	0	1	2	3
5. Poor appetite or overeating	0	1	2	3
6. Feeling bad about yourself — or that you are a failure or have let yourself or your family down	0	1	2	3
7. Trouble concentrating on things, such as reading the newspaper or watching television	0	1	2	3
8. Moving or speaking so slowly that other people could have noticed? Or the opposite — being so fidgety or restless that you have been moving around a lot more than usual	0	1	2	3
9. Thoughts that you would be better off dead or of hurting yourself in some way	0	1	2	3

FOR OFFICE CODING ___0___ + _____ + _____ + _____

=Total Score: _____

If you checked off any problems, how difficult have these problems made it for you to do your work, take care of things at home, or get along with other people?

Not difficult at all	Somewhat difficult	Very difficult	Extremely difficult
☐	☐	☐	☐

Fig. 2. Patient Health Questionnaire-9 (PHQ-9). (*Courtesy of* Drs Robert L. Spitzer, Janet B.W. Williams, Kurt Kroenke and colleagues, with an educational grant from Pfizer Inc.)

Categories/Areas Concerned: Appetite
                               Mood
                               Sleep
                               Activity and Energy
                               Death: thoughts of or feelings of worthlessness/guilt

Date _____   Code (research use only) _____

Gender _____   Age _____ Date of Birth _____ Race _____

Within the past 2 weeks, how many times have you experienced :

1. unexplained change in appetite?

Never	0 points
One day	1 point
More than one day	2 points

2. unexplained lowered mood on a day to day basis?

Never	0 points
One day	1 point
More than one day	2 points

3. unexplained disturbed sleep?

Never	0 points
One day	1 point
More than one day	2 points

4. less energy or not being interested in performing your usual daily activities?

Never	0 points
One day	1 point
More than one day	2 points

5. feelings of worthlessness or guilt or that your life is not worth living?

Never	0 points
One day	1 point
More than one day	2 points

Total score : _____

Fig. 3. Saint Louis University AM SAD depression screening tool. (*From* Chakkamparambil B, Chibnall JT, Graypel EA, et al. Development of a brief validated geriatric depression screening tool: the SLU "AM SAD". Am J Geriatr Psychiatry 2015;23(8):781; with permission.)

Although little evidence exists to support best treatment practices, it is currently recommended to treat depression in dementia using a combination of pharmacologic and aggressive nonpharmacologic measures.[94,99,102] Be mindful of the pharmacologic effects of several antidepressant classes on cognition (discussed elsewhere in this article) and always start at the lowest dose possible and increase at a slow rate to maximize benefits while minimizing side effects. Electroconvulsive therapy is a relatively safe treatment option and should be considered in people with severe depression that is refractory to conventional treatment.

Name_____ Age___ Sex___ Date_____

Inpatient   Nursing Home Resident   Outpatient
Person performing evaluation: Clinician   Nurse   Family Member   Other

Scoring System

A = unable to evaluate   0 = absent   1 = mild or intermittent   2 = severe

Base ratings on symptoms and signs occurring during the week prior to interview.
No score should be given in symptoms resulting from physical disability or illness.

A. Mood-Related Signs

1. Anxiety: anxious expression, ruminations, worrying   a 0 1 2
2. Sadness: sad expression, sad voice, tearfulness   a 0 1 2
3. Lack of reactivity to pleasant events   a 0 1 2
4. Irritability: easily annoyed, short-tempered   a 0 1 2

B. Behavioral Disturbance

5. Agitation: restlessness, handwringing, hairpulling   a 0 1 2
6. Retardation: slow movement, slow speech, slow reactions   a 0 1 2
7. Multiple physical complaints (score 0 if GI symptoms only)   a 0 1 2
8. Loss of interest: less involved in usual activities   a 0 1 2
   (score only if change occurred acutely, i.e., in less than one month)

C. Physical Signs

9. Appetite loss: eating less than usual   a 0 1 2
10. Weight loss (score 2 if greater than 5 lbs. in one month)   a 0 1 2
11. Lack of energy: fatigues easily, unable to sustain activities   a 0 1 2
    (score only if change occurred acutely, i.e., in less than one month)

D. Cyclic Functions

12. Diurnal variation of mood: symptoms worse in morning   a 0 1 2
13. Difficulty falling asleep: later than usual for this individual   a 0 1 2
14. Multiple awakenings during sleep   a 0 1 2
15. Early morning awakening: earlier than usual for this individual   a 0 1 2

E. Ideational Disturbance

16. Suicide: feels life is not worth living, has suicidal wishes or   a 0 1 2
    makes suicide attempt
17. Poor self-esteem: self-blame, self-deprecation, feelings of failure   a 0 1 2
18. Pessimism: anticipation of the worst   a 0 1 2
19. Mood congruent delusions: delusions of poverty, illness, loss   a 0 1 2

A score of ≥8 suggests significant depressive symptoms.

Fig. 4. Cornell scale for depression in dementia. (*From* Alexopoulos GS, Abrams RC, Young RC, et al. Cornell scale for depression in dementia. Biol Psychiatry 1988;23(3):281–3; with permission.)

NORMAL PRESSURE HYDROCEPHALUS

Normal pressure hydrocephalus (NPH) is a neurologic condition in which the cerebrospinal fluid fails to drain properly, leading to enlarged cerebral ventricles, cortical atrophy, dementia, and increased mortality.[113,114] The most common cause of NPH is idiopathic, but it can also be caused by intracranial surgery, trauma, meningitis and subarachnoid hemorrhage.[8] The clinical triad that is required for the diagnosis of NPH is cognitive impairment or confusion (wacky), unsteady and magnetic gait (wobbly), and urinary incontinence (wet). International guidelines state that a probable diagnosis is based on the presence of all 3 features,[7] but even the presence of 1 or 2 features should lead a practitioner to consider NPH in the differential diagnosis.[115,116]

Gait and balance disorders are the most common features of NPH and are usually the first to manifest.[117] Typical NPH gait is described as broad based, slow, short stepped, and magnetic. Patients may complain of feeling like their feet are glued to the floor, difficulty rising from a chair, difficulty walking up a hill or stairs, or dizziness. On examination, clinicians may notice externally rotated feet, difficulty turning, and the lack of apraxia (motor planning). Cognitive deficits are usually frontal subcortical in nature, such as psychomotor slowing, difficulties with concentration and executive function, short-term memory disturbances, and apathy.[115,118,119] Simple clinic-based tools that can be used to identify these features include the 10-m get up and go test, the trails-making A/B test, and the counting backward test.[120] Diagnosis is further corroborated by demonstration of enlarged ventricles on brain imaging via computed tomography scans or MRI (**Figs. 5** and **6**). Definitive treatment for NPH is through the insertion of a ventriculoperitoneal shunt, which has been shown to improve clinical outcomes in 70% to 90% of those with confirmed NPH.[87] Unfortunately, brain pathology, MRI findings, and cerebrospinal fluid markers in idiopathic NPH can look very similar to Alzheimer disease, so confirming the diagnosis can be difficult.[121–124] Because the clinical and imaging findings are not pathognomonic for NPH but treatment can significant improve short-term cognition and function,[125] expert radiologic review and serial lumbar punctures are indicated before undertaking definitive treatment. Testing the various cognitive domains and gait (eg, using the dynamic gait index) before and after cerebrospinal fluid drainage can help to determine which patients would most benefit from definitive shunt placement because evidence shows that initial improvement after drainage can predict long-term impact after shunt placement.[117,126,127] Recent evidence suggests that there are subtle MRI changes in NPH that can help to distinguish this condition from Alzheimer or Lewy body disease, including a decreased corpus callosal angle measure[123,128] and differences in white

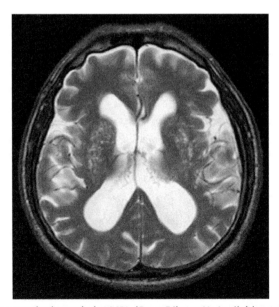

Fig. 5. Normal pressure hydrocephalus MRI. (*From* Dilmen N. Available at: https://commons. wikimedia.org/wiki/File:NPH_MRI_069.png. Accessed February 6, 2018. [CC BY-SA 3.0 (https://creativecommons.org/licenses/by-sa/3.0)].)

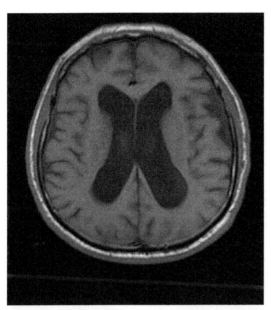

Fig. 6. Normal pressure hydrocephalus MRI. (*From* Dilmen N. Available at: https://commons.wikimedia.org/wiki/File:NPH_MRI_088.png. Accessed February 6, 2018. [CC BY-SA 3.0 (https://creativecommons.org/licenses/by-sa/3.0)].)

matter diffusion patterns.[129,130] Unfortunately, long-term prospective studies indicate that even shunt-responsive people with idiopathic NPH have high rates of cognitive decline and progression to comorbid dementia of an Alzheimer disease, vascular, or frontotemporal type.[119,124,131,132] Shunting may help to delay the deposition of beta-amyloid deposition[133] with initial improvements in memory and gait disturbances,[134] but it does not likely completely halt disease progression.

TUMOR

Similar to NPH, space-occupying lesions caused by benign tumors (meningioma), malignant tumors, or chronic subdural hematomas can lead to stepwise or slow cognitive decline. If caught and treated early, patients may experience reversal of cognitive damage. A comprehensive physical examination with a thorough neurologic and ophthalmologic evaluation as well as computed tomography imaging with and without contrast is warranted in the evaluation of cognitive decline to exclude the presence of tumor or other brain lesions[8] (**Figs. 7** and **8**). The long-term impact of treatments on cognition has not been readily studied or understood but at least partial reversibility has been reported.[6]

INFECTION

Human immunodeficiency virus infection (and associated opportunistic central nervous system infections), syphilis, and Lyme disease are the most common infections to cause neurocognitive damage and cognitive decline. Infectious causes of dementia are not as common in Western countries as in other countries, but should be included in the differential diagnosis, especially in the presence of risk factors or travel to

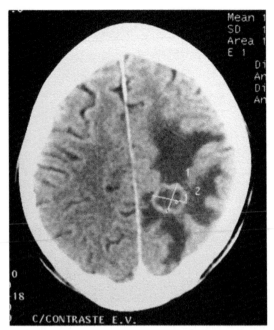

Fig. 7. Brain tumor computed tomography image. (*From* Dilmen N. Available at: https://commons.wikimedia.org/wiki/File:CT_brain_tumor.jpg. Accessed February 6, 2018. [CC BY-SA 3.0 (https://creativecommons.org/licenses/by-sa/3.0)].)

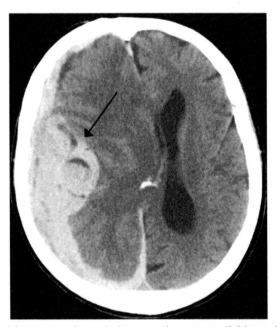

Fig. 8. Intracranial hematoma (*arrow*). (*From* Heilman J. Available at: https://commons.wikimedia.org/wiki/File:Intracranial_bleed_with_significant_midline_shift.png. Accessed February 6, 2018. [CC BY-SA 3.0 (https://creativecommons.org/licenses/by-sa/3.0)].)

endemic areas.[8] Neuroborreliosis has been associated with rapid (over months) cognitive decline, as well as clinical and computed tomography imaging features consistent with NPH. Treatment with appropriate antibiotic therapy has been shown to dramatically improve cognition.[8,135] Risk factors for these infections should be assessed during every cognitive assessment and testing (serum or spinal fluid) may be considered in those with high risk features.

ATRIAL FIBRILLATION

Atrial fibrillation is the most common cardiac arrhythmia and its prevalence increases with age. Multiple studies and metaanalyses have confirmed a link between atrial fibrillation and dementia, even in the absence of a stroke history.[136–142] It is thought that chronic cerebral damage through microembolic and microhemorrhagic events is the leading cause of atrial fibrillation-related dementia.[138,140,143] Several stroke risk factor assessment tools have been developed to guide in the appropriate use of anticoagulation, the most common being the $CHADS_2$ (Congestive heart failure, Hypertension, Age over 75, Diabetes, and Stroke) and CHA_2DS_2 VASc (Congestive heart failure, Hypertension, Age over 65, Age over 75, Diabetes, Stroke, Vascular disease, Sex) scores. It seems that atrial fibrillation and dementia share common risk factors (**Fig. 9**).[139,140] A recent cohort study indicates that these scores not only predict risk of stroke, but also of incident dementia, rendering these assessment tools useful for more aggressive evaluation and management of cognitive impairment in people with atrial fibrillation.[144] In addition, people presenting with cognitive impairment should be assessed for the presence of atrial fibrillation through physical examination, electrocardiogram (**Fig. 10**), and cardiac event monitoring.

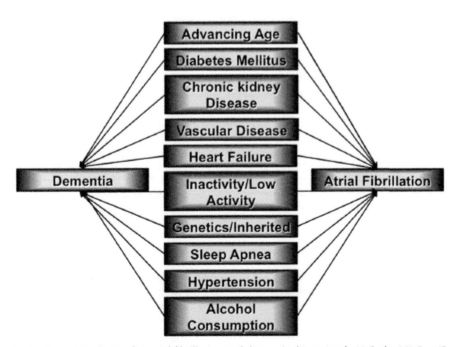

Fig. 9. Shared risk factors for atrial fibrillation and dementia. (*From* Jacobs V, Cutler MJ, Day JD, et al. Atrial fibrillation and dementia. Trends Cardiovasc Med 2015;25(1):46; with permission.)

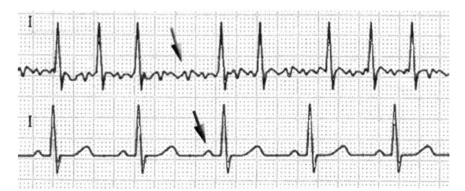

Fig. 10. Electrocardiogram tracing of atrial fibrillation (*top*) and sinus rhythm (*bottom*). The red arrow indicating irregularly irregular P waves in the tracing. The purple arrow indicates a P wave, which is lost in atrial fibrillation. (*From* Heuser J. Available at: https://commons.wikimedia.org/wiki/File:Afib_ecg.jpg#/media/File:Afib_ecg.jpg. Accessed February 6, 2018. [CC BY-SA 3.0 (https://creativecommons.org/licenses/by-sa/3.0)].)

The adequate treatment of atrial fibrillation may help to prevent the onset of both vascular and nonvascular dementia and slow cognitive decline. Anticoagulation is recommended in people with atrial fibrillation to prevent strokes. The incidence of dementia has been shown to be higher in those with indications for anticoagulation who were inadequately treated.[145] There is also evidence that therapeutic doses of warfarin are protective against dementia and anticoagulated individuals who spent more time below the therapeutic range had a greater incidence of dementia.[143] Newer anticoagulant agents that do not require frequent blood monitoring may be preferred for the prevention of cognitive decline, but this strategy has not been studied. Rhythm control was not associated with decreased risk of dementia or mortality in the short-term AFFIRM trial.[140,146] There are even fewer data on the effect of rate control on cognitive impairment and decline but what limited data do exist indicate that those with heart rate averages of less than 75 bpm had a paradoxically higher incidence of dementia.[138] There is emerging evidence that catheter ablation of atrial fibrillation reduces the risk of dementia,[139,140] but ablation has also been associated with short-term postprocedure cognitive impairment. Further studies are needed to confirm these associations and guide appropriate rate or rhythm control (including ablation) therapies. A large, observational, population-based study found that the use of statins in people with chronic atrial fibrillation reduced the risk of nonvascular dementia; therefore, prescribers should consider the use of statin therapy when managing patients with atrial arrhythmias.[136]

ALCOHOLISM

Alcohol use disorders are increasing in those over the age of 65. Interestingly, the effect of alcohol intake on cognition seems to have a J-shaped curve with nonusers and heavy users more likely to experience cognitive decline than those with moderate intake. Several unrelated confounding factors likely contribute to the increased risk seen with nonusers.[147] Excessive alcohol use has long been associated with dementia, particularly affecting the prefrontal and frontal cortices. In addition to the direct neurotoxic effect of alcohol on the brain, other potentially reversible alcohol-related consequences may contribute to potentially reversible cognitive damage, including thiamine deficiency, chronic liver disease, seizures, falls leading to head injury, and other concurrent substance abuse disorders.[147] The brain structures of the affected areas experience shrinkage, which has been shown to reverse to some extent with cessation of drinking. Because normal aging is also associated with prefrontal cortex shrinkage, the effects of alcohol on the brain and cognition may be even more pronounced in older adults.[148,149] All adults over 65 years of age should be asked about alcohol intake and advised to limit intake to 1 to 2 drinks per day. Screening for alcohol abuse should be part of every cognitive evaluation and can be done with rapid screening tests, such as the validated CAGE questionnaire.[150] Individuals who have been identified to have an alcohol use disorder with excessive drinking should be referred to the appropriate rehabilitation services in the area.

SLEEP APNEA

Sleep apnea is defined as the cessation of breathing during sleep lasting 10 seconds or longer and can be classified into obstructive sleep apnea, where there is continued respiratory effort with paradoxic chest wall movement in the absence of air exchange, and central sleep apnea, where there is a complete absence of respiratory effort. Sleep apnea can also be associated with hypopnea events, which are episodes of decreased breathing effort with hypoxia. Severity of disease is measured by the apnea-hypopnea index, with normal being fewer than 5 episodes per hour and severe being more than 30 episodes per hour. Sleep apnea is typically associated with snoring and excessive daytime sleepiness, but can also manifest solely as other systemic complaints, such as hypertension, depression, and memory decline.[151,152]

Extensive literature has linked the presence of sleep apnea with dementia development and cognitive decline[152–161] and excessive daytime sleepiness has recently been associated with increased beta-amyloid deposits in older adults.[162] Not only is sleep apnea associated with memory issues in those without dementia, but apnea/hypopnea episodes in mild to moderate dementia are associated with cognitive decline relative to those without sleep apnea.[163] The exact mechanism that leads to cognitive decline is unclear, but there is evidence that recurrent nighttime hypoxia leads to cerebral vascular changes,[152,160,164,165] mainly in the cerebral areas supplied by the posterior and anterior cerebral arteries,[165] and biomarker changes similar to those seen in Alzheimer disease.[160,166] Hippocampal atrophy and volume loss, similar to that seen with Alzheimer disease, has been seen with chronic sleep apnea.[164,165] Sleep apnea also increases the risk of stroke.[153]

Evaluation for sleep apnea begins with a thorough history that should include questioning any bed partners for the presence of apnea symptoms and performing a screen for excessive daytime sleepiness, such as the EPWORTH sleepiness scale. Referral to a specialized sleep center for overnight polysomnography is the definitive test of choice, but there are increasingly more options for home testing. The latter may be more acceptable when assessing for sleep apnea in home-bound individuals.

Treatment of sleep apnea may improve memory. Studies have shown partial to complete reversal of cognitive symptoms in people effectively treated with continuous positive airway pressure.[153,159,167,168] This outcome has been shown even in people with mild to moderate dementia.[169–171] Two randomized, controlled studies found that treatment with donepezil improved sleep architecture and decreased excessive daytime sleepiness in those with concurrent obstructive sleep apnea and Alzheimer disease.[172,173] The long-term impact of donepezil on cognition in this group requires further study. Other treatments, such as management of obesity, improved bed positioning, elimination of alcohol or tobacco, sleep hygiene training, and surgical intervention, may also improve cognitive outcomes in obstructive sleep apnea, but more research is needed to confirm this in the absence of continuous positive airway pressure use.[153]

SUMMARY

The prevention and treatment of dementia should always begin with a thorough risk factor assessment and evaluation for potentially reversible causes of cognitive impairment. Treatments aimed at ameliorating these conditions may help to improve quality of life, functional status, and cognitive function for months or years after the initial identification of cognitive impairment. The use of the DEMENTIAS mnemonic and standardized screening tools and can help guide practitioners when caring for our rapidly aging population.

REFERENCES

1. Singh-Manoux A, Kivimaki M. The importance of cognitive aging for understanding dementia. Age 2010;32(4):509–12.
2. Rakesh G, Szabo ST, Alexopoulos GS, et al. Strategies for dementia prevention: latest evidence and implications. Ther Adv Chronic Dis 2017;8(8–9):121–36.
3. Cooper C, Sommerlad A, Lyketsos CG, et al. Modifiable predictors of dementia in mild cognitive impairment: a systematic review and meta-analysis. Am J Psychiatry 2015;172(4):323–34.
4. Clarfield AM. The decreasing prevalence of reversible dementias: an updated meta-analysis. Arch Intern Med 2003;163(18):2219–29.
5. Bello VME, Schultz RR. Prevalence of treatable and reversible dementias: a study in a dementia outpatient clinic. Demen Neuropsychol 2011;5(1):44–7.
6. Chari D, Ali R, Gupta R. Reversible dementia in elderly: really uncommon? J Geriatr Ment Health 2015;2:30–7.
7. Sorbi S, Hort J, Erkinjuntti T, et al. EFNS-ENS guidelines on the diagnosis and management of disorders associated with dementia. Eur J Neurol 2012;19(9):1159–79.
8. Ladika DJ, Gurevitz SL. Identifying the most common causes of reversible dementias: a review. JAAPA 2011;24(3):28–31, 57.
9. Swift CG, Ewen JM, Clarke P, et al. Responsiveness to oral diazepam in the elderly: relationship to total and free plasma concentrations. Br J Clin Pharmacol 1985;20(2):111–8.
10. Castleden CM, George CF, Marcer D, et al. Increased sensitivity to nitrazepam in old age. Br Med J 1977;1(6052):10–2.
11. Scott JC, Stanski DR. Decreased fentanyl and alfentanil dose requirements with age. A simultaneous pharmacokinetic and pharmacodynamic evaluation. J Pharmacol Exp Ther 1987;240(1):159–66.
12. Scott JC, Ponganis KV, Stanski DR. EEG quantitation of narcotic effect: the comparative pharmacodynamics of fentanyl and alfentanil. Anesthesiology 1985;62(3):234–41.
13. Vestal RE, Wood AJ, Shand DG. Reduced beta-adrenoceptor sensitivity in the elderly. Clin Pharmacol Ther 1979;26(2):181–6.
14. Evans MD, Shinar R, Yaari R. Reversible dementia and gait disturbance after prolonged use of valproic acid. Seizure 2011;20(6):509–11.
15. Cepeda OA, Morley JE. Polypharmacy, is it another disease?. In: Pathy MS, Sinclair A, Morley JE, editors. Principles and practice of geriatric medicine. 4th edition. London: John Wiley & Sons, Ltd; 2006. p. 215–21.

16. Flaherty JH. Geropharmacology. In: Schmidt PG, Martin KJ, editors. Internal medicine: just the facts. New York: McGraw Hill Medical; 2008. p. 121–8.

17. Britt DM, Day GS. Over-prescribed medications, under-appreciated risks: a review of the cognitive effects of anticholinergic medications in older adults. Mo Med 2016;113(3):207–14.

18. Brooks JO, Hoblyn JC. Neurocognitive costs and benefits of psychotropic medications in older adults. J Geriatr Psychiatry Neurol 2007;20(4):199–214.

19. Ancelin ML, Artero S, Portet F, et al. Non-degenerative mild cognitive impairment in elderly people and use of anticholinergic drugs: longitudinal cohort study. BMJ 2006;332(7539):455–9.

20. Campbell N, Boustani M, Limbil T, et al. The cognitive impact of anticholinergics: a clinical review. Clin Interv Aging 2009;4:225–33.

21. Cardwell K, Hughes CM, Ryan C. The association between anticholinergic medication burden and health related outcomes in the 'oldest old': a systematic review of the literature. Drugs Aging 2015;32(10):835–48.

22. Carriere I, Fourrier-Reglat A, Dartigues JF, et al. Drugs with anticholinergic properties, cognitive decline, and dementia in an elderly general population: the 3-city study. Arch Intern Med 2009;169(14):1317–24.

23. Collamati A, Martone AM, Poscia A, et al. Anticholinergic drugs and negative outcomes in the older population: from biological plausibility to clinical evidence. Aging Clin Exp Res 2016;28(1):25–35.

24. Fox C, Richardson K, Maidment ID, et al. Anticholinergic medication use and cognitive impairment in the older population: the medical research council cognitive function and ageing study. J Am Geriatr Soc 2011;59(8):1477–83.

25. Gray SL, Lai KV, Larson EB. Drug-induced cognition disorders in the elderly: incidence, prevention and management. Drug Saf 1999;21(2):101–22.

26. Jessen F, Kaduszkiewicz H, Daerr M, et al. Anticholinergic drug use and risk for dementia: target for dementia prevention. Eur Arch Psychiatry Clin Neurosci 2010;260(Suppl 2):S111–5.

27. Shah RC, Janos AL, Kline JE, et al. Cognitive decline in older persons initiating anticholinergic medications. PLoS One 2013;8(5):e64111.

28. Moore AR, O'Keeffe ST. Drug-induced cognitive impairment in the elderly. Drugs Aging 1999;15(1):15–28.

29. Billioti de Gage S, Begaud B, Bazin F, et al. Benzodiazepine use and risk of dementia: prospective population based study. BMJ 2012;345:e6231.

30. Gallacher J, Elwood P, Pickering J, et al. Benzodiazepine use and risk of dementia: evidence from the Caerphilly Prospective Study (CaPS). J Epidemiol Community Health 2012;66(10):869–73.

31. Tannenbaum C, Paquette A, Hilmer S, et al. A systematic review of amnestic and non-amnestic mild cognitive impairment induced by anticholinergic, antihistamine, GABAergic and opioid drugs. Drugs Aging 2012;29(8):639–58.

32. Gray SL, Anderson ML, Dublin S, et al. Cumulative use of strong anticholinergics and incident dementia: a prospective cohort study. JAMA Intern Med 2015; 175(3):401–7.

33. Han L, Agostini JV, Allore HG. Cumulative anticholinergic exposure is associated with poor memory and executive function in older men. J Am Geriatr Soc 2008;56(12):2203–10.

34. Starr JM, Whalley LJ. Drug-induced dementia. Incidence, management and prevention. Drug Saf 1994;11(5):310–7.

35. By the American Geriatrics Society 2015 Beers Criteria Update Expert Panel. American Geriatrics Society 2015 updated beers criteria for potentially inappropriate medication use in older adults. J Am Geriatr Soc 2015;63(11):2227–46.

36. O'Mahony D, O'Sullivan D, Byrne S, et al. STOPP/START criteria for potentially inappropriate prescribing in older people: version 2. Age Ageing 2015;44(2):213–8.

37. Campbell NL, Perkins AJ, Bradt P, et al. Association of anticholinergic burden with cognitive impairment and health care utilization among a diverse ambulatory older adult population. Pharmacotherapy 2016;36(11):1123–31.

38. Rudolph JL, Salow MJ, Angelini MC, et al. The anticholinergic risk scale and anticholinergic adverse effects in older persons. Arch Intern Med 2008;168(5):508–13.

39. Yeh YC, Liu CL, Peng LN, et al. Potential benefits of reducing medication-related anticholinergic burden for demented older adults: a prospective cohort study. Geriatr Gerontol Int 2013;13(3):694–700.

40. Potter K, Flicker L, Page A, et al. Deprescribing in frail older people: a randomised controlled trial. PLoS One 2016;11(3):e0149984.

41. Roberts MS, Stokes JA, King MA, et al. Outcomes of a randomized controlled trial of a clinical pharmacy intervention in 52 nursing homes. Br J Clin Pharmacol 2001;51(3):257–65.

42. Iyer S, Naganathan V, McLachlan AJ, et al. Medication withdrawal trials in people aged 65 years and older: a systematic review. Drugs Aging 2008;25(12):1021–31.

43. van der Cammen TJ, Rajkumar C, Onder G, et al. Drug cessation in complex older adults: time for action. Age Ageing 2014;43(1):20–5.

44. Scott IA, Hilmer SN, Reeve E, et al. Reducing inappropriate polypharmacy: the process of deprescribing. JAMA Intern Med 2015;175(5):827–34.

45. Bernabei R, Bonuccelli U, Maggi S, et al. Hearing loss and cognitive decline in older adults: questions and answers. Aging Clin Exp Res 2014;26(6):567–73.

46. Martini A, Castiglione A, Bovo R, et al. Aging, cognitive load, dementia and hearing loss. Audiol Neurootol 2014;19(Suppl 1):2–5.

47. Peracino A. Hearing loss and dementia in the aging population. Audiol Neurootol 2014;19(Suppl 1):6–9.

48. Fortunato S, Forli F, Guglielmi V, et al. A review of new insights on the association between hearing loss and cognitive decline in ageing. Acta Otorhinolaryngol Ital 2016;36(3):155–66.

49. Lin FR, Albert M. Hearing loss and dementia - who is listening? Aging Ment Health 2014;18(6):671–3.

50. Davidson JGS, Guthrie DM. Older adults with a combination of vision and hearing impairment experience higher rates of cognitive impairment, functional dependence, and worse outcomes across a set of quality indicators. J Aging Health 2017. 898264317723407.

51. Behrman S, Chouliaras L, Ebmeier KP. Considering the senses in the diagnosis and management of dementia. Maturitas 2014;77(4):305–10.

52. Chen SP, Bhattacharya J, Pershing S. Association of vision loss with cognition in older adults. JAMA Ophthalmol 2017;135(9):963–70.

53. Davies HR, Cadar D, Herbert A, et al. Hearing impairment and incident dementia: findings from the English longitudinal study of ageing. J Am Geriatr Soc 2017;65(9):2074–81.

54. Deal JA, Betz J, Yaffe K, et al. Hearing impairment and incident dementia and cognitive decline in older adults: the health ABC study. J Gerontol A Biol Sci Med Sci 2017;72(5):703–9.

55. Fischer ME, Cruickshanks KJ, Schubert CR, et al. Age-related sensory impairments and risk of cognitive impairment. J Am Geriatr Soc 2016;64(10):1981–7.

56. Gates GA, Gibbons LE, McCurry SM, et al. Executive dysfunction and presbycusis in older persons with and without memory loss and dementia. Cogn Behav Neurol 2010;23(4):218–23.
57. Golub JS. Brain changes associated with age-related hearing loss. Curr Opin Otolaryngol Head Neck Surg 2017;25(5):347–52.
58. Golub JS, Luchsinger JA, Manly JJ, et al. Observed hearing loss and incident dementia in a multiethnic cohort. J Am Geriatr Soc 2017;65(8):1691–7.
59. Gurgel RK, Ward PD, Schwartz S, et al. Relationship of hearing loss and dementia: a prospective, population-based study. Otol Neurotol 2014;35(5):775–81.
60. Lin FR, Metter EJ, O'Brien RJ, et al. Hearing loss and incident dementia. Arch Neurol 2011;68(2):214–20.
61. Loughrey DG, Kelly ME, Kelley GA, et al. Association of age-related hearing loss with cognitive function, cognitive impairment, and dementia: a systematic review and meta-analysis. JAMA Otolaryngol Head Neck Surg 2018;144(2):115–26.
62. Rizzo M, Sparks J, McEvoy S, et al. Change blindness, aging, and cognition. J Clin Exp Neuropsychol 2009;31(2):245–56.
63. Su P, Hsu CC, Lin HC, et al. Age-related hearing loss and dementia: a 10-year national population-based study. Eur Arch Otorhinolaryngol 2017;274(5):2327–34.
64. Wen YH, Wu SS, Lin CH, et al. A Bayesian approach to identifying new risk factors for dementia: a nationwide population-based study. Medicine 2016;95(21):e3658.
65. Yochim BP, Mueller AE, Kane KD, et al. Prevalence of cognitive impairment, depression, and anxiety symptoms among older adults with glaucoma. J Glaucoma 2012;21(4):250–4.
66. Zheng Y, Fan S, Liao W, et al. Hearing impairment and risk of Alzheimer's disease: a meta-analysis of prospective cohort studies. Neurol Sci 2017;38(2):233–9.
67. Luo Y, He P, Guo C, et al. Association between sensory impairment and dementia in older adults: evidence from China. J Am Geriatr Soc 2018;66(3):480–6.
68. Stahl SM. Does treating hearing loss prevent or slow the progress of dementia? Hearing is not all in the ears, but who's listening? CNS Spectr 2017;22(3):247–50.
69. Sturdivant GG. Top 10 facts you should know about hearing loss and cognitive decline. J Miss State Med Assoc 2016;57(5):142–4.
70. Moore AM, Voytas J, Kowalski D, et al. Cerumen, hearing, and cognition in the elderly. J Am Med Dir Assoc 2002;3(3):136–9.
71. Deal JA, Albert MS, Arnold M, et al. A randomized feasibility pilot trial of hearing treatment for reducing cognitive decline: results from the aging and cognitive health evaluation in elders pilot study. Alzheimers Dement (N Y) 2017;3(3):410–5.
72. Hardy CJ, Marshall CR, Golden HL, et al. Hearing and dementia. J Neurol 2016;263(11):2339–54.
73. Vossel KA, Ranasinghe KG, Beagle AJ, et al. Incidence and impact of subclinical epileptiform activity in Alzheimer's disease. Ann Neurol 2016;80(6):858–70.
74. Tjong E, McHugh W, Peng YY. Reversible dementia: subclinical seizure in early-onset dementia. Clin Case Rep 2017;5(3):321–7.
75. Chen Z, Liang X, Zhang C, et al. Correlation of thyroid dysfunction and cognitive impairments induced by subcortical ischemic vascular disease. Brain Behav 2016;6(4):e00452.

76. Forti P, Olivelli V, Rietti E, et al. Serum thyroid-stimulating hormone as a predictor of cognitive impairment in an elderly cohort. Gerontology 2012;58(1):41–9.

77. Harper PC, Roe CM. Thyroid medication use and subsequent development of dementia of the Alzheimer type. J Geriatr Psychiatry Neurol 2010;23(1):63–9.

78. Pasqualetti G, Caraccio N, Dell Agnello U, et al. Cognitive function and the ageing process: the peculiar role of mild thyroid failure. Recent Pat Endocr Metab Immune Drug Discov 2016;10(1):4–10.

79. Tan ZS, Vasan RS. Thyroid function and Alzheimer's disease. J Alzheimers Dis 2009;16(3):503–7.

80. de Jong FJ, den Heijer T, Visser TJ, et al. Thyroid hormones, dementia, and atrophy of the medial temporal lobe. J Clin Endocrinol Metab 2006;91(7): 2569–73.

81. Yamamoto N, Ishizawa K, Ishikawa M, et al. Cognitive function with subclinical hypothyroidism in elderly people without dementia: one year follow up. Geriatr Gerontol Int 2012;12(1):164–5.

82. Flicker L, Ames D. Metabolic and endocrinological causes of dementia. Int Psychogeriatr 2005;17(Suppl 1):S79–92.

83. de Jong FJ, Masaki K, Chen H, et al. Thyroid function, the risk of dementia and neuropathologic changes: the Honolulu-Asia aging study. Neurobiol Aging 2009;30(4):600–6.

84. Malouf M, Grimley EJ, Areosa SA. Folic acid with or without vitamin B12 for cognition and dementia. Cochrane Database Syst Rev 2003;(4):CD004514.

85. Blasko I, Hinterberger M, Kemmler G, et al. Conversion from mild cognitive impairment to dementia: influence of folic acid and vitamin B12 use in the VITA cohort. J Nutr Health Aging 2012;16(8):687–94.

86. Malouf R, Areosa Sastre A. Vitamin B12 for cognition. Cochrane Database Syst Rev 2003;(3):CD004326.

87. Malouf R, Grimley Evans J. The effect of vitamin B6 on cognition. Cochrane Database Syst Rev 2003;(4):CD004393.

88. Chung MC, Yu TM, Shu KH, et al. Hyponatremia and increased risk of dementia: a population-based retrospective cohort study. PLoS One 2017;12(6): e0178977.

89. Singh H, Selvaraj V, Padala PR. Dementia secondary to hyperparathyroidism. Psychiatry 2010;7(8):13–4.

90. Zheng F, Yan L, Yang Z, et al. HbA1c, diabetes and cognitive decline: the English longitudinal study of ageing. Diabetologia 2018;61(4):839–48.

91. Ben Assayag E, Eldor R, Korczyn AD, et al. Type 2 diabetes mellitus and impaired renal function are associated with brain alterations and poststroke cognitive decline. Stroke 2017;48(9):2368–74.

92. Bennett S, Thomas AJ. Depression and dementia: cause, consequence or coincidence? Maturitas 2014;79(2):184–90.

93. Cherbuin N, Kim S, Anstey KJ. Dementia risk estimates associated with measures of depression: a systematic review and meta-analysis. BMJ Open 2015; 5(12):e008853.

94. Cipriani G, Lucetti C, Carlesi C, et al. Depression and dementia. A review. Eur Geriatr Med 2015;6(5):479–86.

95. Liu YC, Meguro K, Nakamura K, et al. Depression and dementia in old-old population: history of depression may be associated with dementia onset. The Tome Project. Front Aging Neurosci 2017;9:335.

96. Valkanova V, Ebmeier KP, Allan CL. Depression is linked to dementia in older adults. Practitioner 2017;261(1800):11–5.

97. Steenland K, Karnes C, Seals R, et al. Late-life depression as a risk factor for mild cognitive impairment or Alzheimer's disease in 30 US Alzheimer's disease centers. J Alzheimers Dis 2012;31(2):265–75.

98. Kim HK, Nunes PV, Oliveira KC, et al. Neuropathological relationship between major depression and dementia: a hypothetical model and review. Prog Neuro-psychopharmacol biol Psychiatry 2016;67:51–7.

99. Ellison JM, Kyomen HH, Harper DG. Depression in later life: an overview with treatment recommendations. Psychiatr Clin North Am 2012;35(1):203–29.

100. Butters MA, Young JB, Lopez O, et al. Pathways linking late-life depression to persistent cognitive impairment and dementia. Dialogues Clin Neurosci 2008; 10(3):345–57.

101. Ganguli M. Depression, cognitive impairment and dementia: why should clinicians care about the web of causation? Indian J Psychiatry 2009;51(Suppl 1): S29–34.

102. Chu H, Yang CY, Lin Y, et al. The impact of group music therapy on depression and cognition in elderly persons with dementia: a randomized controlled study. Biol Res Nurs 2014;16(2):209–17.

103. Zhang Q, Yang C, Liu T, et al. Citalopram restores short-term memory deficit and non-cognitive behaviors in APP/PS1 mice while halting the advance of Alzheimer's disease-like pathology. Neuropharmacology 2017;131:475–86.

104. Gong WG, Wang YJ, Zhou H, et al. Citalopram ameliorates synaptic plasticity deficits in different cognition-associated brain regions induced by social isolation in middle-aged rats. Mol Neurobiol 2017;54(3):1927–38.

105. Bartels C, Wagner M, Wolfsgruber S, et al, Alzheimer's Disease Neuroimaging Initiative. Impact of SSRI therapy on risk of conversion from mild cognitive impairment to Alzheimer's dementia in individuals with previous depression. Am J Psychiatry 2018;175(3):232–41.

106. Gatt A, Ekonomou A, Somani A, et al. Importance of proactive treatment of depression in Lewy body dementias: the impact on hippocampal neurogenesis and cognition in a post-mortem study. Demen Geriatr Cogn Disord 2018; 44(5–6):283–93.

107. Banerjee S, Hellier J, Romeo R, et al. Study of the use of antidepressants for depression in dementia: the HTA-SADD trial–a multicentre, randomised, double-blind, placebo-controlled trial of the clinical effectiveness and cost-effectiveness of sertraline and mirtazapine. Health Technol Assess 2013;17(7): 1–166.

108. Teri L, Reifler BV, Veith RC, et al. Imipramine in the treatment of depressed Alzheimer's patients: impact on cognition. J Gerontol 1991;46(6):P372–7.

109. Leong C. Antidepressants for depression in patients with dementia: a review of the literature. Consult Pharm 2014;29(4):254–63.

110. Chakkamparambil B, Chibnall JT, Graypel EA, et al. Development of a brief validated geriatric depression screening tool: the SLU "AM SAD". Am J Geriatr Psychiatry 2015;23(8):780–3.

111. Goodarzi ZS, Mele BS, Roberts DJ, et al. Depression case finding in individuals with dementia: a systematic review and meta-analysis. J Am Geriatr Soc 2017; 65(5):937–48.

112. Alexopoulos GS, Abrams RC, Young RC, et al. Cornell scale for depression in dementia. Biol Psychiatry 1988;23(3):271–84.

113. Jaraj D, Wikkelso C, Rabiei K, et al. Mortality and risk of dementia in normal-pressure hydrocephalus: a population study. Alzheimers Dement 2017;13(8): 850–7.

114. Mori E, Ishikawa M, Kato T, et al. Guidelines for management of idiopathic normal pressure hydrocephalus: second edition. Neurol Med-Chir 2012; 52(11):775–809.

115. Kiefer M, Unterberg A. The differential diagnosis and treatment of normal-pressure hydrocephalus. Dtsch Arztebl Int 2012;109(1–2):15–25 [quiz: 26].

116. Olazaran J, Martinez MD, Rabano A. Normal pressure hydrocephalus mimicking Alzheimer's disease: such an infrequent case? Clin Neuropathol 2013;32(6):502–7.

117. Rosseau G. Normal pressure hydrocephalus. Dis Mon 2011;57(10):615–24.

118. Kito Y, Kazui H, Kubo Y, et al. Neuropsychiatric symptoms in patients with idiopathic normal pressure hydrocephalus. Behav Neurol 2009;21(3):165–74.

119. Koivisto AM, Alafuzoff I, Savolainen S, et al. Poor cognitive outcome in shunt-responsive idiopathic normal pressure hydrocephalus. Neurosurgery 2013; 72(1):1–8 [discussion: 8].

120. Kanno S, Saito M, Hayashi A, et al. Counting-backward test for executive function in idiopathic normal pressure hydrocephalus. Acta Neurol Scand 2012; 126(4):279–86.

121. Hiraoka K, Narita W, Kikuchi H, et al. Amyloid deposits and response to shunt surgery in idiopathic normal-pressure hydrocephalus. J Neurol Sci 2015; 356(1–2):124–8.

122. Graff-Radford NR. Alzheimer CSF biomarkers may be misleading in normal-pressure hydrocephalus. Neurology 2014;83(17):1573–5.

123. Hoza D, Vlasak A, Horinek D, et al. DTI-MRI biomarkers in the search for normal pressure hydrocephalus aetiology: a review. Neurosurg Rev 2015;38(2):239–44 [discussion: 244].

124. Koivisto AM, Kurki MI, Alafuzoff I, et al. High risk of dementia in ventricular enlargement with normal pressure hydrocephalus related symptoms1. J Alzheimers Dis 2016;52(2):497–507.

125. Peterson KA, Savulich G, Jackson D, et al. The effect of shunt surgery on neuropsychological performance in normal pressure hydrocephalus: a systematic review and meta-analysis. J Neurol 2016;263(8):1669–77.

126. Chaudhry P, Kharkar S, Heidler-Gary J, et al. Characteristics and reversibility of dementia in normal pressure hydrocephalus. Behav Neurol 2007;18(3):149–58.

127. Chivukula S, Tempel ZJ, Zwagerman NT, et al. The dynamic gait index in evaluating patients with normal pressure hydrocephalus for cerebrospinal fluid diversion. World Neurosurg 2015;84(6):1871–6.

128. Cagnin A, Simioni M, Tagliapietra M, et al. A simplified callosal angle measure best differentiates idiopathic-normal pressure hydrocephalus from neurodegenerative dementia. J Alzheimers Dis 2015;46(4):1033–8.

129. Horinek D, Stepan-Buksakowska I, Szabo N, et al. Difference in white matter microstructure in differential diagnosis of normal pressure hydrocephalus and Alzheimer's disease. Clin Neurol Neurosurg 2016;140:52–9.

130. Kang K, Choi W, Yoon U, et al. Abnormal white matter integrity in elderly patients with idiopathic normal-pressure hydrocephalus: a tract-based spatial statistics study. Eur Neurol 2016;75(1–2):96–103.

131. Korhonen VE, Solje E, Suhonen NM, et al. Frontotemporal dementia as a comorbidity to idiopathic normal pressure hydrocephalus (iNPH): a short review of literature and an unusual case. Fluids Barriers CNS 2017;14(1):10.

132. Pomeraniec IJ, Bond AE, Lopes MB, et al. Concurrent Alzheimer's pathology in patients with clinical normal pressure hydrocephalus: correlation of high-volume lumbar puncture results, cortical brain biopsies, and outcomes. J Neurosurg 2016;124(2):382–8.

133. Moriya M, Miyajima M, Nakajima M, et al. Impact of cerebrospinal fluid shunting for idiopathic normal pressure hydrocephalus on the amyloid cascade. PLoS One 2015;10(3):e0119973.

134. Yasar S, Jusue-Torres I, Lu J, et al. Alzheimer's disease pathology and shunt surgery outcome in normal pressure hydrocephalus. PLoS One 2017;12(8): e0182288.

135. Topakian R, Artemian H, Metschitzer B, et al. Dramatic response to a 3-week course of ceftriaxone in late neuroborreliosis mimicking atypical dementia and normal pressure hydrocephalus. J Neurol Sci 2016;366:146–8.

136. Chao TF, Liu CJ, Chen SJ, et al. Statins and the risk of dementia in patients with atrial fibrillation: a nationwide population-based cohort study. Int J Cardiol 2015; 196:91–7.

137. de Bruijn RF, Heeringa J, Wolters FJ, et al. Association between atrial fibrillation and dementia in the general population. JAMA Neurol 2015;72(11):1288–94.

138. Jacobs V, Cutler MJ, Day JD, et al. Atrial fibrillation and dementia. Trends Cardiovasc Medicine 2015;25(1):44–51.

139. Kalantarian S, Stern TA, Mansour M, et al. Cognitive impairment associated with atrial fibrillation: a meta-analysis. Ann Intern Med 2013;158(5 Pt 1):338–46.

140. Kanmanthareddy A, Vallakati A, Sridhar A, et al. The impact of atrial fibrillation and its treatment on dementia. Curr Cardiol Rep 2014;16(8):519.

141. Kwok CS, Loke YK, Hale R, et al. Atrial fibrillation and incidence of dementia: a systematic review and meta-analysis. Neurology 2011;76(10):914–22.

142. Santangeli P, Di Biase L, Bai R, et al. Atrial fibrillation and the risk of incident dementia: a meta-analysis. Heart Rhythm 2012;9(11):1761–8.

143. Jacobs V, Woller SC, Stevens S, et al. Time outside of therapeutic range in atrial fibrillation patients is associated with long-term risk of dementia. Heart Rhythm 2014;11(12):2206–13.

144. Graves KG, May HT, Jacobs V, et al. Atrial fibrillation incrementally increases dementia risk across all CHADS2 and CHA2DS2VASc strata in patients receiving long-term warfarin. Am Heart J 2017;188:93–8.

145. Viscogliosi G, Ettorre E, Chiriac IM. Dementia correlates with anticoagulation underuse in older patients with atrial fibrillation. Arch Gerontol Geriatr 2017; 72:108–12.

146. Wyse DG, Waldo AL, DiMarco JP, et al. A comparison of rate control and rhythm control in patients with atrial fibrillation. N Engl J Med 2002;347(23):1825–33.

147. Ballard C, Lang I. Alcohol and dementia: a complex relationship with potential for dementia prevention. Lancet Public Health 2018;3(3):e103–4.

148. Sullivan EV, Zahr NM, Sassoon SA, et al. The role of aging, drug dependence, and hepatitis c comorbidity in alcoholism cortical compromise. JAMA Psychiatry 2018;75(5):474–83.

149. Koob GF. Age, alcohol use, and brain function: Yoda says, "with age and alcohol, confused is the force". JAMA Psychiatry 2018;75(5):422.

150. Ewing JA. Detecting alcoholism. The CAGE questionnaire. Jama 1984;252(14): 1905–7.

151. Paul GAHD. Sleep apnea. In: Ferri F, editor. Ferri's clinical advisor 2018. Elsevier; 2018. p. 1189–91.

152. Shastri A, Bangar S, Holmes J. Obstructive sleep apnoea and dementia: is there a link? Int J Geriatr Psychiatry 2016;31(4):400–5.

153. Buratti L, Luzzi S, Petrelli C, et al. Obstructive sleep apnea syndrome: an emerging risk factor for dementia. CNS Neurol Disord Drug Targets 2016; 15(6):678–82.

154. Chang WP, Liu ME, Chang WC, et al. Sleep apnea and the risk of dementia: a population-based 5-year follow-up study in Taiwan. PLoS One 2013;8(10):e78655.
155. Winer JR, Mander BA. Waking up to the importance of sleep in the pathogenesis of Alzheimer disease. JAMA Neurol 2018;75(6):654–6.
156. Bubu OM, Brannick M, Mortimer J, et al. Sleep, cognitive impairment, and Alzheimer's disease: a systematic review and meta-analysis. Sleep 2017;40(1).
157. Ding X, Kryscio RJ, Turner J, et al. Self-reported sleep apnea and dementia risk: findings from the prevention of Alzheimer's disease with vitamin E and selenium trial. J Am Geriatr Soc 2016;64(12):2472–8.
158. Grigg-Damberger M, Ralls F. Cognitive dysfunction and obstructive sleep apnea: from cradle to tomb. Curr Opin Pulm Med 2012;18(6):580–7.
159. Osorio RS, Gumb T, Pirraglia E, et al. Sleep-disordered breathing advances cognitive decline in the elderly. Neurology 2015;84(19):1964–71.
160. Pan W, Kastin AJ. Can sleep apnea cause Alzheimer's disease? Neurosci Biobehav Rev 2014;47:656–69.
161. Yaffe K, Laffan AM, Harrison SL, et al. Sleep-disordered breathing, hypoxia, and risk of mild cognitive impairment and dementia in older women. JAMA 2011; 306(6):613–9.
162. Carvalho DZ, St Louis EK, Knopman DS, et al. Association of excessive daytime sleepiness with longitudinal beta-amyloid accumulation in elderly persons without dementia. JAMA Neurol 2018;75(6):672–80.
163. Aoki K, Matsuo M, Takahashi M, et al. Association of sleep-disordered breathing with decreased cognitive function among patients with dementia. J Sleep Res 2014;23(5):517–23.
164. Daulatzai MA. Quintessential risk factors: their role in promoting cognitive dysfunction and Alzheimer's disease. Neurochem Res 2012;37(12):2627–58.
165. Buratti L, Viticchi G, Falsetti L, et al. Vascular impairment in Alzheimer's disease: the role of obstructive sleep apnea. J Alzheimers Dis 2014;38(2):445–53.
166. Liguori C, Mercuri NB, Izzi F, et al. Obstructive sleep apnea is associated with early but possibly modifiable Alzheimer's disease biomarkers changes. Sleep 2017;40(5).
167. Rosenzweig I, Glasser M, Crum WR, et al. Changes in neurocognitive architecture in patients with obstructive sleep apnea treated with continuous positive airway pressure. EBioMedicine 2016;7:221–9.
168. Gagnon K, Baril AA, Gagnon JF, et al. Cognitive impairment in obstructive sleep apnea. Pathol Biol (Paris) 2014;62(5):233–40.
169. Ancoli-Israel S, Palmer BW, Cooke JR, et al. Cognitive effects of treating obstructive sleep apnea in Alzheimer's disease: a randomized controlled study. J Am Geriatr Soc 2008;56(11):2076–81.
170. Cooke JR, Ayalon L, Palmer BW, et al. Sustained use of CPAP slows deterioration of cognition, sleep, and mood in patients with Alzheimer's disease and obstructive sleep apnea: a preliminary study. J Clin Sleep Med 2009;5(4):305–9.
171. Troussiere AC, Charley CM, Salleron J, et al. Treatment of sleep apnoea syndrome decreases cognitive decline in patients with Alzheimer's disease. J Neurol Neurosurg Psychiatry 2014;85(12):1405–8.
172. Moraes W, Poyares D, Sukys-Claudino L, et al. Donepezil improves obstructive sleep apnea in Alzheimer disease: a double-blind, placebo-controlled study. Chest 2008;133(3):677–83.
173. Sukys-Claudino L, Moraes W, Guilleminault C, et al. Beneficial effect of donepezil on obstructive sleep apnea: a double-blind, placebo-controlled clinical trial. Sleep Med 2012;13(3):290–6.

Mild Cognitive Impairment in Geriatrics

Eric G. Tangalos, MD*, Ronald C. Petersen, MD, PhD

KEYWORDS

- MCI • Mild cognitive impairment • Biomarkers in Alzheimer disease • Cognition
- Functional impairment

KEY POINTS

- Mild cognitive impairment is an intermediate state between normal cognition and dementia. It is an important construct in understanding cognitive decline.
- Mild cognitive impairment is the most predominant form and is the best predictor of future dementia, including Alzheimer disease.
- Mild cognitive impairment has predictive value for conversion to Alzheimer disease. Biomarkers may have value in determining disease-modifying therapy.
- The genetics of Alzheimer disease apply to rates of conversion from mild cognitive impairment to Alzheimer disease. This link will benefit future tailored therapies.
- In long-term care settings the condition is common and it is particularly problematic in assisted living if a resident's cognitive capacity is not correctly identified.

INTRODUCTION

The concept of mild cognitive impairment (MCI) as an intermediate state between normal cognition and dementia entered into the vernacular of geriatric medicine more than 30 years ago. Geriatric fellowship programs teach to the condition and primary care providers all have a passing understand that somewhere between normal and dementia there resides a population that fits the definition. In long-term care settings, the condition is common and it is particularly problematic in assisted living if a resident's cognitive capacity is not correctly identified. Incorrect placement or movement to a higher level of care for additional services shortly after a move in destabilizes the resident and family all the more at a most critical time of transition.

MCI as a term was introduced into the literature in 1988 by Reisberg and colleagues,[1] but referred to a severity index of stage 3 as identified on the Global Deterioration Scale. Another instrument, the Clinical Dementia Rating scale sought to

Disclosure Statement: Dr E.G. Tangalos is a paid consultant for BCAT and Brain Test.
Department of Medicine, Division of Community Internal Medicine, Mayo Clinic, 200 First Street Southwest, Rochester, MN 55905, USA
* Corresponding author.
E-mail address: tangalos@mayo.edu

Clin Geriatr Med 34 (2018) 563–589
https://doi.org/10.1016/j.cger.2018.06.005
0749-0690/18/© 2018 Elsevier Inc. All rights reserved.

identify very early dementia given the possibility of identifying disease early and intervening as soon as possible.[2] By 1999, MCI had been proposed as a prodromal condition for Alzheimer disease with the focus on memory as a chief clinical complaint for incipient disease.[3] Not all forms of MCI evolve into Alzheimer disease.

Although a misclassification may be a disservice to the diagnosis of MCI, the greater disservice is to the patient. Geriatricians need to use the diagnosis appropriately for patient care, understand the treatment limitations, apply appropriate management strategies, and prepare for a biomarker approach to diagnosis that makes MCI a valuable construct at looking at the spectrum of Alzheimer disease.

A COMMON UNDERSTANDING

MCI refers to cognitive impairment that does not meet the criteria for dementia. Several criteria for, and subtypes of, MCI have been proposed.[4–6] For our purposes, there must be a measurable deficit in cognition in at least 1 domain, there cannot be a dementia diagnosis, and the individual should have no functional impairment in their activities of daily living.

MCI has a number of different clinical presentations and etiologies, although the prognosis and prevalence[6–8] varies depending on the starting point of decline. The usefulness of the diagnosis now allows extending the early detection of other dementias in their prodromal stages.[9–11] Current criteria were developed to encompass the cognitive domains most commonly affected in the disorders (eg, memory problems and Alzheimer disease).[11,12]

MCI fits between the cognitive changes of aging and the impact of dementia. Considerable judgment is required in making the distinction between impairments that are normal for the elderly population and, at the other extreme, do not represent dementia. What constitutes impairment in daily living is always contextual. Patients with spouses, good financial resources, or attentive families do better. They display fewer functional difficulties because of their socioeconomic environment. The astute geriatrician is well aware that changes in the living environment have great impact on revealing significant limitations. Subjective cognitive complaints and even activities of daily living have been challenged as criteria in establishing the diagnosis.[3,13,14]

Amnestic Mild Cognitive Impairment

Amnestic MCI (aMCI) is often thought of as a precursor to Alzheimer disease.[15] aMCI is the most common subtype, with a ratio of 2:1 compared with non-aMCI (naMCI), although relative prevalence of MCI subtypes has varied among studies.[16,17]

Initially, MCI was used to refer to the amnestic subtype, but other subtypes have since been recognized (see Nonamnestic Mild Cognitive Impairment).

- Single domain aMCI refers to those individuals with significantly impaired memory who do not meet the criteria for dementia. The criteria originally outlined for MCI are understood to identify specifically this type[4,9]:
  - Memory complaint, preferably corroborated by an informant;
  - Objective memory impairment (for age and education);
  - Preserved general cognitive function;
  - Intact activities of daily living; and
  - Not demented.

Memory impairments that qualify for MCI are generally represented by defects that are 1.5 standard deviations or more below age-corrected norms. This threshold is not absolute, however, because individuals can experience a significant loss of memory without satisfying that criterion. Different tests of memory likely have different sensitivity and specificity and norms are not available for all populations; this lack further justifies the necessity of clinical judgment.[7]

Multiple Domains

Many individuals with aMCI complain only of memory loss; however, they may have additional subtle impairments in other cognitive domains that are revealed with careful neuropsychological testing.[10,18–20] Such persons may also manifest subtle problems with activities of daily living, but do not meet the criteria for a formal diagnosis of dementia.[8] The multiple domains are, by definition, only slightly impaired (ie, <0.5–1.0 standard deviations below age- and education-matched normal participants). These individuals often progress to meet criteria for Alzheimer disease dementia; in a minority of cases, the cognitive profile may simply reflect normal aging.[8] The prognostic usefulness of the multiple domain form of aMCI remains unclear, because some studies have identified this as the highest risk category for conversion to dementia, whereas others have exposed instability with some individuals returning to baseline level of function over time.[10,21,22] Much of this variability derives from different sources of subjects, for example, specialty clinics versus population cohorts.

Nonamnestic Mild Cognitive Impairment

Single domain

The concept of single domain naMCI is similar to aMCI, except that this form of MCI is characterized by a relatively isolated impairment in a single nonmemory domain, such as executive functioning, language, or visual spatial skills.[8] Depending on the domain, individuals with this subtype of MCI may progress to other syndromes, such as frontotemporal dementia (FTD), primary progressive aphasia, dementia with Lewy bodies, progressive supranuclear palsy, or corticobasal degeneration. Individuals within this group seem to be at less of a risk of conversion to dementia, although supporting evidence is limited.[12,23]

In certain disorders such as behavioral variant FTD, cognitive complaints are often preceded by significant alterations in behavior and comportment. Thus, some investigators have proposed the concept of mild behavioral impairment as a similar paradigm to recognize an additional group with increased risk of dementia.[24]

Multiple domains

Patients who meet these criteria are affected in multiple domains with a relative sparing of memory problems. The substrate of multidomain naMCI is felt to be that of degenerative disorders associated with tau, TAR DNA binding protein and alpha-synuclein such as FTD and dementia with Lewy bodies.[2,25] Other studies have linked MCI in multiple domains to other types of dementia.[26]

The *Diagnostic and Statistical Manual of Mental Disorders, fifth edition* has included mild neurocognitive disorder since 2013.[27] Age-associated memory impairment and age-associated cognitive decline are also widely used terms but represent normal age-associated memory and cognitive changes in older adults as referenced to young normal adult individuals.[4,28,29] Age-associated cognitive decline was developed to better define the cognitive changes in elderly patients compared with age-adjusted norms, but has more recently been recognized as identifying a state of impairment similar to MCI.[30]

MAKING THE CASE

Cognitive impairment is prevalent in American nursing homes and assisted living facilities; 70% or more of residents have some type of cognitive impairment.[31–34] In both settings, studies estimate that approximately 50% to 60% of all residents meet criteria for dementia[35–38] and approximately 20% to 25% of residents meet criteria for MCI.[33] The concept is now accepted for clinical care[39,40] and has been adopted in Europe. The ability to identify residents in long-term care settings with cognitive impairment is critical to effective care plans and interventions and can facilitate appropriate staff interactions so important to residents' quality of life.[41] There is ample evidence that, when cognitive impairment is not identified accurately, the management of medical conditions can be adversely affected.[42,43]

An International Association of Gerontology and Geriatrics–Global Aging Research Network consensus conference in St. Louis in early 2015 identified that cognitive impairment creates significant challenges for patients, their families and friends, and the clinicians who provide their health care. Early recognition allows for diagnosis and appropriate treatment, education, psychosocial support, and engagement in shared decision making regarding life planning, health care, involvement in research, and financial matters. The consensus panel examined the importance of early recognition of impaired cognitive health. Their major conclusion was that case finding by physicians and health professionals is an important step toward enhancing brain health for aging populations throughout the world. This conclusion is in keeping with the position of the United States' Centers for Medicare and Medicaid Services, which reimburses for the detection of cognitive impairment as part the of Medicare Annual Wellness Visit and with the international call for early detection of cognitive impairment as a patient's right. The panel agreed on the following specific findings:

1. Validated screening tests are available that take 3 to 7 minutes to administer;
2. A combination of patient- and informant-based screens is the most appropriate approach for identifying early cognitive impairment;
3. Early cognitive impairment may have treatable components; and
4. Emerging data support a combination of medical and lifestyle interventions as a potential way to delay or reduce cognitive decline.[44]

TOOLS OF THE TRADE

Currently, the Brief Interview for Mental Status[45] is the mandated cognitive assessment tool included in the Minimum Data Set 3.0 for skilled care nursing home residents. The Brief Interview for Mental Status is an efficient measure that has strong reliability and convergent validity, can be rapidly administered (average time is about 3 minutes), and is suitable for paraprofessional use.[46] The Brief Interview for Mental Status was never intended to be sensitive to the full cognitive continuum and does not stage dementia levels. The cut scores differentiating residents with and without cognitive impairments are based, in part, on the Modified Mini-Mental State Examination,[47] a measure that seems to have poor sensitivity to MCI.[48] Cut scores were not based on broader and potentially more powerful assessments, such as a neuropsychological battery, imaging analyses, or biomarkers. Consequently, reported test scores may be inaccurate. Memory is assessed using a simple word list (3 words), with no story recall component, and executive function is only addressed minimally.[33,49] The Brief Cognitive Assessment Tool has been proposed to address these shortcomings. The Brief Cognitive Assessment Tool is a 21-item instrument that can be administered in approximately 10 to 15 minutes by paraprofessionals and clinicians, contains a strong multilevel verbal memory component (inclusive of story recall items), and has a broadly complex executive function component. Another purported advantage of the Brief Cognitive Assessment Tool is that it has been shown to specifically differentiate between MCI and dementia.[31]

Geriatricians also have available to them a wide assortment of additional cognitive screens, including the informant-based AD8.[50–54] Each can have its place in a busy primary care practice to screen at-risk populations of patients, especially those who find themselves transitioning into some higher level of service with less independence. Assisted living and nursing homes come quickly to mind. The Mini Mental State Examination (MMSE), which was published in 1975[23] and the Kokmen Short Test of Mental Status[55] are now mostly relegated to research/drug protocols that rely on these baseline measures. All are validated, some have been translated into many languages (the AD8 is available in >100 languages), and each carries with it enough sensitivity and specificity when used in populations at risk to provide good stratification from normal to abnormal once the age and education is taken into account.

The Gerontological Society of America also looked at brief instruments that were nonproprietary. Their comprehensive toolkit is focused on the KAER model developed by the GSA Workgroup on Cognitive Impairment Detection and Earlier Diagnosis.[56] The workgroup identified valuable tools and resources to implement the 4 steps in the *KAER* model. The resulting toolkit provides options for each of the steps so that primary care providers, health plans and health care systems can select the approaches and tools that fit best with their existing primary care structure, organization, and procedures.

The toolkit is broken down by each section of the *KAER* model to allow quick and easy access:

- *Kickstart* the cognition conversation,
- *Assess* for cognitive impairment,
- *Evaluate* for dementia, and
- *Refer* for community resources.

THE AGING PATIENT

Although specific changes in cognition are frequently observed in normal aging, there is increasing evidence that some forms of cognitive impairment are recognizable as an early manifestation of dementia.[3] MCI is a heterogeneous syndrome and there remains controversy over aspects of the construct. However, the usefulness of this paradigm is the recognition that dementia is not a dichotomous state and thus refining our understanding of the layers of transition will improve the understanding of cognitive decline and ultimately benefit patients. Appropriate diagnosis lets us address our patient needs with the best available therapies, be they drug or nondrug interventions.

Unfortunately, all too often MCI is used to soften a diagnosis of what should really be dementia. In 2003, Winblad and colleagues[57] sought to expand and revise the criteria.[58] From that conference the criteria now used by the National Institute on Aging-sponsored Alzheimer Disease Centers Program Uniform Data Set and the Alzheimer Disease Neuroimaging Initiative[59] have helped us design protocols to improve our understanding of the dementing process. The clinical phenotypes as we have now discussed include aMCI and naMCI with the subtypes of single and multiple domain classifications.

In general, our shortcomings in approaching patients with cognitive decline have been to avoid a diagnosis and delay our interventions. The reasons are multiple, although taking the time to make a diagnosis means that much more time will be needed to explain the diagnosis and take action. Any assault on our independence with special concern regarding the loss of driving privileges plays poorly to the American mindset. We live in a land where our first right of passage is the driver's license and where all roads lead to the shopping mall. We do not live in walking communities and the last thing we give up is our driver's license. There have also been financial disincentives in the past when clinicians used a psychiatric code to define cognitive disease though MCI and the dementing syndromes now can be classified with *International Classification of Diseases*-10 medical codes.

MCI has been studied more extensively in ambulatory patients, but both nursing homes and assisted living facilities have a high reported prevalence of cognitive impairment.[36,37] Questions remain regarding whether MCI subtypes found in community-dwelling patients are mirrored in long-term care settings and how selected impairment thresholds might impact probable diagnosis. The work by Mansbach and associates[60] identified 3 clear MCI subtypes in the long term care setting: amnestic, single domain; nonamnestic, single domain (executive); and amnestic, multidomain (memory and executive). A fourth category (undifferentiated) was identified in patients who did not meet the criteria for a distinct MCI subtype, but still had cognitive impairments.

Given the difficulty in identifying state by state assisted living facilities (conservative estimate of 1 million) as compared with skilled care (1.4 million, 2014 National Center for Health Statistics), the long-term care population should command the interest and respect of geriatricians. Generally, the only separation of these 2 populations is their functional impairment. Attempts have been made in assisted living to test the performance of various instruments given the high prevalence of disease. In a North Carolina sample of assisted living residents, 55 of 146 participants (38%) were diagnosed with probable dementia and 76 (52%) met criteria for MCI (most nonamnestic). Both the Mini-Cog and the MMSE showed high sensitivity and negative predictive value for dementia, but had relatively low sensitivity and negative predictive value for MCI. The Mini-Cog had low specificity and was less accurate as a dementia screen than either the MMSE or MMX. Reliability and validity data for testing the MMX, a 50-point test based on expanding selected MMSE items, were satisfactory and it performed better as a screening test for MCI than either the MMSE or Mini-Cog.[61] Additional studies have also indicated that amnestic and executive deficits are particularly common in long-term care patients,[36,62] whereas amnestic and executive subtypes have been identified in community samples of the elderly.[63]

FRAILTY AS A CONFOUNDER

Geriatricians may be confronted by those who are extremely old (90 in a male, 95 in a female) where sudden near complete failure includes a rapidly progressing dementia. It is unlikely that this is Alzheimer disease alone and there is rarely a classic presentation of MCI as prodromal. Cognitive frailty is a term that has recently emerged in the geriatrics literature, inspired by potential parallel links to and possible common underlying mechanisms with the physical frailty syndrome.

Physical frailty has been defined as "a medical syndrome with multiple causes and contributors that is, characterized by diminished strength, endurance, and reduced physiologic function that increases an individual's vulnerability for developing increased dependency and/or death."[64] Recently, it has been recognized that a subgroup of persons with cognitive impairment have a decreased resilience and functional decline that interacts with physical frailty. Converging evidence suggests that the cognitive status represents an important dimension of the frailty syndrome.

Epidemiologic studies have shown an association between frailty and late-life cognitive decline, incident MCI and Alzheimer disease, and non-Alzheimer disease dementias.[65] It has been suggested that cognitive frailty can be defined as a reduced cognitive function (Clinical Dementia Rating score of 0.5) with the cognitive impairment being due to either physical or brain disease[2,66] or accelerated brain aging in the absence of evident brain disease. Physical frailty has to coexist to evoke the term cognitive frailty. It manifests commonly with executive dysfunction (frontal cortex) and less with pure amnestic defects (mesial temporal cortex). Others have suggested that the deficits in frail and prefrail patients in executive function and memory may be similar in size.[67]

There is some evidence that, even with normal aging, both cognitive decline and physical frailty often coexist.[68–70] Cross-sectional studies find a high level of coexistence between rates of cognitive impairment and dementia and physical frailty.[71] Frailty predicts cognitive decline and incident dementia[72,73] and cognitive impairment predicts frailty[74,75] in longitudinal studies. Loss of executive function and poor attention are particularly associated with slow gait.[76] There is increasing evidence that persons with white matter hyperintensities have poor balance, poor get up and go performance, slow gait speed, and increased falls.[77–79] White matter hyperintensities also predict functional decline.[80] In a Spanish study, fall risk factors did not hold a direct correlation with the level of cognitive impairment among elderly nursing home care residents.[81]

HOME-BASED AND COMMUNITY-BASED CARE

- The vast majority—80%—of elderly people receiving assistance, including many with several functional limitations, live in private homes in the community and not in institutions.[82]
- Elderly people with limitations in 3 or more activities of daily living who live in the community receive an average of 9 hours of assistance per day (counting both formal and informal sources of care) and people age 85 or older with that degree of impairment typically receive about 11 hours of assistance per day.[83]
- The trend toward community-based services as opposed to nursing home placement was formalized with the Olmstead Decision (July, 1999), a court case in which the Supreme Court upheld the right of individuals to receive care in the community as opposed to an institution whenever possible.
- The proportion of Americans aged 65 and over with disabilities who rely entirely on formal care for their personal assistance needs has increased to 9% in 1999 from 5% in 1984.
- Between 2000 and 2002, the number of licensed assisted living and board and care facilities increased from 32,886 to 36,399 nationally, reflecting the trend toward community-based care as opposed to nursing homes.[84] Most assisted living facilities, however, are unlicensed.
- Most assisted living facilities discharge residents whose cognitive impairments become moderate or severe or who need help with transfers (eg, moving from a wheelchair to a bed). This factor limits the ability of these populations to find appropriate services outside of nursing homes or other institutions.[85]

WHY DOES IT MATTER?

If we wait for functional decline to define dementia, it may be too late to treat the underlying disease process.[4] Moreover, because functional decline is in the definition of dementia, it is best to work with a construct that would allow intervention sooner rather than later. With this theoretic framework, many studies have been conducted to investigate the usefulness and prognostic outcome of the diagnoses.[4]

In addition, the concept of MCI plays extremely well as we design hypothesis-driven research, be it with regard to clinical markers, psychological assessment, neuroimaging, biomarkers, or drug and nondrug interventions.[13] This point is perhaps equally as important as the clinical diagnosis and has generated research opportunities worldwide. The construct of MCI has been incorporated into research on aging from multiple perspectives including clinical research, epidemiology, neuroimaging, mechanisms of disease, clinical trials, and caregiving.[13]

Numerous investigations worldwide have used these criteria as an infrastructure for estimating the frequency of MCI and its subtypes.[5–8] Both prospective[5,9] and retrospective studies[10] have helped to define the subtleties of the diagnosis. A major factor in determining outcome depends on the source of the patient being studied. The closer one is to a community sample, the lower the annual rates of progression (6%–10%).[11] With referral-based studies, such as those that come from sampling a memory disorders clinic or Alzheimer disease center, the progression rates increases to 10% to 15% per year, particularly for Alzheimer disease.[12] These differences reflect the probability of having an underlying disorder such as MCI when a participant or concerned family member seeks treatment at a referral clinic. The same phenomenon occurs at dementia screening clinics that advertise their services and claim diagnostic rates approaching 50%. This finding is in the face of baseline incidence rates of dementia and Alzheimer disease of 1% to 2% per year.[3]

EPIDEMIOLOGY

The Mayo Clinic Study of Aging was designed as a population-based study in Olmsted County, Minnesota, involving a random sample of nearly 3000 participants aged 70 through 89 years who were nondemented and cognitively normal or who had MCI at entry.[14] The prevalence of MCI from this study is estimated at approximately 15% of the nondemented population, with a 2:1 ratio of aMCI to naMCI. The most common putative cause is degenerative[86] and this cause predominates to a greater extent for aMCI than for naMCI. There is also strong evidence that these rates tend to hold up throughout the world at about 14% to 18% for individuals aged 70 and older.[13]

In early 2018, the American Academy of Neurology published its "Practice Guideline Update: Mild Cognitive Impairment."[86] The guideline focuses on the prevalence and treatment of MCI and finds that there is strong evidence that MCI prevalence is high in the general population, with prevalence increasing for every 4-year age group starting at the age of 60 years. Overall, in persons 65 and older, the pooled prevalence of MCI is about 15% to 20%, and that compares with a population prevalence of dementia of about 10% to 12%. Furthermore, strong evidence shows that the natural history for many MCI cases can progress to dementia so a thorough evaluation to determine the underlying cause is important because some causes are treatable (**Figs. 1** and **2**).

ASSESSING THE PATIENT

Patients with MCI, particularly the amnestic subtype, complain primarily of impaired memory, or at least their families make the case that there is a new problem. It is also likely that the changes have been progressive over time, subtle but taken as a whole a change from a former level of function. Subjective memory complaints have been demonstrated to predict cognitive decline, even when patients seems to be unimpaired on testing.[87–91] The 1 free pass, such as recalling names, is frequently reported by normal elderly patients. The patient that arrives worried and reports memory complaints can be found to have impaired concentration with a mood or affective disorder.[87,92] Some individuals who meet neuropsychological test criteria for MCI deny having any significant memory problems.[93]

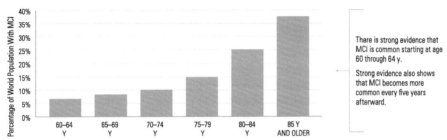

Fig. 1. Mild cognitive impairment (MCI) is common. (Practice guideline update: Mild cognitive impairment [patient summary]. Minneapolis, MN: American Academy of Neurology; Epub 2017 Dec 27. https://www.aan.com/Guidelines/Home/GetGuidelineContent/883. Accessed August 16, 2018. © 2017 American Academy of Neurology Institute. Reproduced with permission.)

In contrast with the impaired awareness of deficits commonly present in patients with Alzheimer disease, younger patients with MCI are often troubled by their symptoms.[89,94,95] However, as the patient ages and develops more overt disease, including Alzheimer disease, informant-reported symptoms over self-reported symptoms predominate.[96] As with dementia, mood and behavioral symptoms are more common in patients with MCI than in cognitively unimpaired, age-matched controls.[97–102] The prevalence of depression ranges from 25% to 40%[103]; other common symptoms include irritability, anxiety, aggression, and apathy.[99] Patients with MCI and behavioral symptoms may be more impaired on cognitive measures than those without behavioral symptoms.[99]

Population-based studies comparing MCI and patients with Alzheimer disease find a similar range of neuropsychiatric symptoms, with patients with Alzheimer disease having them in somewhat higher frequency and severity.[100,104,105] The end stage for nursing home patients is often the overt manifestation of behavioral symptoms, although this population continues to receive antidepressant therapy and treatment with atypical antipsychotics, although in lesser numbers and amounts than a decade ago.

Cognitive impairment may be a presenting symptom of depression, so-called pseudodementia. Depression may also be an early manifestation of cognitive impairment. A number of population-based studies have found an association between various measure of depression and the presence of MCI.[97,106,107] However, follow-up data have yielded somewhat mixed results:

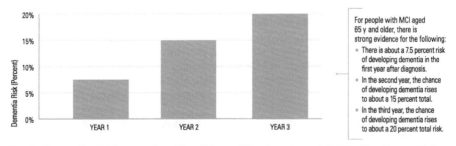

Fig. 2. Dementia risk in people with mild cognitive impairment (MCI). (Practice guideline update: Mild cognitive impairment [patient summary]. Minneapolis, MN: American Academy of Neurology; Epub 2017 Dec 27. https://www.aan.com/Guidelines/Home/GetGuidelineContent/883. Accessed August 16, 2018. © 2017 American Academy of Neurology Institute. Reproduced with permission.)

- Among 500 persons who were 85 years old, impaired cognition at baseline was associated with increasing depressive symptoms over 4 years of follow-up, but baseline depression was not associated with accelerated cognitive decline.[106]
- In contrast, other large cohort studies have found that depressed mood and/or anxiety are associated with increased risk of MCI in patients with normal cognition, and with progression to dementia in patients with MCI.[97,107–110]
- Finally, an analysis of MCI diagnostic criteria used in 6 clinical trials found that excluding patients with depression significantly decreased the sensitivity rates of MCI diagnosis for a future diagnosis of Alzheimer disease.[111]

ESTABLISHING THE DIAGNOSIS

A work group on diagnostic guidelines from the National Institute on Aging-Alzheimer's Association identified the following core clinical features that indicate MCI owing to Alzheimer disease.[112] These criteria only refer to the majority of MCI that is likely to progress to Alzheimer disease and not to MCI owing to other etiologies, for example, vascular disease, other neurodegenerative conditions, or psychiatric conditions.[58]

- Cognitive concern reflecting a change in cognition reported by patient or informant or observed by clinician;
- Objective evidence of impairment in 1 or more cognitive domains, typically including memory;
- Preservation of independence in functional abilities; and
- Not demented.

In addition, the etiology of MCI should be evaluated to identify the cause as most likely to be Alzheimer disease:

- Rule out vascular, traumatic, and medical causes of cognitive decline, where possible;
- Provide evidence of longitudinal decline in cognition, when feasible; and
- Report history consistent with Alzheimer disease genetic factors, where relevant.

As part of the MCI owing to Alzheimer disease criteria, biomarkers are used to augment clinical suspicions that the clinical syndrome of MCI is due to Alzheimer disease.[112] The geriatrician needs to be familiar with the concept of biomarkers. Future therapies will depend on the construct of prodromal MCI, MCI, and early Alzheimer disease and the vast array of testing now becoming available to segment the population for disease-modifying therapies based on genotype, amyloid or tau imaging on PET, and even cerebrospinal fluid evaluation.

One of the first biomarkers for MCI and Alzheimer disease was apolipoprotein E (APOE) genotypes. Generally, the E4 phenotype conveys a higher likelihood of disease, whereas the E2 genotype is somewhat protective.[113] The APOE e4 allele remains as an important predictor in MCI conversion to Alzheimer disease for patients with single domain MCI and multiple domains MCI from onset to disease progression. Among those with MCI, e4 carriers had the lowest level of plasma APOE as well **(Fig. 3)**.[114]

The geriatrician must evaluate the patient for the potential of other conditions that can present with MCI:

- Depression or other disorders of mood that may present with cognitive complaints.
- Medications including anticholinergics, antihistamines, benzodiazepines, and the nonbenzodiazepine Z-class of sedative hypnotics.[115,116]

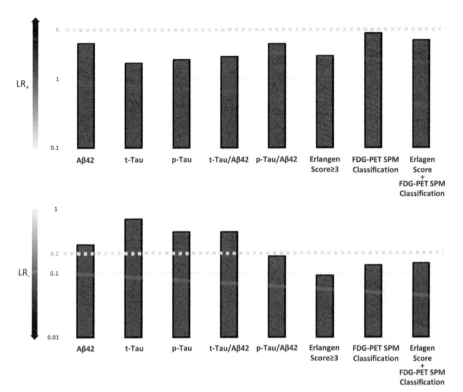

Fig. 3. Positive and negative likelihood ratio (LR$_+$ and LR$_-$) for correct classification or patients with mild cognitive impairment (MCI) converting to Alzheimer disease (AD) dementia. A LR$_+$ of greater than 5 indicates that the biomarker positive classification is associated with the disease occurrence. A LR$_-$ of less than 0.2 indicates a relevant association between the negative biomarker classification and the absence of the dementia condition at follow-up. LR values are represented on a logarithmic scale. FDG, fludeoxyglucose F 18; SPM, statistical parametrical. (*From* Scarabino D, Broggio E, Gambina G, et al. Apolipoprotein E genotypes and plasma levels in mild cognitive impairment conversion to Alzheimer's disease: a follow-up study. Am J Med Genet B Neuropsychiatr Genet 2016;171(8):1135; with permission.)

- Vitamin B$_{12}$ deficiency and hypothyroidism are always looked for and seldom found.
- Alcohol use and abuse and, as the boomers age, other recreational drug use as well.

In a community sample, patients with "cognitive impairment, no dementia" were diagnosed with depression and other psychiatric disease (10.2%), alcohol- and drug-related causes (6.9%), and delirium (1%).[117] Approximately one-quarter of patients had neurologic disease (brain tumor, Parkinson disease, multiple sclerosis, cerebrovascular disease, and epilepsy). Among the remaining 57.5% of patients, most (31.7%) had circumscribed memory impairment.

The story of beta amyloid is also intricately locked with our understanding of Alzheimer disease and, likewise, MCI. The role of beta amyloid in neurodegeneration has been thought to be seminal to the progression of disease. Unfortunately, all targeted therapies to date to clear beta amyloid, prevent its aggregation, or limit its impact on cellular function have not resulted in new drug interventions. Nonetheless, as a biomarker it clearly reflects disease progression (**Fig. 4**).[118]

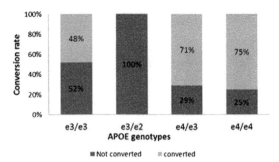

Fig. 4. Conversion rate of patients with mild cognitive impairment (MCI) according to apolipoprotein (APOE) genotypes. (*From* Doraiswamy PM, Sperling RA, Coleman RE, et al. Amyloid-beta assessed by florbetapir F 18 PET and 18-month cognitive decline: a multicenter study. Neurology 2012;79(16):1638; with permission.)

APPROACHING THE PATIENT AND THEIR CAREGIVER

The clinical history remains the mainstay in making a diagnosis of MCI. It is all about what insight the patient maintains in understanding their memory deficit. However, obtaining a history from both the patient and an informant may provide further support that a cognitive decline does exist.[21] Questions about cognition should address all major domains, including memory, attention–executive functioning, visuospatial skills, and language. Common memory symptoms include the tendency to repeat oneself or forgetfulness for recent events.

Patients with attention–executive functioning impairment may have problems in making decisions, planning activities, and multitasking. Visuospatial difficulties may be elicited by asking about a tendency to get lost while driving or an inability track the lines on a page while reading. Word finding difficulty, paraphasias, and/or anomia may indicate language dysfunction. The history taking should also focus on functional status, including the ability to drive, manage finances, and maintain basic activities of daily living. Possible neuropsychiatric, motor, and sleep issues should be addressed, because the presence of these symptoms may suggest a possible etiology of an MCI subtype.

Language difficulties, disinhibition, or socially inappropriate behavior may be seen in those with FTD; REM sleep behavior disorder, characterized by a tendency to act out dreams, has been associated with dementia with Lewy bodies. A past medical history may reveal cerebrovascular disease, seizures, head trauma, or systemic cancer or infections that may be contributing to the cognitive impairment.

The time course of symptoms is also important. A gradual, insidious progression of symptoms may suggest a degenerative cause, whereas a more acute onset may indicate a vascular, inflammatory, or infectious etiology. The loss of concentration may be a presenting symptom, but it is more often associated with depression than with cognitive impairment. Good screening tests for depression are readily available and the Patients Health Questionnaire (PHQ)-9 has found its way into many office practices.[22] The PHQ-9 is the 9-item depression scale of the Patient Health Questionnaire. It is a powerful tool for assisting primary care clinicians in diagnosing depression as well as selecting and monitoring treatment.

The primary care clinician and/or office staff should discuss with the patient the reasons for completing the questionnaire and how to fill it out. It can be done by intact patients or used as a survey instrument and done by just about anyone. After the patient has completed the PHQ-9 questionnaire, it is simply scored. There are 2 components of the PHQ-9: (1) assessing symptoms and functional impairment to make a tentative depression diagnosis, and (2) deriving a severity score to help select and monitor treatment. It also responds to treatment initiatives with clinically validated changes in the patient's response.

After a history has been obtained that will also evaluate the impact of decline, a general neurologic examination should be performed. Any practitioner with appropriate experience can do the examination. Although the examination may be normal, abnormalities could suggest a potential etiology for the cognitive deficits. Parkinsonism may be seen with dementia with Lewy bodies as well as other neurodegenerative disorders, motor neuron signs may be associated with FTD, and focal deficits consistent with a specific vascular distribution may suggest a vascular cause for the cognitive impairment.

In addition to a general neurologic examination, a screening mental status examination, such as the MMSE, 3MS, or Kokmen Short Test of Mental Status, should be administered.[23–25] The severity of symptoms may be determined using assessments such as the Clinical Dementia Rating scale.[2] A formal neuropsychological battery also can be performed and should include tests that sufficiently challenge a patient in each cognitive domain.

After adjusting for age and education, scores below 1.0 to 1.5 standard deviations below the mean typically indicate cognitive impairment on neuropsychological testing.[26,119] Learning and recall tasks may differentiate subjects with MCI from those experiencing normal aging. On measures of general cognitive function such as the MMSE and full-scale IQ, the individual with MCI performs more similar to a normal elderly subject, whereas memory function on delayed verbal recall (Logical Memory II) and nonverbal delayed recall (Visual Reproductions II) more closely resembles mild Alzheimer disease.[3]

Although the screening mental status examination and neuropsychological battery may be useful, it is important to remember that these tests may not be sensitive to cognitive impairment. Individuals may score within the normal range, particularly those with high premorbid intellectual functioning. Despite normal scores, these patients may have MCI if the clinician determines that there has been a change from baseline functioning. In these circumstances, it is usually best to follow these patients clinically, with repeat evaluations at regular intervals.

Laboratory tests used in the evaluation of dementia may identify medical issues that could affect cognitive function.[120] Basic laboratory tests that look for reversible causes of cognitive impairment include a complete blood count, basic metabolic panel, thyroid function tests, vitamin B_{12} levels, and folate levels. Neuroimaging with MRI or computed tomography of the brain is also recommended to look for any structural abnormalities that may be contributing to symptoms.

Information from the history, screening mental status examination, neuropsychological testing, and ancillary studies should be used to determine if cognitive function is changing, normal, or impaired. Functional status can be obtained from the individual, the informant, or both. If the patient has experienced cognitive decline but has maintained most daily activities, then that individual can be given an MCI diagnosis. Once an individual has been diagnosed as having MCI, the clinician can determine the MCI subtype based on which cognitive domains are impaired. From this determination, the MCI subtype can be determined. If memory impairment is present, then the individual has an aMCI subtype. If memory is preserved but evidence of decline is seen in other cognitive domains, then the subtype is naMCI.

After indicating the subtype as aMCI or naMCI, the next step is to determine if 1 or more cognitive domains are affected. If memory is the only domain affected, then the subtype would be aMCI single domain; if at least 1 other cognitive domain is also affected, then the subtype would be an aMCI multiple domain. If the impairment was isolated to one of the nonmemory domains, then the subtype would be naMCI single domain; if 2 or more nonmemory domains were affected, then the subtype would be naMCI multiple domains. Again, function must be essentially preserved to differentiate multiple domain MCI from dementia.

The goal of such subtyping in clinical practice is to accurately describe the individual's clinical syndrome and to determine the possible etiology of the patient's symptoms. Using the history, examination, and ancillary data, the clinician can begin to deduce whether the cause of impairment is degenerative, vascular, psychiatric, or secondary to concomitant medical disorders. Such deductions may assist in providing treatment options for each patient.

NATURAL PROGRESSION OF DISEASE AND OUTCOMES

Because MCI is considered to be a transitional state between normal aging and dementia, the etiologies for dementia theoretically could be applied to MCI. Although the construct has yet to be validated, aMCI owing to a degenerative etiology is thought to progress most likely to Alzheimer disease, an assertion that has been endorsed in a practice parameter from the American Academy of Neurology.[121]

Our earliest work in the Mayo Alzheimer's Disease Research Center taught us that even normal individuals change as they get older. Not only does reaction time slow, but on measures of Verbal IQ and measures of Performance IQ the things we do day in and day out are better preserved.[122–124] In all of our attempts at providing care to the elderly, these are the principles that shaped us early and continue to play out in the advice we give out every day. Overlearned behaviors, repetitive tasks, and rehearsed activities make it easy and comfortable for us to go about the routines of the day. The things we are confronted with that take an element of problem solving become all the more difficult as we age.

Although a diagnosis of MCI places an individual at higher risk for developing dementia, it does not indicate that the patient necessarily will progress to a dementia state. Although the majority of the patients with MCI in 1 large prospective trial progressed to Alzheimer disease at a rate of 7% to 10% per year, a small percentage of these individuals improved to normal.[5] Others have been known to remain clinically stable for many years and may not develop dementia.[125] These potential outcomes should be discussed with patients and their families after a diagnosis of MCI has been made.

Pathology

Studies of preclinical Alzheimer disease should be distinguished from studies of MCI.[126] In MCI studies, patients meet cognitive criteria for the diagnosis and are then followed prospectively to assess for conversion to Alzheimer disease. In contrast, preclinical Alzheimer disease refers to individuals with normal cognition who possess positive biomarkers for Alzheimer disease, such as a positive amyloid PET scan or evidence of Alzheimer disease biomarkers in the cerebrospinal fluid.[127]

The Religious Orders Study has followed a group of nuns and priests for many years and has an achieved high autopsy rates. The study reports that approximately 60% of the participants with MCI have neuropathologic evidence of Alzheimer disease, but that vascular disease also accounts for significant pathology.[15] Other studies have implicated the importance and the findings of neurofibrillary tangle density to account for the symptoms of MCI.[16,128] The best summary of outcomes after diagnosis of MCI was the results of a large autopsy series published in 2017. Of the 874 individuals ever diagnosed with MCI, final clinical diagnoses were varied: 39.2% died with an MCI diagnosis, 46.8% with a dementia diagnosis, and 13.9% with intact cognition. The MCI diagnosis was usually associated with comorbid neuropathologies; fewer than one-quarter of MCI cases showed pure Alzheimer disease pathology.[128]

Two additional studies come from our own early investigations. We evaluated participants who died while their clinical classification was MCI and found that most had a low probability of having the neuropathologic features of Alzheimer disease at that point in time.[17] A second study observed participants who had been previously diagnosed with MCI and had progressed to dementia, and characterized these participants as having diagnostic pathology. This study indicated that, although most of the participants with aMCI developed Alzheimer disease, another sizable group (20%–30%) developed another type of dementing disorder.[18] These studies remain in contrast with opinions that the discoverable pathology of MCI, albeit more advanced MCI, is only Alzheimer disease.[19,20]

PET with fludeoxyglucose F 18 and cerebrospinal fluid biomarkers also play a role in predicting conversion to different dementias in patients with MCI. Even in prodromal MCI (before clinical relevance), the array of diagnostic tools will help us in determining whether to use cerebrospinal fluid biomarkers or the expanding array of biomarker images to help us predict what therapy might work best with what precondition (**Fig. 5**).[129]

Erlangen scores refers to an algorithm that divides cerebrospinal fluid biomarker patterns into 5 groups, covering all possible cerebrospinal fluid result combinations based on the presence of pathologic tau and/or amyloid-β cerebrospinal fluid values. The PET with fludeoxyglucose F 18 statistical parametrical classification uses statistical parametrical maps to normalize how scans are read and thus interpreted from one research center to another.

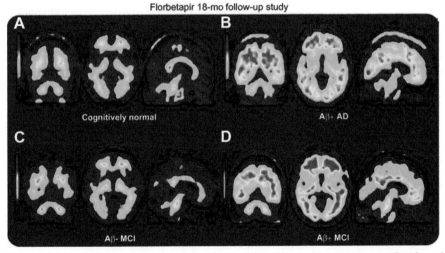

Fig. 5. Florbetapir PET scans in controls, patients with mild cognitive impairment (MCI), and patients with Alzheimer disease. Florbetapir PET images for an amyloid-negative Aβ− cognitively normal subject (*A*), an amyloid-positive (Aβ+) patient with Alzheimer disease (AD) (*B*), an amyloid-negative (Aβ−) patient with MCI (*C*), and an Aβ+ patient with MCI who converted to dementia during the course of this study (*D*). Aβ+ was determined per the majority of 3 raters. Color scale is shown in standardized uptake value ratio (SUVr) units. (*From* Caminiti SP, Ballarini T, Sala A, et al. FDG-PET and CSF biomarker accuracy in prediction of conversion to different dementias in a large multicentre MCI cohort. Neuroimage Clin 2018;18:173; with permission.)

Most likely, aMCI owing to a degenerative cause has similar features to clinically probable Alzheimer disease, with risk factors such as age, hypertension, and diabetes.[27–29] APOE4 carrier status is a recognized genetic risk factor for the development of Alzheimer disease,[30] but its value for detecting progression to cognitive impairment is less clear. It has been a consistent predictor but has not found a useful way into clinical practice.

Some studies have suggested that APOE4 carrier status may have assist in predicting those more likely to convert from MCI to Alzheimer disease[126,127,130] and a synergistic effect with depression has been seen in cognitively normal individuals at risk for developing MCI. APOE4 carrier status also may be associated both with hippocampal atrophy in patients with MCI and with higher rates of cognitive decline in cognitively normal adults.[131,132] However, others have shown that APOE4 carrier status itself has not been shown to predict cognitive decline or conversion to Alzheimer disease[133] and its routine use is not recommended[134]; the diagnosis of MCI is made clinically.

Suspected non-Alzheimer disease pathology MCI is a term that is increasingly used in research studies to denote individuals who meet the clinical criteria for MCI and show no evidence of amyloid pathology based on cerebrospinal fluid biomarker and/or amyloid PET imaging, but have evidence of neuronal injury as measured by either medial temporal lobe atrophy or hypometabolism on PET with fludeoxyglucose F 18.[130,131] In MCI with suspected non-Alzheimer disease pathology, low APOE e4 and high APOE e2 carrier prevalence may account for differences in neurodegeneration patterns when measuring beta amyloid peptide load using florbetpir F-18 PET scanning and hippocampal volume determined by MRI.[135]

TREATMENT

The early detection of cognitive decline theoretically may lead to the implementation of therapies that slow the progression of impairment. However, there currently is no treatment approved by the US Food and Drug Administration for MCI likely owing to Alzheimer disease. Because the etiologies of MCI can be heterogeneous, medications targeting a neurodegenerative cause theoretically would be different than those targeting cognitive impairment owing to vascular, psychiatric, or other medical disorders. Clinical trials nevertheless have focused on the aMCI subtype, with the goal of slowing the progression to Alzheimer disease.

The evidence is low that targeted cognitive interventions, taken as a group, may help to improve performance on some cognitive measures but with no evidence of functional benefit. The concept has further expanded to include a population of patients where the condition may be reversible owing to a combination of disease, medical stressors, and acute illness. An Italian study evaluated the proportion of MCI subjects who revert to normal cognition in a memory clinic context, focusing on the role of comorbidities. Between 2004 and 2013, 374 patients with MCI were recruited. During a mean time of 32 ± 25.5 months, 21 (5.6%) reverted to normal control. Subjects who reverted to normal cognition were younger ($P = .0001$), more educated ($P = .0001$), had a better global cognition ($P = .0001$), as assessed by the MMSE, and suffered from more comorbidities ($P = .002$), as assessed by Cumulative Illness Rating Scale than those who developed dementia.[136] There remain no known pharmacologic therapies for which evidence of lasting benefit has been demonstrated in well-designed studies for patients with static or progressive conditions. Moderate evidence shows that people diagnosed with MCI can benefit from regular physical exercise. Conceivably, if MCI were due to depression, it could also be treated with a drug.

A number of studies have targeted medications used in the symptomatic treatment of clinically probable Alzheimer disease. These medications have included 3 of the cholinesterase inhibitors, namely, donepezil, galantamine, and rivastigmine.[137–139] Additionally, vitamin E and rofecoxib have been studied,[137,140] because both oxidative damage and inflammation have been implicated in the pathophysiology of Alzheimer disease.[141–144] Unfortunately, none of these interventions have shown a significant decrease in conversion rates of aMCI to Alzheimer disease, ranging from 6% to 17% in the medication arms versus 4% to 21% with placebo. However, 1 study did find that donepezil reduced the progression risk for 12 months in those with aMCI, an effect that persisted for up to 24 months in APOE4 carriers.[137]

Despite the results of clinical trial data, these studies do support the construct of MCI as a transitional state between normal cognition and Alzheimer disease. The overall progression rates for MCI in these studies ranged from 5% to 16%, which are higher than the incidence rate for Alzheimer disease in the general population.[3,137] These rates suggest that patients who meet MCI criteria are at a higher risk of developing Alzheimer disease. Because not all of those with MCI develop Alzheimer disease pathology, more accurate identification of these subjects is essential. Incorporating potential predictive biomarkers in clinical trials may assist in testing compounds that target the underlying disease process of Alzheimer disease.[145]

A variety of nondrug interventions has also been tried on this population. Not surprisingly, cognitive training has been the most studied.[86] There may even be some benefit from exercise.[86] The environment of care has been addressed and lifestyle management has been included. Interventions range from individualized therapy to group programs that additionally address activity planning, self-assertiveness training, relaxation techniques, stress management, use of external memory aids, and motor exercise. Multicomponent interventions seem to benefit activities of daily living, mood, and memory performance. A standardized cognitive training manual has been proposed as well further studies using a larger sample size and more robust experimental designs.[146–148]

Although no symptomatic or disease-modifying drug therapies are available for MCI owing to Alzheimer disease, there is much that can be done. The domains of cognition, function, and behavior define this population and where they reside in the spectrum of disease. Their preserved abilities can also serve as markers for how the disease is progressing and how well they are living within a defined environment. Even without a drug treatment for MCI, understanding the environment that surrounds every one of these patients and how they function within their universe is most important. Overlearned behaviors and an environment that limits or prohibits excess disabilities should be stressed, even for patients with MCI. Much can be done and running toward a diagnosis is better than running away from it.

ADVANCE CARE PLANNING

Cognitive impairment, be it MCI or dementia, can still be defined by the capacities that are preserved and the capacities that are lost. This is where the issue of driving comes into play, although the concept applies to all kinds of tasks and opportunities. We counsel that a diagnosis is not an all or none phenomenon and many individuals with MCI or even early dementia sit on advisory boards to provide a patient voice in better understanding the needs of the patient. Unfortunately, explaining these concepts and what is both retained and what is lost takes time, especially for the primary care provider.

As our understanding of disease advances, the triad of cognition, function, and behavior not only defines the type of care that may be appropriate, but also contributes to our understanding of where the best site of care might be. Our ability to address the environment early in the care of patients with MCI or other age-dependent deficiencies may improve the quality of life for our patients, avoid common pitfalls and provide for more cost-effective and successful management of the person, and not just the disease they may have. A goal set by the Alzheimer's Association back in 1987 was to create an environment where a person can function with minimal failure and maximal use of retained abilities. There is even more opportunity today to create this success with earlier diagnosis and earlier intervention.

Patients and families should be aware that those who have aMCI owing to a degenerative cause may have a 10% to 15% chance of developing dementia; however, it also should be noted that MCI is heterogeneous with a number of potential outcomes.[125] Although some patients may not develop dementia, the label of "mild cognitive impairment" nevertheless may lead to psychological consequences, such as a feeling of uncertainty or concerns of becoming burdensome to others.[149] Neuropsychiatric symptoms such as depression, anxiety, apathy, and/or irritability also may be seen in those with MCI and may be associated with progression to Alzheimer disease.[104]

Encouraging patients and their families and caregivers to consider decisions about advance directives, future planning, and finances is essential, especially if the cognitive impairment is thought to be due to a degenerative cause. Although preventative strategies remain elusive, patients should be encouraged to follow a heart healthy diet, control for diabetes mellitus and hypertension, remain physically active, and engage intellectually and socially without frustration. Participation in a cognitive rehabilitation program also may be useful in patients with MCI, with improvements in activities of daily living, mood, and memory. Although these modifications may improve their overall quality of life, there has not been enough research to support that a decreased progression from aMCI to Alzheimer disease.

SUMMARY

The MCI construct implies an intermediate state between normal cognition and dementia. Individuals with MCI have (a) a subjective cognitive complaint that is usually corroborated by an informant, (b) preserved general cognitive functioning, (c) impairment in 1 or more of the cognitive domains (memory, attention–executive function, visuospatial skills, and/or language), and (d) essentially normal activities of daily living. Once the diagnosis of MCI has been made, the specific subtype can be determined, with aMCI referring to the presence of memory impairment and naMCI referring to the presence of impairment in 1 or more of the other domains with relative preservation of memory.

MCI remains a clinical diagnosis, aided by a thorough history, neurologic examination, screening mental status examination, and formal neuropsychological testing. Although an individual with high premorbid intellectual functioning may score within the normal range on bedside and formal testing, that patient may still be considered to have MCI based on the judgment of the clinician. Because there is subjectivity in the clinical diagnosis, creating an operational definition for clinical trials has been a challenge. In addition, a number of etiologies can be associated with MCI, including degenerative and vascular processes, psychiatric causes, and comorbid medical conditions. Treatable medical conditions may also present as MCI and have reversible outcomes.

Our goal with the geriatric patient remains the preservation of function and the amelioration of symptoms. Accurate diagnosis of MCI allows us to advise patients and families regarding placement, level of care needs, and quite possibly predict the future. Limiting transitions is in the best interest of all parties and allows for the maximal use of retained abilities while limiting the frustrations that accrue with cognitive and functional decline. We urge practitioners, providers, patients, and their family to be as precise as possible in evaluating cognitive and memory complaints given the wealth of information and diagnostic testing available regarding MCI. The accuracy of the diagnosis affects the outcome and experience of each individual and family that seek our opinion.

REFERENCES

1. Reisberg B, Ferris SH, de Leon MJ, et al. Stage-specific behavioral, cognitive, and in vivo changes in community residing subjects with age-associated memory impairment and primary degenerative dementia of the Alzheimer type. Drug Dev Res 1988;15(2–3):101–14.
2. Morris JC. The Clinical Dementia Rating (CDR): current version and scoring rules. Neurology 1993;43(11):2412–4.
3. Petersen RC, Smith GE, Waring SC, et al. Mild cognitive impairment: clinical characterization and outcome. Arch Neurol 1999;56(3):303–8.
4. Gauthier S, Reisberg B, Zaudig M, et al. Mild cognitive impairment. Lancet 2006;367(9518):1262–70.
5. Busse A, Hensel A, Guhne U, et al. Mild cognitive impairment: long-term course of four clinical subtypes. Neurology 2006;67(12):2176–85.
6. Ganguli M, Dodge HH, Shen C, et al. Mild cognitive impairment, amnestic type: an epidemiologic study. Neurology 2004;63(1):115–21.
7. Larrieu S, Letenneur L, Orgogozo JM, et al. Incidence and outcome of mild cognitive impairment in a population-based prospective cohort. Neurology 2002;59(10):1594–9.
8. DeCarli C. Mild cognitive impairment: prevalence, prognosis, aetiology, and treatment. Lancet Neurol 2003;2(1):15–21.
9. Lopez OL, Jagust WJ, DeKosky ST, et al. Prevalence and classification of mild cognitive impairment in the cardiovascular health study cognition study: part 1. Arch Neurol 2003;60(10):1385–9.
10. Ritchie K, Artero S, Touchon J. Classification criteria for mild cognitive impairment: a population-based validation study. Neurology 2001;56(1):37–42.
11. Fischer P, Jungwirth S, Zehetmayer S, et al. Conversion from subtypes of mild cognitive impairment to Alzheimer dementia. Neurology 2007;68(4):288–91.
12. Farias ST, Mungas D, Reed BR, et al. Progression of mild cognitive impairment to dementia in clinic- vs community-based cohorts. Arch Neurol 2009;66(9):1151–7.
13. Petersen RC, Roberts RO, Knopman DS, et al. Mild cognitive impairment: ten years later. Arch Neurol 2009;66(12):1447–55.
14. Roberts RO, Geda YE, Knopman DS, et al. The Mayo Clinic Study of Aging: design and sampling, participation, baseline measures and sample characteristics. Neuroepidemiology 2008;30(1):58–69.
15. Bennett DA, Schneider JA, Bienias JL, et al. Mild cognitive impairment is related to Alzheimer disease pathology and cerebral infarctions. Neurology 2005;64(5):834–41.
16. Guillozet AL, Weintraub S, Mash DC, et al. Neurofibrillary tangles, amyloid, and memory in aging and mild cognitive impairment. Arch Neurol 2003;60(5):729–36.

17. Petersen RC, Parisi JE, Dickson DW, et al. Neuropathologic features of amnestic mild cognitive impairment. Arch Neurol 2006;63(5):665–72.

18. Jicha GA, Parisi JE, Dickson DW, et al. Neuropathologic outcome of mild cognitive impairment following progression to clinical dementia. Arch Neurol 2006; 63(5):674–81.

19. Morris JC. Mild cognitive impairment is early-stage Alzheimer disease: time to revise diagnostic criteria. Arch Neurol 2006;63(1):15–6.

20. Markesbery WR, Schmitt FA, Kryscio RJ, et al. Neuropathologic substrate of mild cognitive impairment. Arch Neurol 2006;63(1):38–46.

21. Daly E, Zaitchik D, Copeland M, et al. Predicting conversion to Alzheimer disease using standardized clinical information. Arch Neurol 2000;57(5):675–80.

22. Nease DE Jr, Nutting PA, Dickinson WP, et al. Inducing sustainable improvement in depression care in primary care practices. Jt Comm J Qual Patient Saf 2008; 34(5):247–55.

23. Folstein MF, Folstein SE, McHugh PR. "Mini-mental state". A practical method for grading the cognitive state of patients for the clinician. J Psychiatr Res 1975; 12(3):189–98.

24. Teng E, Lu PH, Cummings JL. Neuropsychiatric symptoms are associated with progression from mild cognitive impairment to Alzheimer's disease. Dement Geriatr Cogn Disord 2007;24(4):253–9.

25. Kokmen E, Smith GE, Petersen RC, et al. The short test of mental status. Correlations with standardized psychometric testing. Arch Neurol 1991;48(7):725–8.

26. Ivnik RJ, Malec JF, Smith GE, et al. Mayo's older Americans normative studies: WAIS-R norms for ages 56 to 97. Clin Neuropsychol 1992;6(sup001):1–30.

27. Reitz C, Tang MX, Manly J, et al. Hypertension and the risk of mild cognitive impairment. Arch Neurol 2007;64(12):1734–40.

28. Luchsinger JA, Reitz C, Patel B, et al. Relation of diabetes to mild cognitive impairment. Arch Neurol 2007;64(4):570–5.

29. Kryscio RJ, Schmitt FA, Salazar JC, et al. Risk factors for transitions from normal to mild cognitive impairment and dementia. Neurology 2006;66(6):828–32.

30. Corder EH, Saunders AM, Strittmatter WJ, et al. Gene dose of apolipoprotein E type 4 allele and the risk of Alzheimer's disease in late onset families. Science 1993;261(5123):921–3.

31. Mansbach WE, Mace RA. A comparison of the diagnostic accuracy of the AD8 and BCAT-SF in identifying dementia and mild cognitive impairment in long-term care residents. Neuropsychol Dev Cogn B Aging Neuropsychol Cogn 2016; 23(5):609–24.

32. Department of Health and Human Services Centers for Medicare and Medicaid Studies. Nursing home data compendium: Washington (DC). 2013. Available at: https://www.cms.gov/Medicare/Provider-Enrollment-and-Certification/Certification andCompliance/downloads/nursinghomedatacompendium_508.pdf. Accessed December 14, 2017.

33. Mansbach WE, MacDougall EE, Rosenzweig AS. The Brief Cognitive Assessment Tool (BCAT): a new test emphasizing contextual memory, executive functions, attentional capacity, and the prediction of instrumental activities of daily living. J Clin Exp Neuropsychol 2012;34(2):183–94.

34. Zimmerman S, Sloane PD, Reed D. Dementia prevalence and care in assisted living. Health Aff (Millwood) 2014;33(4):658–66.

35. Magaziner J, German P, Zimmerman SI, et al. The prevalence of dementia in a statewide sample of new nursing home admissions aged 65 and older:

diagnosis by expert panel. Epidemiology of Dementia in Nursing Homes Research Group. Gerontologist 2000;40(6):663–72.

36. Mansbach WE, MacDougall EE, Clark KM, et al. Preliminary investigation of the Kitchen Picture Test (KPT): a new screening test of practical judgment for older adults. Neuropsychol Dev Cogn B Aging Neuropsychol Cogn 2014;21(6): 674–92.

37. Rosenblatt A, Samus QM, Steele CD, et al. The Maryland Assisted Living Study: prevalence, recognition, and treatment of dementia and other psychiatric disorders in the assisted living population of central Maryland. J Am Geriatr Soc 2004;52(10):1618–25.

38. Zimmerman S, Sloane PD, Williams CS, et al. Residential care/assisted living staff may detect undiagnosed dementia using the minimum data set cognition scale. J Am Geriatr Soc 2007;55(9):1349–55.

39. Petersen RC. Mild cognitive impairment. Continuum (Minneap Minn) 2016;22(2 Dementia):404–18.

40. Roberts JS, Karlawish JH, Uhlmann WR, et al. Mild cognitive impairment in clinical care: a survey of American Academy of Neurology members. Neurology 2010;75(5):425–31.

41. Singer C, Luxenberg J. Diagnosing dementia in long-term care facilities. J Am Med Dir Assoc 2003;4(6 Suppl):S134–40.

42. Cohen-Mansfield J. Nursing staff members' assessments of pain in cognitively impaired nursing home residents. Pain Manag Nurs 2005;6(2):68–75.

43. Cohen-Mansfield J, Creedon M. Nursing staff members' perceptions of pain indicators in persons with severe dementia. Clin J Pain 2002;18(1):64–73.

44. Morley JE, Morris JC, Berg-Weger M, et al. Brain health: the importance of recognizing cognitive impairment: an IAGG consensus conference. J Am Med Dir Assoc 2015;16(9):731–9.

45. Chodosh J, Edelen MO, Buchanan JL, et al. Nursing home assessment of cognitive impairment: development and testing of a brief instrument of mental status. J Am Geriatr Soc 2008;56(11):2069–75.

46. Saliba D, Buchanan J, Edelen MO, et al. MDS 3.0: brief interview for mental status. J Am Med Dir Assoc 2012;13(7):611–7.

47. Teng EL, Chui HC. The modified mini-mental state (3MS) examination. J Clin Psychiatry 1987;48(8):314–8.

48. McDowell I, Kristjansson B, Hill GB, et al. Community screening for dementia: the Mini Mental State Exam (MMSE) and modified mini-mental state exam (3MS) compared. J Clin Epidemiol 1997;50(4):377–83.

49. Mansbach WE, Mace RA, Clark KM. Differentiating levels of cognitive functioning: a comparison of the Brief Interview for Mental Status (BIMS) and the Brief Cognitive Assessment Tool (BCAT) in a nursing home sample. Aging Ment Health 2014;18(7):921–8.

50. Galvin JE, Roe CM, Powlishta KK, et al. The AD8: a brief informant interview to detect dementia. Neurology 2005;65(4):559–64.

51. Galvin JE, Roe CM, Xiong C, et al. Validity and reliability of the AD8 informant interview in dementia. Neurology 2006;67(11):1942–8.

52. Tariq SH, Tumosa N, Chibnall JT, et al. Comparison of the Saint Louis University mental status examination and the mini-mental state examination for detecting dementia and mild neurocognitive disorder–a pilot study. Am J Geriatr Psychiatry 2006;14(11):900–10.

53. Borson S, Scanlan J, Brush M, et al. The Mini-COG: a cognitive 'vital signs' measure for dementia screening in multi-lingual elderly. Int J Geriatr Psychiatry 2000; 15(11):1021–7.

54. Nasreddine ZS, Phillips NA, Bedirian V, et al. The Montreal Cognitive Assessment, MoCA: a brief screening tool for mild cognitive impairment. J Am Geriatr Soc 2005;53(4):695–9.

55. Kokmen E, Naessens JM, Offord KP. A short test of mental status: description and preliminary results. Mayo Clin Proc 1987;62(4):281–8.

56. Gerontological Society of America. Cognitive impairment detection and earlier diagnosis: KAER Toolkit: 4-step process to detecting cognitive impairment and earlier diagnosis of dementia: the Gerontological Society of America, Washington (DC). 2018. Available at: https://www.geron.org/programs-services/alliances-and-multi-stakeholder-collaborations/cognitive-impairment-detection-and-earlier-diagnosis. Accessed July 25, 2018.

57. Winblad B, Palmer K, Kivipelto M, et al. Mild cognitive impairment–beyond controversies, towards a consensus: report of the international working group on mild cognitive impairment. J Intern Med 2004;256(3):240–6.

58. Petersen RC. Mild cognitive impairment as a diagnostic entity. J Intern Med 2004;256(3):183–94.

59. Petersen RC, Aisen PS, Beckett LA, et al. Alzheimer's Disease Neuroimaging Initiative (ADNI): clinical characterization. Neurology 2010;74(3):201–9.

60. Mansbach WE, Mace RA, Clark KM. Mild cognitive impairment (MCI) in long-term care patients: subtype classification and occurrence. Aging Ment Health 2016;20(3):271–6.

61. Kaufer DI, Williams CS, Braaten AJ, et al. Cognitive screening for dementia and mild cognitive impairment in assisted living: comparison of 3 tests. J Am Med Dir Assoc 2008;9(8):586–93.

62. Mansbach WE, MacDougall EE. Development and validation of the short form of the Brief Cognitive Assessment Tool (BCAT-SF). Aging Ment Health 2012;16(8): 1065–71.

63. Reinvang I, Grambaite R, Espeseth T. Executive dysfunction in MCI: subtype or early symptom. Int J Alzheimers Dis 2012;2012:936272.

64. Morley JE, Vellas B, van Kan GA, et al. Frailty consensus: a call to action. J Am Med Dir Assoc 2013;14(6):392–7.

65. Panza F, Solfrizzi V, Barulli MR, et al. Cognitive frailty: a systematic review of epidemiological and neurobiological evidence of an age-related clinical condition. Rejuvenation Res 2015;18(5):389–412.

66. Lin JS, O'Connor E, Rossom RC, et al. Screening for cognitive impairment in older adults: an evidence update for the US preventive services task force. Rockville (MD): U.S. Preventive Services Task Force Evidence Syntheses, formerly Systematic Evidence Reviews; 2013.

67. Robertson DA, Savva GM, Coen RF, et al. Cognitive function in the prefrailty and frailty syndrome. J Am Geriatr Soc 2014;62(11):2118–24.

68. Malmstrom TK, Morley JE. The frail brain. J Am Med Dir Assoc 2013;14(7): 453–5.

69. Shimada H, Makizako H, Doi T, et al. Combined prevalence of frailty and mild cognitive impairment in a population of elderly Japanese people. J Am Med Dir Assoc 2013;14(7):518–24.

70. Nishiguchi S, Yamada M, Fukutani N, et al. Differential association of frailty with cognitive decline and sarcopenia in community-dwelling older adults. J Am Med Dir Assoc 2015;16(2):120–4.

71. Mitnitski A, Fallah N, Rockwood MR, et al. Transitions in cognitive status in relation to frailty in older adults: a comparison of three frailty measures. J Nutr Health Aging 2011;15(10):863–7.

72. Avila-Funes JA, Pina-Escudero SD, Aguilar-Navarro S, et al. Cognitive impairment and low physical activity are the components of frailty more strongly associated with disability. J Nutr Health Aging 2011;15(8):683–9.

73. Auyeung TW, Lee JS, Kwok T, et al. Physical frailty predicts future cognitive decline - a four-year prospective study in 2737 cognitively normal older adults. J Nutr Health Aging 2011;15(8):690–4.

74. Parihar R, Mahoney JR, Verghese J. Relationship of gait and cognition in the elderly. Curr Transl Geriatr Exp Gerontol Rep 2013;2(3):167–73.

75. Halil M, Cemal Kizilarslanoglu M, Emin Kuyumcu M, et al. Cognitive aspects of frailty: mechanisms behind the link between frailty and cognitive impairment. J Nutr Health Aging 2015;19(3):276–83.

76. McGough EL, Kelly VE, Logsdon RG, et al. Associations between physical performance and executive function in older adults with mild cognitive impairment: gait speed and the timed "up & go" test. Phys Ther 2011;91(8):1198–207.

77. Ogama N, Sakurai T, Shimizu A, et al. Regional white matter lesions predict falls in patients with amnestic mild cognitive impairment and Alzheimer's disease. J Am Med Dir Assoc 2014;15(1):36–41.

78. Bolandzadeh N, Liu-Ambrose T, Aizenstein H, et al. Pathways linking regional hyperintensities in the brain and slower gait. Neuroimage 2014;99:7–13.

79. Callisaya ML, Beare R, Phan T, et al. Progression of white matter hyperintensities of presumed vascular origin increases the risk of falls in older people. J Gerontol A Biol Sci Med Sci 2015;70(3):360–6.

80. Prins ND, Scheltens P. White matter hyperintensities, cognitive impairment and dementia: an update. Nat Rev Neurol 2015;11(3):157–65.

81. Seijo-Martinez M, Cancela JM, Ayan C, et al. Influence of cognitive impairment on fall risk among elderly nursing home residents. Int Psychogeriatr 2016; 28(12):1975–87.

82. Congressional Budget Office. 2013. Rising demand for long-term services and supports for elderly people: Washington (DC). Rising demand for long-term services and supports for elderly people. Available at: https://www.cbo.gov/publication/44363. Accessed July 25, 2018.

83. LaPlante MP, Harrington C, Kang T. Estimating paid and unpaid hours of personal assistance services in activities of daily living provided to adults living at home. Health Serv Res 2002;37(2):397–415.

84. Monica RL. State assisted living policy. Portland (OR): National Academy for State Health Policy; 2002.

85. Hawes RM, Rose M, Phillips CD. 1999. A national study of assisted living for the frail elderly: results of a national survey of facilities Washington (DC). 2017. Available at: https://aspe.hhs.gov/system/files/pdf/73016/facres.pdf. Accessed July 25, 2018.

86. Petersen RC, Lopez O, Armstrong MJ, et al. Practice guideline update summary: mild cognitive impairment: report of the guideline development, dissemination, and implementation subcommittee of the American Academy of Neurology. Neurology 2018;90(3):126–35.

87. Tobiansky R, Blizard R, Livingston G, et al. The Gospel Oak Study stage IV: the clinical relevance of subjective memory impairment in older people. Psychol Med 1995;25(4):779–86.

88. Geerlings MI, Jonker C, Bouter LM, et al. Association between memory complaints and incident Alzheimer's disease in elderly people with normal baseline cognition. Am J Psychiatry 1999;156(4):531–7.

89. van Norden AG, Fick WF, de Laat KF, et al. Subjective cognitive failures and hippocampal volume in elderly with white matter lesions. Neurology 2008;71(15): 1152–9.

90. Scheef L, Spottke A, Daerr M, et al. Glucose metabolism, gray matter structure, and memory decline in subjective memory impairment. Neurology 2012;79(13): 1332–9.

91. Mitchell AJ, Beaumont H, Ferguson D, et al. Risk of dementia and mild cognitive impairment in older people with subjective memory complaints: meta-analysis. Acta Psychiatr Scand 2014;130(6):439–51.

92. Riedel-Heller SG, Matschinger H, Schork A, et al. Do memory complaints indicate the presence of cognitive impairment? Results of a field study. Eur Arch Psychiatry Clin Neurosci 1999;249(4):197–204.

93. Mitchell AJ. Is it time to separate subjective cognitive complaints from the diagnosis of mild cognitive impairment? Age Ageing 2008;37(5):497–9.

94. Petersen RC, Doody R, Kurz A, et al. Current concepts in mild cognitive impairment. Arch Neurol 2001;58(12):1985–92.

95. Stewart R, Dufouil C, Godin O, et al. Neuroimaging correlates of subjective memory deficits in a community population. Neurology 2008;70(18):1601–7.

96. Tabert MH, Albert SM, Borukhova-Milov L, et al. Functional deficits in patients with mild cognitive impairment: prediction of AD. Neurology 2002;58(5):758–64.

97. Palmer K, Berger AK, Monastero R, et al. Predictors of progression from mild cognitive impairment to Alzheimer disease. Neurology 2007;68(19):1596–602.

98. Feldman H, Scheltens P, Scarpini E, et al. Behavioral symptoms in mild cognitive impairment. Neurology 2004;62(7):1199–201.

99. Geda YE, Roberts RO, Knopman DS, et al. Prevalence of neuropsychiatric symptoms in mild cognitive impairment and normal cognitive aging: population-based study. Arch Gen Psychiatry 2008;65(10):1193–8.

100. Okura T, Plassman BL, Steffens DC, et al. Prevalence of neuropsychiatric symptoms and their association with functional limitations in older adults in the United States: the aging, demographics, and memory study. J Am Geriatr Soc 2010; 58(2):330–7.

101. Gabryelewicz T, Styczynska M, Pfeffer A, et al. Prevalence of major and minor depression in elderly persons with mild cognitive impairment–MADRS factor analysis. Int J Geriatr Psychiatry 2004;19(12):1168–72.

102. Kumar R, Jorm AF, Parslow RA, et al. Depression in mild cognitive impairment in a community sample of individuals 60-64 years old. Int Psychogeriatr 2006; 18(3):471–80.

103. Ismail Z, Elbayoumi H, Fischer CE, et al. Prevalence of depression in patients with mild cognitive impairment: a systematic review and meta-analysis. JAMA Psychiatry 2017;74(1):58–67.

104. Lyketsos CG, Lopez O, Jones B, et al. Prevalence of neuropsychiatric symptoms in dementia and mild cognitive impairment: results from the cardiovascular health study. JAMA 2002;288(12):1475–83.

105. Lopez OL, Becker JT, Sweet RA. Non-cognitive symptoms in mild cognitive impairment subjects. Neurocase 2005;11(1):65–71.

106. Vinkers DJ, Gussekloo J, Stek ML, et al. Temporal relation between depression and cognitive impairment in old age: prospective population based study. BMJ 2004;329(7471):881.

107. Wilson RS, Schneider JA, Boyle PA, et al. Chronic distress and incidence of mild cognitive impairment. Neurology 2007;68(24):2085–92.

108. Geda YE, Knopman DS, Mrazek DA, et al. Depression, apolipoprotein E genotype, and the incidence of mild cognitive impairment: a prospective cohort study. Arch Neurol 2006;63(3):435–40.

109. Goveas JS, Espeland MA, Woods NF, et al. Depressive symptoms and incidence of mild cognitive impairment and probable dementia in elderly women: the Women's Health Initiative Memory Study. J Am Geriatr Soc 2011;59(1): 57–66.

110. Caracciolo B, Backman L, Monastero R, et al. The symptom of low mood in the prodromal stage of mild cognitive impairment and dementia: a cohort study of a community dwelling elderly population. J Neurol Neurosurg Psychiatry 2011; 82(7):788–93.

111. Visser PJ, Scheltens P, Verhey FR. Do MCI criteria in drug trials accurately identify subjects with predementia Alzheimer's disease? J Neurol Neurosurg Psychiatry 2005;76(10):1348–54.

112. Albert MS, DeKosky ST, Dickson D, et al. The diagnosis of mild cognitive impairment due to Alzheimer's disease: recommendations from the National Institute on Aging-Alzheimer's Association workgroups on diagnostic guidelines for Alzheimer's disease. Alzheimers Dement 2011;7(3):270–9.

113. Verghese PB, Castellano JM, Holtzman DM. Apolipoprotein E in Alzheimer's disease and other neurological disorders. Lancet Neurol 2011;10(3):241–52.

114. Scarabino D, Broggio E, Gambina G, et al. Apolipoprotein E genotypes and plasma levels in mild cognitive impairment conversion to Alzheimer's disease: a follow-up study. Am J Med Genet B Neuropsychiatr Genet 2016;171(8): 1131–8.

115. Boustani M, Hall KS, Lane KA, et al. The association between cognition and histamine-2 receptor antagonists in African Americans. J Am Geriatr Soc 2007;55(8):1248–53.

116. Carriere I, Fourrier-Reglat A, Dartigues JF, et al. Drugs with anticholinergic properties, cognitive decline, and dementia in an elderly general population: the 3-city study. Arch Intern Med 2009;169(14):1317–24.

117. Graham JE, Rockwood K, Beattie BL, et al. Prevalence and severity of cognitive impairment with and without dementia in an elderly population. Lancet 1997; 349(9068):1793–6.

118. Doraiswamy PM, Sperling RA, Coleman RE, et al. Amyloid-beta assessed by florbetapir F 18 PET and 18-month cognitive decline: a multicenter study. Neurology 2012;79(16):1636–44.

119. Smith GE, Petersen RC, Parisi JE, et al. Definition, course, and outcome of mild cognitive impairment. Aging Neuropsychol Cogn 1996;3(2):141–7.

120. Knopman DS, DeKosky ST, Cummings JL, et al. Practice parameter: diagnosis of dementia (an evidence-based review). Report of the quality standards subcommittee of the American Academy of Neurology. Neurology 2001;56(9): 1143–53.

121. Petersen RC, Stevens JC, Ganguli M, et al. Practice parameter: early detection of dementia: mild cognitive impairment (an evidence-based review). Report of the Quality Standards Subcommittee of the American Academy of Neurology. Neurology 2001;56(9):1133–42.

122. Ivnik RJ, Malec JF, Tangalos EG, et al. The Auditory-Verbal Learning Test (AVLT): norms for ages 55 years and older. Psychol Assess 1990;2(3):304–12.

123. Ivnik RJ, Smith GE, Tangalos EG, et al. Wechsler memory scale: IQ-dependent norms for persons ages 65 to 97 years. Psychol Assess 1991;3(2):156–61.

124. Smith G, Ivnik RJ, Petersen RC, et al. Age-associated memory impairment diagnoses: problems of reliability and concerns for terminology. Psychol Aging 1991; 6(4):551–8.

125. Panza F, D'Introno A, Colacicco AM, et al. Current epidemiology of mild cognitive impairment and other predementia syndromes. Am J Geriatr Psychiatry 2005;13(8):633–44.

126. Petersen RC, Smith GE, Ivnik RJ, et al. Apolipoprotein E status as a predictor of the development of Alzheimer's disease in memory-impaired individuals. JAMA 1995;273(16):1274–8.

127. Tierney MC, Szalai JP, Snow WG, et al. A prospective study of the clinical utility of ApoE genotype in the prediction of outcome in patients with memory impairment. Neurology 1996;46(1):149–54.

128. Abner EL, Kryscio RJ, Schmitt FA, et al. Outcomes after diagnosis of mild cognitive impairment in a large autopsy series. Ann Neurol 2017;81(4):549–59.

129. Caminiti SP, Ballarini T, Sala A, et al. FDG-PET and CSF biomarker accuracy in prediction of conversion to different dementias in a large multicentre MCI cohort. Neuroimage Clin 2018;18:167–77.

130. Aggarwal NT, Wilson RS, Beck TL, et al. The apolipoprotein E epsilon4 allele and incident Alzheimer's disease in persons with mild cognitive impairment. Neurocase 2005;11(1):3–7.

131. Jak AJ, Houston WS, Nagel BJ, et al. Differential cross-sectional and longitudinal impact of APOE genotype on hippocampal volumes in nondemented older adults. Dement Geriatr Cogn Disord 2007;23(6):382–9.

132. Caselli RJ, Reiman EM, Locke DE, et al. Cognitive domain decline in healthy apolipoprotein E epsilon4 homozygotes before the diagnosis of mild cognitive impairment. Arch Neurol 2007;64(9):1306–11.

133. Devanand DP, Pelton GH, Zamora D, et al. Predictive utility of apolipoprotein E genotype for Alzheimer disease in outpatients with mild cognitive impairment. Arch Neurol 2005;62(6):975–80.

134. Farrer LA, Cupples LA, Haines JL, et al. Effects of age, sex, and ethnicity on the association between apolipoprotein E genotype and Alzheimer disease. A meta-analysis. APOE and Alzheimer Disease Meta Analysis Consortium. JAMA 1997; 278(16):1349–56.

135. Schreiber S, Schreiber F, Lockhart SN, et al. Alzheimer disease signature neurodegeneration and APOE genotype in mild cognitive impairment with suspected non-Alzheimer disease pathophysiology. JAMA Neurol 2017;74(6):650–9.

136. Grande G, Cucumo V, Cova I, et al. Reversible mild cognitive impairment: the role of comorbidities at baseline evaluation. J Alzheimers Dis 2016;51(1):57–67.

137. Petersen RC, Thomas RG, Grundman M, et al. Vitamin E and donepezil for the treatment of mild cognitive impairment. N Engl J Med 2005;352(23):2379–88.

138. Winblad B, Gauthier S, Scinto L, et al. Safety and efficacy of galantamine in subjects with mild cognitive impairment. Neurology 2008;70(22):2024–35.

139. Feldman HH, Ferris S, Winblad B, et al. Effect of rivastigmine on delay to diagnosis of Alzheimer's disease from mild cognitive impairment: the InDDEx study. Lancet Neurol 2007;6(6):501–12.

140. Thal LJ, Ferris SH, Kirby L, et al. A randomized, double-blind, study of rofecoxib in patients with mild cognitive impairment. Neuropsychopharmacology 2005; 30(6):1204–15.

141. Goodwin JS, Goodwin JM, Garry PJ. Association between nutritional status and cognitive functioning in a healthy elderly population. JAMA 1983;249(21): 2917–21.
142. Gale CR, Martyn CN, Cooper C. Cognitive impairment and mortality in a cohort of elderly people. BMJ 1996;312(7031):608–11.
143. La Rue A, Koehler KM, Wayne SJ, et al. Nutritional status and cognitive functioning in a normally aging sample: a 6-y reassessment. Am J Clin Nutr 1997; 65(1):20–9.
144. Morris MC, Beckett LA, Scherr PA, et al. Vitamin E and vitamin C supplement use and risk of incident Alzheimer disease. Alzheimer Dis Assoc Disord 1998; 12(3):121–6.
145. Cummings JL, Doody R, Clark C. Disease-modifying therapies for Alzheimer disease: challenges to early intervention. Neurology 2007;69(16):1622–34.
146. Belleville S. Cognitive training for persons with mild cognitive impairment. Int Psychogeriatr 2008;20(1):57–66.
147. Jean L, Bergeron ME, Thivierge S, et al. Cognitive intervention programs for individuals with mild cognitive impairment: systematic review of the literature. Am J Geriatr Psychiatry 2010;18(4):281–96.
148. Kurz A, Pohl C, Ramsenthaler M, et al. Cognitive rehabilitation in patients with mild cognitive impairment. Int J Geriatr Psychiatry 2009;24(2):163–8.
149. Joosten-Weyn Banningh L, Vernooij-Dassen M, Rikkert MO, et al. Mild cognitive impairment: coping with an uncertain label. Int J Geriatr Psychiatry 2008;23(2): 148–54.

Alzheimer Disease

John E. Morley, MB,BCh[a],*, Susan A. Farr, PhD[a,b],
Andrew D. Nguyen, PhD[a]

KEYWORDS

- Amyloid-β • Cognitive stimulation therapy • Progranulin • SAMP8 • Biomarkers
- Olive oil

KEY POINTS

- Both amyloid-β protein and progranulin play central roles in Alzheimer disease.
- PET scanning for amyloid-β and phosphorylated tau are key to the diagnosis of Alzheimer disease.
- Available drugs for Alzheimer disease have limited efficacy.
- Cognitive stimulation therapy should be available to all persons with moderate Alzheimer disease.

Alzheimer's is a disease for which there is no effective treatment whatsoever. To be clear, there is no pharmaceutical agent, no magic pill that a doctor can prescribe that will have any significant effect on the progressive downhill course of this disease.

—*David Perlmutter*

Unfortunately, this quotation is a fairly accurate summary of the state of the art for Alzheimer disease at the beginning of 2018. To help elucidate the problems in the understanding of Alzheimer disease, this article traces its origins, where it was inappropriately named Alzheimer disease by Emil Kraepelin[1] in his *Handbook of Psychiatry* to give credit to his university in Munich, through modern times, where failure to understand how neurotransmitters enhance and inhibit memory is broadly seen in the approaches to its treatment.

The first description of plaques in the brain was in 1892 by Paul Blocq and George Mannesco in Paris, who found "round heaps in an aged patient."[2] In 1898, Emil Redlich reported that these plaques were common in persons with "senile dementia."[1] In the same year as Alzheimer reported his single case of young-onset dementia (1901),

Disclosures: The authors have nothing to disclose.
[a] Division of Geriatric Medicine, Saint Louis University School of Medicine, 1402 South Grand Boulevard, M238, St Louis, MO 63104, USA; [b] Research and Development Service, VA Medical Center, St Louis, MO, USA
* Corresponding author. Division of Geriatric Medicine, Saint Louis University School of Medicine, 1402 South Grand Boulevard, M238, St Louis, MO 63104.
E-mail address: john.morley@health.slu.edu

Koichi Miyaki from Japan and Solomon Carter Fuller from Liberia reported the presence of plaques associated with dementia. The following year Oskar Fischer reported an extensive series of older persons with dementia who had plaques at postmortem.

Pathologically, Alzheimer disease consists of amyloid-β plaques, neurofibrillary tangles containing phosphorylated tau (p-tau), and cerebral angiopathy. Although there is a crude correlation between cognitive performance and mean plaque count,[3] at least a quarter of persons dying with significant amounts of plaque in their brain are not cognitively impaired.[4,5] Tau consists of 3-repeat or 4-repeat isoforms. The 4 binding domains stabilize microtubules. With progression of Alzheimer disease there is a shift from 4-repeat tau to 3-repeat tau. Disassembly of microtubules occurs when tau is hyperphosphorylated, leading to the formation of tangles.[6] In addition, in Alzheimer disease, there is evidence of mitochondrial dysfunction with impaired fusion/fission, disruption of the electron transfer chain, and increased reactive oxygen species, leading to oxidative damage to neurons and apoptosis.[7]

Recent evidence has suggested a protective role for progranulin in Alzheimer disease as well as frontotemporal dementia.[8] Progranulin is a glycosylated peptide precursor that regulates cell growth. Loss of function mutations in the progranulin gene (GRN) increases the possibility of an individual developing Alzheimer disease.[9] Progranulin brain levels are low in persons with Alzheimer disease.[10] Progranulin seems to improve neuronal survival and decrease neuroinflammation.[9] In addition, upregulation of cyclin-dependent kinases with progranulin deficiency can lead to hyperphosphorylation of tau. **Fig. 1** provides a potential role of how progranulin deficiency can accelerate Alzheimer disease.

AMYLOID-β AND ALZHEIMER DISEASE

Injecting pathologic amounts of amyloid-β peptide directly into the mouse brain causes amnesia.[11,12] These high doses also increase glycogen synthase kinase 3β, which phosphorylates tau, increases neuronal oxidative damage, disrupts the blood-brain barrier, and eventually leads to the accumulation of amyloid plaques.[13–15]

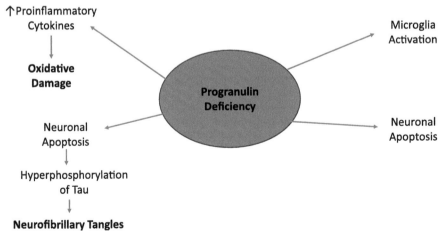

Fig. 1. The putative role of progranulin deficiency in Alzheimer disease.

In contradistinction, physiologic amounts of amyloid-β peptide improve memory.[16] These doses also increase the release of acetylcholine in the hippocampus. Inhibiting amyloid-β with antibodies or its production with antisenses blocking the mRNA for amyloid precursor protein in young animals leads to impairment of memory. These findings suggest that the physiologic role of amyloid-β is to enhance memory and it is only when levels become pathologic that they inhibit memory. The primary effect of overproduction (pathologic) of amyloid-β seems to be amnesia, with its other effects being later (**Fig. 2**). This is a revised version of the amyloid hypothesis.

NEUROPSYCHOLOGICAL SYMPTOMS OF ALZHEIMER DISEASE

The neuropsychological symptoms of Alzheimer disease include

1. Episodic memory impairment (amnesia)
2. Abnormally rapid forgetting (delayed recall failure)
3. Intrusion errors (paraphasias)
4. Deficits in language abilities
   - Verbal fluency (number of words produced on a given category in a given time [eg, animal naming])
   - Semantic categorization (not recognizing objects [words that belong together])
   - Inability to recall over-learned facts
5. Executive function (inability to recognize blue when printed in another color)
6. Working memory (inability to name the country when given a town in the country)
7. Failure of dual tasking (inability to answer a simple question while walking)
8. Attention deficits
9. Visuospatial deficits (clock drawing failure)
10. Functional impairment (decline in instrumental and basic activities of daily living)

In addition, persons with Alzheimer disease may develop apathy early in the disease and agitation and other behavioral disturbances later in the disease. Higher levels of amyloid-β in older persons are linked to anxiety.[17]

Initial screening for Alzheimer disease originally involved the Mini-Mental State Examination (MMSE). In modern times, both the St. Louis University Mental Status examination and the Montreal Cognitive Assessment are better tests.[18-20]

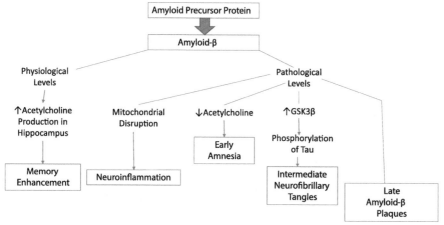

Fig. 2. The effects of physiologic and pathologic levels of amyloid-β.

The Rapid Cognitive Survey is a quick test that is at least as good as the MMSE.[21] The AD8 screening test, which uses a family informant, is also a good screening test.[22]

GENES AND ALZHEIMER DISEASE

Onset of Alzheimer disease before the age of 65 years (like Auguste Deter) is a rare form of the disease, which is inherited in an autosomal dominant fashion. There are mutations in any of 3 genes, namely amyloid precursor protein (chromosome 21), presenilin 1 (chromosome 14), and presenilin 2 (chromosome 1), that cause early-onset disease. Two mutations with amyloid precursor protein are the Swedish mutation (at the β-secretase site) and the arctic mutation, which change the form of amyloid-β, increasing protofibril formation. Presenilin 1 and presenilin 2 cause an overproduction in amyloid precursor protein by increasing γ-secretase activity, perhaps through the Notch signaling pathway.

ApoE4 is the gene most commonly associated with late-onset Alzheimer disease.[23] Persons homozygous for ApoE4 have a 50% chance of developing Alzheimer disease. Its major effects are to alter clearance of the amyloid-β protein from the central nervous system and to have neurotoxic effects.

In general, Alzheimer disease in older persons has a major genetic component, with at least 30 genes identified.[24] An example is TREM2, which activates the transmembrane receptor protein in the microglia membrane. It plays a role in decreasing plaque formation. Several other genes associated with microglial and immune activation have also been identified: SYK is a gene regulating amyloid-β and tau hyperphosphorylation. ADAM10 is an α-secretase that cleaves to amyloid precursor protein. TYROBP triggers TREM2 and likewise plays a role in amyloid-β clearance. As precision medicine (P4[predictive, preventive, personalized, participatory]) begins to be used, it will be realized that many variants of Alzheimer disease exist, which may require specific treatment to obtain an optimum response.

BRAIN IMAGING

A variety of imaging techniques are available to help confirm a diagnosis of Alzheimer disease. These include

- Structural MRI: classically, Alzheimer disease has a decrease in hippocampal volume, which can be detected before a person has clear-cut dementia.[25] This is coupled with a reduction in gray matter density. Synaptic damage results in neurodegeneration, leading to atrophy in the temporal lobe and angulate gyrus and the hippocampus.
- Functional MRI examines blood flow to areas of the brain using detection of oxygen levels in the brain. Abnormalities in the default mode network (areas active in the brain during rest, for example, connections with the posterior angulate gyrus) are commonly found in Alzheimer disease.[26]
- Diffusion tensor maximum signal intensity ratio measures water diffusion in the brain, allowing reconstruction of neural connections. There is a breakdown of the brain barriers that regulate fluid diffusion in Alzheimer disease.[27]
- PET identifies glucose metabolism in the brain. Using an 18-18-fludeoxyglucose PET scan in persons with Alzheimer disease show that the glucose metabolic rate is most consistently reduced in the posterior cingulate cortex and temporal and parietal cortices and less commonly in the frontal cortex.[28]

- Amyloid PET: amyloid load in the brain can be measured by a variety of carbon or fluoride labeled tracers. These methods are becoming popular to find increased amyloid burden in persons with Alzheimer disease.[29]
- Tau PET: several selective tracers have been developed to measure hyperphosphorylated tau in paired helical fragments. There is evidence to suggest that these tau PET scans and the areas in which hyperphosphorylated tau is found correlates with clinical findings.[30,31]
- Retinal scans: neurodegenerative changes occur in the retina in concert with changes in the brain of persons with Alzheimer disease. These include a decrease in retinal nerve fiber layer, choroidal thinning, and optic nerve volume. In addition, amyloid-β is present in drusen, which occur in greater amounts in the retina of persons with Alzheimer disease. Retinal vascular changes as seen by photographic changes can be used to assess amyloid burden in the brain. Curcumin, which binds to amyloid-β, has been used with fluorescence imaging to detect amyloid-β plaques in the retina.[32]

BIOMARKERS

Several biomarkers have been developed to correlate with Alzheimer disease. Classically, a low amyloid-β42 in the cerebrospinal fluid (CSF), perhaps due to amyloid-β deposition in the plaque, together with elevated hyperphosphorylated tau, is considered a diagnostic hallmark of Alzheimer disease.[33] Peripheral measurement of amyloid-β or p-tau have had poor sensitivity and specificity for Alzheimer disease.

Neurogranin levels are increased in the CSF of Alzheimer disease[34] and, as previously alluded to, progranulin levels are decreased in both the CSF and plasma in some cases of Alzheimer disease.[35,36] Using precision medicine approaches some multianalyte panels has been developed.[37]

MANAGEMENT

Management of cognitive dysfunction in Alzheimer disease can involve medications or nutritional and behavioral approaches. On the whole, the success of any of these approaches is limited.

Medications

Cholinesterase inhibitors have been the mainstay of drugs available to treat Alzheimer disease. Tacrine, the original cholinesterase inhibitor, improved memory but in a study where the optimal dose for each individual was determined.[38] It was removed from the market because of liver toxicity. These drugs have not been shown useful for preventing cognitive decline or for treating mild cognitive impairment.[39]

At present, 3 cholinesterase inhibitors, namely donepezil, rivastigmine, and galantamine, are approved by the US Food and Drug Administration. They are indicated for mild to moderate dementia. Most clinical trials have been for 6 months to 12 months. The Cochrane database suggested that these agents improved cognition by −2.7 points in the 70-point Alzheimer's Disease Assessment Scale–Cognitive Subscale.[40] The Health Technology Assessment suggested that these drugs are effective at a cost of $41,100 per quality-adjusted life year.[41] Donepezil was considered more cost-effective than the others. These drugs increased side effects, in particular nausea, vomiting, and diarrhea. As it stands, the data for high-dose (23-mg) donepezil show questionable effectiveness.

Memantine is an antagonist of the N-methyl-D-aspartate receptor, which is a glutamate receptor. It prevents excessive neuronal cell death.[42] In a meta-analysis, memantine, like acetylcholinesterase inhibitors, shows a small effect in improving cognitive function and behavioral disturbance scores.[43,44] In the authors' clinical experience, it can cause severe hypotension, leading to fainting and falls.[45]

The effects of the nootropics (piracetam and vinpocetine) were nonsignificant.[46,47] Both hydergine[48] and nicergoline,[49] however, showed effects suggestive of the same magnitude as cholinesterase inhibitors. The measurements used were not those now accepted for clinical trials.

Nutrition

Numerous epidemiologic studies have suggested that a Mediterranean diet is protective against developing Alzheimer disease.[50,51] Extra virgin olive oil improved memory in an animal model of Alzheimer—the SAMP8[52] and in the PREDIMED study (Prevención con Dieta Mediterránea) in humans.[53] Dietary n-3 polyunsaturated fatty acids also improve memory in the SAMP8.[54] No effects of omega-3 fatty acids have been shown for the treatment of dementia in humans.[55,56]

Souvenaid (Danone, Paris) is a supplement containing omega-3 polyunsaturated fatty acids, uridine, and phospholipids. It may show some effects in verbal recall in early Alzheimer disease but otherwise the results of human studies have been disappointing.[57]

Physical activity may improve outcomes in persons with Alzheimer disease, but the evidence is limited.[58]

Other nutritional approaches that may have some benefit include ketone bodies,[59] α-lipoic acid,[60] and polyphenols.[61,62] So far, however, there are inadequate human studies to support these approaches.

BEHAVIORAL INTERVENTIONS

Several behavioral interventions to improve memory have been developed. Of these, cognitive stimulation therapy (CST) has the most support. CST is a 12-week therapy developed at the University College London. It has a solid evidence base[63–69] and the National Institute for Health Care Excellence guidelines recommend its use in groups for persons with moderate dementia. (More information is available at www.cstdementia.com.)

Several other behavioral approaches at improving memory exist. They include SAIDO[70] and Staff Training in Assisted Living Residences (STAR).[71–73] In addition, reminiscence therapy can be helpful.[74] Sports reminiscence, for example, baseball and soccer, seems a particularly enjoyable approach for older persons with cognitive problems.[75–77]

SUMMARY

Alzheimer disease clearly represents a complex condition with a variety of molecular abnormalities, leading to the eventual presentation of the disease. In the past decade, a variety of immunotherapy approaches from an active immunization trial against amyloid[78] to passive immunization strategies, for example, bapineuzumab and solanezumab,[79,80] have failed to improve cognition in persons with Alzheimer disease. This could be related to the fact that lowering amyloid-β levels too low would be expected to interfere with memory. An antibody to tau has also failed.[81] These studies suggest that an individualized approach may be needed.

Other approaches that have yet to be explored, but are successful in animals, are antisense oligonucleotides, stem cell therapy,[82] and possibly metformin[83] or glucagon-like peptide I enhancers.[84] It is likely that in the next decade highly effective drugs to treat Alzheimer disease will be found. An ethical question for the future will be the question of cost of therapy, particularly if these drugs are only partially cost-effective.

REFERENCES

1. Morley JE, Farr SA. Alzheimer mythology: a time to think out of the box. J Am Med Dir Assoc 2016;17:769–74.
2. Blocq P, Marinesco G. Sur les lesions et la pathologenie de l'epilepsie dite essentiele. Sem Med 1892;12:445–6.
3. Roth M, Tomlinson BE, Blessed G. Correlation between scores for dementia and counts of 'senile plaques' in cerebral grey matter of elderly subjects. Nature 1966; 209:109–10.
4. Crystal H, Dickson D, Fuld P, et al. Clinico-pathologic studies in dementia: nondemented subjects with pathologically confirmed Alzheimer's disease. Neurology 1988;38:1682–7.
5. Knopman DS, Parisi JE, Salviati A, et al. Neuropathology of cognitively normal elderly. J Neuropathol Exp Neurol 2003;62:1087–95.
6. Uematsu M, Nakamura A, Ebashi M, et al. Brain stem tau pathology in Alzheimer's disease is characterized by increase of three repeat tau and independent of amyloid β. Acta Neuropathol Commun 2018;6:1.
7. Onyango IG, Khan SM, Bennett JP Jr. Mitochondria in the pathophysiology of Alzheimer's and Parkinson's diseases. Front Biosci (Landmark Ed) 2017;22:854–72.
8. Nguyen AD, Nguyen TA, Martens LH, et al. Progranulin: at the interface of neurodegenerative and metabolic diseases. Trends Endocrinol Metab 2013;24:597–606.
9. Jing H, Tan MS, Yu JT, et al. The role of PGRN in Alzheimer's disease. Mol Neurobiol 2016;53:4189–96.
10. Mao Q, Wang D, Li Y, et al. Disease and region specificity of granulin immunopositivities in Alzheimer disease and frontotemporal lobar degeneration. J Neuropathol Exp Neurol 2017;76:957–68.
11. Flood JF, Morley JE, Roberts E. Amnestic effects in mice of four synthetic peptides homologous to amyloid beta protein from patients with Alzheimer disease. Proc Natl Acad Sci U S A 1991;88:3363–6.
12. Flood JF, Roberts E, Sherman MA, et al. Topography of a binding site for small amnestic peptides deduced from structure-activity studies: relation to amnestic effect of amyloid beta protein. Proc Natl Acad Sci U S A 1994;91:380–4.
13. Farr SA, Sandoval KE, Niehoff ML, et al. Central and peripheral administration of antisense oligonucleotide targeting amyloid-β protein precursor improves learning and memory and reduces neuroinflammatory cytokines in Tg2576 (AβPPswe) mice. J Alzheimers Dis 2014;40:1005–16.
14. Morley JE, Farr SA, Kumar VB, et al. The SAMP8 mouse: a model to develop therapeutic interventions for Alzheimer's disease. Curr Pharm Des 2012;18:1123–30.
15. Kumar VB, Farr SA, Flood JF, et al. Site-directed antisense oligonucleotide decreases the expression of amyloid precursor protein and reverses deficits in learning and memory in aged SAMP8 mice. Peptides 2000;21:1769–75.
16. Morley JE, Farr SA, Banks WA, et al. A physiological role for amyloid-beta protein: enhancement of learning and memory. J Alzheimers Dis 2010;19:441–9.
17. Donovan NJ, Locascio JJ, Marshall GA, et al. Longitudinal association of Amyloid Beta and anxious-depressive symptoms I cognitively normal older adults. Am J Psychol 2018. https://doi.org/10.1176/appi.ajp.2017.17040442.
18. Tariq SH, Tumosa N, Chibnall JT, et al. Comparison of the Saint Louis University mental status examination and the mini-mental state examination for detecting

dementia and mild neurocognitive disorder—a pilot study. Am J Geriatr Psychiatry 2006;14:900–10.

19. Cummings-Vaughn LA, Chavakula NN, Malmstrom TK, et al. Veterans affairs Saint Louis University Mental Status examination compared with the Montreal Cognitive Assessment and the short test of mental status. J Am Geriatr Soc 2014;62:1341–6.

20. Malmstrom TK, Voss VB, CRUZ-Oliver DM, et al. The rapid cognitive screen (RCS): a point-of-care screening for dementia and mild cognitive impairment. J Nutr Health Aging 2015;19:741–4.

21. Shaik MA, Chan QL, Xue J, et al. Risk factors of cognitive impairment and brief cognitive tests to predict cognitive performance determined by a formal neuropsychological evaluation of primary health care patients. J Am Med Dir Assoc 2016;17:343–7.

22. Galvin JE, Roe CM, Powlishta KK, et al. The AD8: a brief informant interview to detect dementia. Neurology 2005;65(4):559–64.

23. Scheltens P, Blennow K, Breteler MMB, et al. Alzheimer's disease. Lancet 2016; 388:505–17.

24. Lambert JC, Ibrahim-Verbaas CA, Harold D, et al. Meta-analysis of 74,046 individuals identifies 11 new susceptibility loci for Alzheimer's disease. Nat Genet 2013;45:1452–8.

25. Rathore S, Habes M, Iftikhar MA, et al. A review on neuroimaging-based classification studies and associated feature extraction methods for Alzheimer's disease and its prodromal stages. Neuroimage 2017;155:530–48.

26. Buckner RL, Andrews-Hanna JR, Schacter DL. The brain's default network: anatomy, function, and relevance to disease. Ann N Y Acad Sci 2008;1124:1–38.

27. Xie S, Xiao JX, Gong GL, et al. Voxel-based detection of white matter abnormalities in mild Alzheimer disease. Neurology 2006;66:1845–9.

28. Mosconi L, Tsui WH, Herholz K. Multicenter standardized 18F-FDG PET diagnosis of mild cognitive impairment, Alzheimer's disease, and other dementias. J Nucl Med 2008;49:390–8.

29. Klunk WE, Engler H, Nordberg A, et al. Imaging brain amyloid in Alzheimer's disease with Pittsburgh Compound-B. Ann Neurol 2004;55:306–19.

30. Xia C, Makaretz SJ, Caso C, et al. Association of in vivo [18F]AV-1451 Tau PET imaging results with cortical atrophy and symptoms in typical and atypical Alzheimer disease. JAMA Neurol 2017;74:427–36.

31. Masdeu JC. Tau and cortical thickness in Alzheimer's disease. JAMA Neurol 2017;74:390–2.

32. Mahajan D, Votruba M. Can the retina be used to diagnose and plot the progression of Alzheimer's disease? Acta Ophthalmol 2017;95:768–77.

33. Henriques AD, Benedet AL, Camargos EF, et al. Fluid and imaging biomarkers for Alzheimer's disease: where we stand and where to head to. Exp Gerontol 2018. https://doi.org/10.1016/j.exger.2018.01.002.

34. De Vos A, Struyfs H, Jacobs D, et al. The cerebrospinal fluid neurogranin/BACE1 ratio is a potential correlate of cognitive decline in Alzheimer's disease. J Alzheimers Dis 2016;53:1523–38.

35. Finch M, Backer M, Crook R, et al. Plasma progranulin levels predict progranulin mutation status in frontotemporal dementia patients and asymptomatic family members. Brain 2009;132:583–91.

36. Perry DC, Lehmann M, Yokoyama JS, et al. Progranulin mutations as risk factors for Alzheimer disease. JAMA Neurol 2013;70(6):774–8.

37. Galasko D, Golde TE. Biomarkers for Alzheimer's disease in plasma, serum and blood – conceptual and practical problems. Alzheimers Res Ther 2013;5(2):10.

38. Davis KL, Thal LJ, Gamzu ER, et al. A double-blind, placebo-controlled multicenter study of tacrine for Alzheimer's disease. The Tacrine Collaborative Study Group. N Engl J Med 1992;327:1253–9.

39. Fink HA, Jutkowitz E, McCarten JR, et al. Pharmacologic interventions to prevent cognitive decline, mild cognitive impairment, and clinical Alzheimer-type dementia. Ann Intern Med 2018;168:39–51.

40. Birks J. Cholinesterase inhibitors for Alzheimer's disease. Cochrane Database Syst Rev 2006;(1):CD005593.

41. Bond M, Rogers G, Peters J, et al. The effectiveness and cost-effectiveness of donepezil, galantamine, rivastigmine and memantine for the treatment of Alzheimer's disease (review of Technology Appraisal No. 111): a systematic review and economic model. Health Technol Assess 2012;16:1–470.

42. Folch J, Busquets O, Ettcheto M, et al. Memantine for the treatment of dementia: a review on its current and future applications. J Alzheimers Dis 2017. https://doi.org/10.3233/JAD-170672.

43. Kishi T, Matsuaga S, Oya K, et al. Memantine for Alzheimer's disease: an updated systematic review and meta-analysis. J Alzheimers Dis 2017;60:401–25.

44. Matsunaga S, Kishi T, Iwata N. Memantine monotherapy for Alzheimer's disease: a systematic review and meta-analysis. PLoS One 2015;10(4):e012329.

45. Gallini A, Sommet A, Montastruc JL, French PharmacoVigilance Network. Does memantine induce bradycardia? A study in the French PharmacoVigilance database. Pharmacoepidemiol Drug Saf 2008;17:877–81.

46. Flicker L, Grimley Evans G. Piracetam for dementia or cognitive impairment. Cochrane Databse Syst Rev 2001;(2):CD001011.

47. Szatmari SZ, Whitehouse PJ. Vinpocetine for cognitive impairment and dementia. Cochrane Database Syst Rev 2003;(1):CD003119.

48. Olin J, Schneider L, Novit A, et al. Hydergine for dementia. Cochrane Database Syst Rev 2001;(2):CD000359.

49. Fioravanti M, Flicker L. Efficacy of nicergoline in dementia and other age associated forms of cognitive impairment. Cochrane Database Syst Rev 2001;(4):CD003159.

50. Anastasiou CA, Yannakoulia M, Kosmidis MH, et al. Mediterranean diet and cognitive health: initial results from the Hellenic longitudinal investigation of ageing and diet. PLoS One 2017;12(8):e0182048.

51. Petersson SD, Philippou E. Mediterranean diet. Cognitive function, and dementia: a systematic review of the evidence. Adv Nutr 2016;7:889–904.

52. Farr SA, Price TO, Dominguez LJ, et al. Extra virgin olive oil improves learning and memory in SAMP8 mice. J Alzheimers Dis 2012;28:81–92.

53. Martinez-Lapiscina EH, Clavero P, Toledo E, et al. Virgin olive oil supplementation and long-term cognition: the PREDIMED-NAVARRA randomized, trial. J Nutr Health Aging 2013;17:544–52.

54. Petursdottir AL, Farr SA, Morley JE, et al. Effect of dietary n-3 polyunsaturated fatty acids on brain lipid fatty acid composition, learning ability, and memory of senescence-accelerated mouse. J Gerontol A Biol Sci Med Sci 2008;63:1153–60.

55. Hooper C, De Souto Barreto P, Coley N, et al. Cognitive changes with omega-3 polyunsaturated fatty acids in non-demented older adults with low omega-3 index. J Nutr Health Aging 2017;21:988–93.

56. De Souto Barreto P, Andrieu S, Rolland Y, et al. Physical activity domains and cognitive function over three years in older adults with subjective memory complaints: secondary analysis from the MAPT trial. J Sci Med Sport 2018;21:52–7.

57. Onakpoya IJ, Heneghan CJ. The efficacy of supplementation with the novel medical food, Souvenaid, in patients with Alzheimer's disease: a systematic review and meta-analysis of randomized clinical trials. Nutr Neurosci 2017;20:219–27.

58. Stephen R, Hongisto K, Solomon A, et al. Physical activity and Alzheimer's disease: a systematic review. J Gerontol A Biol Sci Med Sci 2017;72:733–9.

59. Ciavardelli D, Piras F, Consalvo A, et al. Medium-chain plasma acylcarnitines, ketone levels, cognition, and gray matter volumes in healthy elderly, mildly cognitively impaired, or alzheimer's disease subjects. Neurobiol Aging 2016;43:1–12.

60. Farr SA, Price TO, Banks WA, et al. Effect of alpha-lipoic acid on memory, oxidation, and lifespan in SAMP8 mice. J Alzheimers Dis 2012;32:447–55.

61. Farr SA, Niehoff ML, Ceddia MA, et al. Effect of botanical extracts containing carnosic acid or rosmarinic acid on learning and memory in SAMP8 mice. Physiol Behav 2016;165:328–38.

62. Syarifah-Noratiqah S, Naina-Mohamed I, Zulfarina MS, et al. Natural polyphenols in the treatment of Alzheimer's disease. Curr Drug Targets 2017. https://doi.org/10.2174/1389450118666170328122527.

63. Spector A, Woods B, Orrell M. Cognitive stimulation for the treatment of Alzheimer's disease. Expert Rev Neurother 2008;8:751–7.

64. Spector A, Thorgrimsen L, Woods B, et al. Efficacy of an evidence-based cognitive stimulation therapy programme for people with dementia: randomised controlled trial. Br J Psychiatry 2003;183:248–54.

65. Woods B, Aguirre E, Spector AE, et al. Cognitive stimulation to improve cognitive functioning in people with dementia. Cochrane Database Syst Rev 2012;(2):CD005562.

66. Orgeta V, Leung P, Yates L, et al. Individual cognitive stimulation therapy for dementia: a clinical effectiveness and cost-effectiveness pragmatic, multicenter, randomized controlled trial. Health Technol Assess 2015;19:1–108.

67. Morley JE, Cruz-Oliver DM. Cognitive stimulation therapy. J Am Med Dir Assoc 2014;15:689–91.

68. Loraine J, Taylor S, McAllister M. Cognitive and physical stimulation therapy. J Am Med Dir Assoc 2014;15:140–1.

69. Berg-Weger M, Tebb S, Henderson-Kalb J, et al. Cognitive stimulation therapy: a tool for your practice with persons with dementia? J Am Med Dir Assoc 2015;16:795–6.

70. Kawashima R, Hiller DL, Sereda SL, et al. SAIDO learning as a cognitive intervention for dementia care: a preliminary study. J Am Med Dir Assoc 2015;16:56–62.

71. Teri L, Huda P, Gibbons L, et al. STAR: a dementia-specific training program for staff in assisted living residences. Gerontologist 2005;45:686–93.

72. Karlin BE, Visnic S, McGee JS, et al. Results from the multisite implementation of STAR-VA: a multicomponent psychosocial intervention for managing challenging dementia-related behaviors of veterans. Psychol Serv 2014;11:200–8.

73. Karel MJ, Teri L, McConnell E, et al. Effectiveness of expanded implementation of STAR-VA for managing dementia-related behaviors among veterans. Gerontologist 2016;56:126–34.

74. Woods B, Spector A, Jones C, et al. Reminiscence therapy for dementia. Cochrane Database Syst Rev 2005;(2):CD001120.

75. Coll-Planas L, Watchman K, Domenech S, et al. Developing evidence for football (soccer) reminiscence interventions within long-term care: a co-operative approach applied in Scotland and Spain. J Am Med Dir Assoc 2017;18:355–60.
76. Wingbermuehle C, Bryer D, Berg-Weger M, et al. Baseball reminiscence league: a model for supporting persons with dementia. J Am Med Dir Assoc 2014;15:85–9.
77. Tolson D, Schofield I. Football reminiscence for men with dementia: lessons from a realistic evaluation. Nurs Inq 2012;19:63–70.
78. Pohanka M. Vaccination to Alzheimer disease. Is it a promising tool or a blind way? Curr Med Chem 2016;23:1432–41.
79. Mehta D, Jackson R, Paul G, et al. Why do trials for Alzheimer's disease drugs keep failing? A discontinued drug perspective for 2010-2015. Expert Opin Investig Drugs 2017;26:735–9.
80. Abushouk AI, Elmaraezy A, Aglan A, et al. Bapineuzumab for mild to moderate Alzheimer's disease: a meta-analysis of randomized controlled trials. BMC Neurol 2017;17:66.
81. West T, Hu Y, Verghese PB, et al. Preclinical and clinical development of ABBV-8E12, a humanized anti-tau antibody, for treatment of Alzheimer's disease and other tauopathies. J Prev Alzheimers Dis 2017;4:236–41.
82. Armbrecht HJ, Siddiqui AM, Green M, et al. Antisense against Amyloid-β protein precursor reverses memory deficits and alters gene expression in neurotropic and insulin-signaling pathways in SAMP8 mice. J Alzheimers Dis 2015;46: 535–48.
83. Ng TP, Feng L, Yap KB, et al. Long-term metformin usage and cognitive function among older adults with diabetes. J Alzheimers Dis 2014;41:61–8.
84. Hansen HH, Fabricius K, Barkholt P, et al. The GLP-1 receptor agonist liraglutide improves memory function and increases hippocampal CA1 neuronal numbers in a senescence-accelerated mouse model of Alzheimer's disease. J Alzheimers Dis 2015;46:877–88.

Lewy Body Dementia

Angela M. Sanford, MD

KEYWORDS

- Dementia • Lewy body dementia • Dementia with Lewy bodies • Synucleinopathy
- Parkinson's disease with dementia

KEY POINTS

- Dementia with Lewy bodies (DLB) is the second most common neurodegenerative dementia after Alzheimer disease.
- DLB is considered an α-synucleinopathy and results from the accumulation of α-synuclein into Lewy bodies, which accumulate in various parts of the brain and nervous system and result in neuronal cell death.
- The core features for diagnosis of DLB are cognitive impairment plus fluctuations in mental status, visual hallucinations, rapid eye movement (REM) sleep behavioral disorder, and Parkinsonian motor symptoms.
- DLB is often underdiagnosed and misdiagnosed.
- There are no disease-modifying treatments or cures for DLB and treatment is targeted at ameliorating symptoms.

INTRODUCTION

Lewy bodies were first discovered in neurons by the German neurologist Dr Friedrich Lewy in 1912 while he was studying the neuropathology of Parkinson disease (PD) in the laboratory of Dr Alois Alzheimer.[1] It was not until the 1990s that the key constituent of Lewy bodies, the protein α-synuclein, was elucidated.[2] The function of α-synuclein is not certain, but it is thought to function in cell membrane remodeling at neuronal terminals.[3] When aggregates of misfolded, overexpressed α-synuclein accumulate in neurons or surrounding glial cells, Lewy bodies are formed (**Fig. 1**). There are 3 main types of "α-synucleinopathies": PD, Lewy body dementia (LBD), and multiple system atrophy.[4] This article primarily focuses on one type of α-synucleinopathy: LBD.

LBD is an "umbrella" term that encompasses dementia with Lewy bodies (DLB) and PD with dementia (PDD) (**Fig. 2**). DLB and PDD have many overlapping symptoms, and in later stages of their disease courses, can be virtually impossible to distinguish from one another and from other forms of dementia. Both result from the aggregation of α-synuclein into Lewy bodies, but where in the brain and body these Lewy body deposits occur is what clinically differentiates these similar disease processes.

Disclosure Statement: The author has nothing to disclose.
Division of Geriatrics, Saint Louis University School of Medicine, 1402 South Grand Boulevard, M238, St Louis, MO 63104, USA
E-mail address: angela.sanford@health.slu.edu

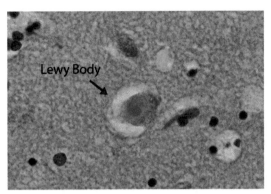

Fig. 1. A Lewy body inclusion formed by aggregation of α-synuclein. (*Courtesy of* George T. Grossberg, MD, Saint Louis University School of Medicine Department of Psychiatry, St Louis, MO.)

Additionally, although DLB and PDD lie along the same clinicopathological spectrum, their diagnoses are differentiated based on the temporal relationship of cognitive decline and deficits in motor functioning, with cognitive function deficits occurring earlier in the DLB course. In general, symptoms of LBD include deficits in motor function, behavioral abnormalities, mood disorders, and cognitive impairment. It is important to correctly diagnose DLB because many of the pharmacologic treatments used for the treatment of behavioral and cognitive symptoms in other forms of dementia dramatically worsen the symptoms of DLB.

EPIDEMIOLOGY

LBD affects an estimated 1.4 million Americans, making it the second most common neurodegenerative dementia after Alzheimer disease. The largest risk factor for developing DLB is age, with most cases becoming clinically evident at approximately 70 to 85 years of age. Men have a higher risk of developing DLB than women. One recent epidemiologic study found that nearly 70% of the diagnoses of DLB and 49% of the diagnoses of PDD occurred in men and that the clinical onset of DLB occurred almost 5 years earlier than PDD (77 years vs 82 years of age at onset).[5] Up to 80% of patients with PD go on to develop dementia at some point in their disease course, which can make distinguishing DLB and PDD challenging.[6]

It is commonly accepted that DLB is widely underdiagnosed, as there is a large discrepancy in the number of cases diagnosed clinically versus those diagnosed via neuropathology at the time of postmortem autopsy. In fact, it is thought that more than 50% of DLB cases are never diagnosed as LBD.[7] One article reviewing the prevalence of DLB in clinical-based studies found the mean prevalence of DLB to be 7.5% of all dementia cases.[8] This is in striking contrast to autopsy findings from research centers, which identify Lewy body pathology in 20% to 25% of patients with a history of dementia undergoing autopsy after death.[9] An additional complicating factor is that there is considerable overlap in brain pathology among vascular dementia, Alzheimer disease, and LBD. Nearly 50% of patients with a primary diagnosis of Alzheimer disease were found to have some degree of α-synuclein pathology on autopsy in addition to the typically expected findings of neurofibrillary tangles and amyloid-β plaques.[10,11] It is suspected that these overlapping pathologies have an additive effect on cognition and motor functioning, but it is often difficult to determine the primary diagnosis.[12]

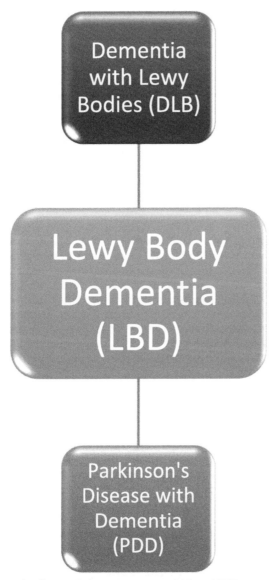

Fig. 2. LBD is an "umbrella term" that encompasses DLB and PDD.

Other risk factors for developing DLB in addition to age and male sex include some established genetic mutations and likely many that have not yet been discovered. Although most cases of DLB occur sporadically, the most common genetic mutations in DLB occur in the leucine-rich receptor kinase 2, synuclein-alpha, and glucocerebrosidase A genes. Other rarer genetic alterations are seen in the microtubule-associated protein tau, scavenger receptor class B member 2, and apolipoprotein E (APOE) genes.[13] The ε4 allele of the APOE gene is the strongest genetic risk factor predisposing to Alzheimer disease, conferring with the idea that there often is an overlap in the neuropathology of Alzheimer disease and LBD. APOE gene mutations are overrepresented in patients with LBD but are seen less commonly than those patients with

Alzheimer disease.[14] Because of lack of evidence, there is currently no role in genetic testing for DLB outside of research studies.

PATHOPHYSIOLOGY

The neuropathology of DLB is centered around the aggregation of overexpressed protein oligomers of α-synuclein into Lewy bodies. In DLB, Lewy bodies deposit primarily in the cytoplasm of neurons. This is in contrast to multiple system atrophy, where the Lewy bodies deposit in the cytoplasm of both glial cells and neurons. Lewy body formation and accumulation lead to mitochondrial damage and fragmentation, ultimately inciting the cascade of cellular apoptosis and death.[15] This process is thought, but not proven, to originate in the enteric nervous system and progress into the central nervous system, specifically through the vagus nerve, and then into the brain stem and higher cortical regions.[16] The dissemination of Lewy bodies in DLB is thought to follow a similar pattern as proposed for PD by Braak and colleagues.[17] In this pathologic staging system, Lewy body deposition first occurs in the ninth and tenth cranial nerves and reticular system and then spreads caudally into the brainstem and limbic system and then upward into the neocortex. In stages 1 and 2, symptoms usually include autonomic and olfactory dysfunction; in stages 3 and 4, sleep and motor disturbances occur; and in stages 5 and 6, emotional and cognitive dysfunction is predominant. Currently, it has not been elucidated as to why α-synuclein has an initial predilection for neurons in the vagus nerve, olfactory nerve, and brainstem nuclei, but deposition of Lewy bodies in these locations lead to the nonspecific symptoms seen early in the disease course, such as anosmia (caused by neuronal death in the olfactory nerve) and constipation (caused by neuronal death in the vagus nerve). Another early symptom often occurring years before diagnosis of DLB is rapid eye movement (REM) sleep behavior disorder (RBD), which results from Lewy body accumulation in the hypothalamus and reticular activation system.

Interestingly, autopsies reveal the presence of Lewy bodies in approximately 10% to 15% of all brains examined in individuals older than 60, despite the absence of symptoms in most of these individuals.[18] This indicates that there is likely a preclinical, asymptomatic period or, perhaps, some Lewy body aggregation can be considered as a normal, age-related variant. Additionally, as referenced previously, the brain pathology is often mixed with a prevalence of α-synuclein, amyloid beta plaques, and tau-containing neurofibrillary tangles in addition to small vessel vascular changes, indicating relative ischemia. One study revealed that 61% of patients with Lewy body deposition and a primary diagnosis of LBD also had a pathologic diagnosis of Alzheimer disease.[19] When α-synuclein deposits occur in acetylcholine esterase-rich producing neurons (ie, the nucleus basalis of Meynert) causing neuronal loss, acetylcholine esterase deficiencies occur, which can lead to symptoms consistent with Alzheimer dementia. Likewise, when Lewy body deposits occur in dopamine-rich nuclei such as the substantia nigra, parkinsonian symptoms result.

DIAGNOSIS

DLB is frequently underdiagnosed and misdiagnosed.[20] The average patient is examined by 3 to 4 physicians before an accurate diagnosis is made. The diagnosis of DLB is based largely on obtaining an accurate clinical history and timeline of symptoms, as well as a thorough physical examination. Cognitive testing is essential, although there may be only small, if any, deficits early in the disease course. Neuropsychiatric testing frequently reveals deficits in visuospatial, executive function, and attention cognitive domains. There is a definitive role for imaging, although the most sensitive imaging studies are not readily available outside of academic institutions. Postmortem autopsy is the only way to make a conclusive diagnosis and even then, overlapping pathology is often seen and it is difficult to know which type of dementia was the primary diagnosis.

Clinical Presentation

Differentiating Alzheimer dementia from DLB and PDD can be a challenging clinical conundrum. To assist in this, diagnostic criteria for DLB were first established in 1996 and then updated again in 2005.[21] An arbitrary 1-year rule was proposed to differentiate DLB and PDD. DLB is diagnosed if cognitive deficits precede or accompany the first motor symptoms and PDD is diagnosed if motor symptoms precede cognitive decline by at least 1 year. The separation of DLB and PDD is controversial, as many feel that there are too many clinical, pathologic, and genetic overlaps between the 2 diagnoses for them to be considered 2 distinct disease entities.[22]

The diagnosis of DLB also requires the presence of dementia significant enough to interfere with activities of daily living, in addition to 2 or more core clinical features including fluctuating cognition, visual hallucinations, Parkinsonism, and REM behavioral sleep disorder (**Fig. 3**). The prevalence of these core symptoms in individuals with DLB at some point in their disease course is as follows: Parkinsonism, 94.4%; REM sleep behavioral disorder, 76.4%; visual hallucinations, 65.2%; and fluctuations in cognition, 45.8%.[23] The pattern of cognitive impairment in DLB differs from that seen in Alzheimer disease in that short-term memory loss is less prominent (as seen predominantly with Alzheimer disease), but deficits in visuospatial, attention, and executive cognitive domains are more pronounced. Tiraboschi and colleagues[24] found that visuospatial impairment was present in 74% of patients with pathologically confirmed early-stage LBD but only seen in 45% of those with pathologically confirmed Alzheimer disease.

The first core feature that may be present and aid in diagnostic certainty is parkinsonism. The parkinsonism motor symptoms seen in DLB include resting tremor, stooped posture, bradykinesia, and postural instability and are thought to result from LB deposition in dopamine-rich neuronal foci. Resting tremors are often less conspicuous in individuals with DLB than in those with PDD, whereas axial symptoms (eg, postural instability) are more frequent.[25]

A second core feature that may be present is hallucinations. Hallucinations in DLB are typically detailed, recurrent visual hallucinations featuring people, children, or animals. They are perhaps the most distressing symptom of DLB for the patient and caregiver and are difficult to treat. Additionally, patients will often develop delusions

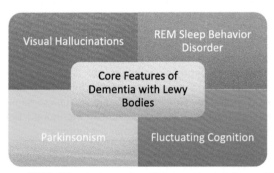

Fig. 3. Core features of DLB. Diagnosis requires the presence of dementia and at least 2 of the core features.

and paranoia constructed around the hallucinations. It is thought that the hallucinations in LBD result from the deposition of Lewy bodies in the occipital cortex, optic nerve, and are also due to the loss of dopaminergic neurotransmission in the eye itself.[26] Interestingly, visual hallucinations in early or prodromal dementia are highly specific for autopsy-proven DLB and one study found them to be the most specific clinical feature differentiating DLB from Alzheimer disease.[24]

The third core feature often present in DLB is fluctuating mental status. Fluctuation in alertness, attention, and cognition is frequently difficult to elicit in clinical history taking, but may manifest as staring spells similar to absence seizures, periods of decreased attention and awareness, frequent daytime napping, and periods of seemingly unprovoked confusion. Some liken this fluctuation to "low-grade" delirium and it is thought to be secondary to cholinergic deficits caused by Lewy body deposition in cholinergic-rich neuronal foci.[19]

The final core diagnostic feature in DLB is RBD. With RBD, those afflicted physically act out their dreams because of lack of muscle paralysis (loss of muscle atonia) during REM sleep. Bed partners of patients with RBD often report that the patient will thrash about the bed, kicking, punching, screaming, and/or grunting. The frequency of these episodes varies greatly, possibly occurring several times per night or every few months.[27] In one study, patients with "idiopathic" RBD were followed for nearly 4 years and 45% went on to develop disease processes meeting the criteria for PD and DLB. Of the 45% developing neurodegenerative processes, 55% developed PD and 44% developed DLB; 93% of those who progressed into DLB had cognitive impairment at baseline compared with only 42% of those who went on to develop PD.[28] The etiology of RBD is suspected to be from the formation of Lewy bodies in various nuclei in the reticular activating system in the brainstem. This can often occur in the very early stages of DLB with symptoms of RBD manifesting years before the disease is clinically diagnosed. When RBD is suspected, an overnight sleep polysomnography should be done, and will reveal increased electromyography activity during REM sleep (ie, lack of atonia).[27]

In addition to the core features of DLB, there are many supporting symptoms that when present, may be suggestive of the diagnosis. These include visuospatial deficits, neuroleptic sensitivity, changes in mood, autonomic dysfunction, and recurrent falls. Visuospatial deficits can manifest as difficulty judging distances when driving, walking, or sitting. For example, individuals may have difficulty parking in a parking spot, may frequently trip over curbs while walking, or may miss the edge of a chair while sitting down. Visuospatial deficits can be detected on cognitive screening examinations that involve clock drawing, as the numbers drawn in by the patient will often be confined to one side of the clock and not evenly spaced out. Patients with DLB frequently are extremely sensitive to neuroleptics and develop increased confusion and parkinsonianlike motor symptoms when administered atypical or typical antipsychotics. Mood symptoms in patients with DLB can be characterized by depression, apathy, and anxiety. Delusions and paranoia may be centered around visual hallucinations and this can further expound depression and anxiety. Autonomic dysfunction is common and can be detected by orthostatic hypotension, bradycardia, syncope, constipation, and erectile dysfunction. Recurrent falls are multifactorial in nature and likely occur because of a combination of the previously mentioned parkinsonian motor symptoms, visuospatial deficits, and autonomic dysfunction.

Imaging

At this time, there is no way to directly image α-synuclein deposits or Lewy bodies, but the currently available imaging modalities can provide indirect evidence of α-synuclein pathology. There are several imaging studies that can help distinguish between DLB and Alzheimer disease, but the distinction between DLB and PD is more difficult to make. Brain MRI is the most commonly used and widely available imaging tool and often reveals a mild decrease in cerebral volume in the temporal, occipital, and parietal lobes along with mild enlargement of the lateral ventricles, which parallels with the volume loss seen in age-matched controls. This is, however, in striking contrast to the moderate to severe global atrophy seen with the later stages of Alzheimer disease.[29] MRI also may show focal atrophy of the midbrain, hypothalamus, and substantia innominata (location of the acetylcholine-rich basal nucleus of Meynert) indicating neuronal death presumably from LB deposition.[23] Of note, the hippocampi in patients with DLB are of normal size, which is another finding on imaging that can be used to distinguish DLB from Alzheimer disease.[30] Presently, there is no reliable way to differentiate DLB and PD using MRI.

Functional brain imaging is available with positron emission tomography (PET) or single-photon emission computed tomography (SPECT) scans. The most commonly used type of PET scan uses a fluorodeoxyglucose (FDG) isotope to bind to regions of the brain where glucose uptake is occurring, providing an overview of metabolic activity. FDG PET scans done in DLB reveal occipital lobe hypometabolism, indicating neuronal death in the region.[31] They also often reveal a distinctive pattern of preserved activity in the posterior cingulate, which is typically affected in Alzheimer disease. This radiographic finding is called the "cingulate island" sign and can be helpful in distinguishing between Alzheimer disease and DLB.[32]

There are 2 methods of imaging with SPECT scans: dopamine transporter uptake studies and brain perfusion studies. In the dopamine transporter SPECT scans, an imaging ligand that binds directly to dopamine transporters is used, and lack of activity indicates neuronal degeneration in these areas. In DLB, dopamine transporter activity is often nearly absent in putamen and reduced in the caudate, but normal dopamine transporter activity is seen in those with Alzheimer disease.[33] Similar to PET scans, in the brain perfusion SPECT scans, radioligands bind to metabolically active areas in the brain. In DLB, there often is a prominent occipital hypoperfusion on SPECT that is not seen in patients with Alzheimer disease.[34] Unfortunately, likewise to MRI, SPECT scans are not yet able to distinguish between DLB and PD on imaging alone.[35] The choice between which imaging modalities to use while evaluating for a potential diagnosis of DLB largely depends on cost, insurance coverage, and regional availability of the imaging study.

Cerebrospinal Fluid Biomarkers

Currently, cerebrospinal fluid (CSF) biomarkers are not routinely used outside of clinical studies to aid in diagnosis of DLB, and there are no biomarkers available that are specifically diagnostic of DLB. Multiple studies have found reduced levels of α-synuclein in CSF in the synucleinopathies compared with Alzheimer disease, but there is no way to differentiate between the synucleinopathies based on CSF findings.[36] CSF levels of β-amyloid 1 to 42 are typically decreased in both DLB and Alzheimer disease, whereas total tau is increased in DLB and Alzheimer disease.[37] Extremely low levels of tau in the CSF have been associated with faster rates of cognitive decline in DLB.[38] These cases may indicate mixed DLB and Alzheimer disease pathology, and individuals with mixed disease are known to have more accelerated cognitive decline.[39] At the present time, it is not possible to accurately differentiate between neurodegenerative disorders by using only CSF biomarkers because of the high number of cases with overlapping disease pathology and additionally because a highly sensitive and specific biomarker has not yet been developed.

TREATMENT

Currently, there are no disease-modifying treatments available and no high-level evidence to support any forms of treatment.[40] Most trials for the pharmacologic management of symptoms of DLB include very small numbers of participants. The present focus is on alleviating symptoms, which is challenging in DLB because while improving one symptom, many medications may worsen another. Multiple medications may be needed to target different symptoms and the risk of side effects and drug-drug interactions is quite high. Generally, one medication should be started at a time at the lowest dose and slowly titrated upward. Medications should be tapered (if necessary) and discontinued if significant side effects occur or if no efficacy is noted after a reasonable trial period.

The most troublesome symptom in DLB is often visual hallucinations, and these can be very difficult to treat because of the neuroleptic sensitivity many patients exhibit. Mild, nonthreatening hallucinations should be managed nonpharmacologically. There have been several small studies done looking at atypical and typical antipsychotics and their effect on visual hallucinations specifically in DLB. One study looking at quetiapine found a reduction in delusions, hallucinations, and agitation in patients taking moderate doses of quetiapine, but 33% of study participants withdrew because of orthostatic hypotension or oversedation.[41] A study using moderately dosed olanzapine again showed some benefit in the reduction of delusions and hallucinations,[42] but another study did not replicate similar results because of a dropout rate of nearly 40% due to adverse side effects.[43] A randomized-controlled trial using risperidone actually showed a deterioration in cognition (reduction of Mini-Mental Status Examination scores of −2.3 points), worsening psychiatric symptoms, and a 65% withdrawal rate.[44] Frequently, antipsychotics worsen parkinsonian symptoms because of their dopamine antagonistic properties. Additionally, antipsychotics carry a black box warning issued by the US Food and Drug Administration regarding the risk of sudden death in the elderly, so the decision to use them in any elderly individual should be made after carefully weighing the risks and benefits.

Acetylcholinesterase inhibitors (AChEIs), such as donepezil, rivastigmine, and galantamine, are frequently administered in patients with Alzheimer disease in hopes to positively augment the disease course and improve cognitive function. There have been many studies done in DLB and most suggest that AChEIs may improve cognition and behavioral symptoms while having no adverse effect on motor symptoms. In one meta-analysis, donepezil was the most effective, followed by rivastigmine. Galantamine was not found to have any significant effect when compared with placebo. There were higher rates of drug discontinuation with AChEIs for adverse events in comparison with placebo, but rates were much smaller than those seen in studies using antipsychotics in DLB.[45] Memantine, an N-methyl-D-aspartate receptor antagonist, is also frequently used to improve cognition in patients with Alzheimer disease. Studies done in DLB with memantine have shown mixed results, with some positive effects on cognition,[46] and some studies showing no effects.[47] A meta-analysis revealed no differences on improvement or absence of cognitive deterioration.[40]

Dopamine agonists, such as carbidopa/levodopa, are frequently used to improve motor symptoms in PD. They also can be used in DLB to reduce tremors and motor symptoms but the clinical response is not as pronounced as in patients with PD. Studies have shown that improvement on the Unified Parkinson's Disease rating scale motor section after steady administration of carbidopa/levodopa occurs in 65% to 70% of patients with PD and only 32% to 50% of patients with DLB.[48,49] Unfortunately, in one study, approximately 33% of patients who experienced an improvement in their motor symptoms with the medication developed worsening psychosis.[50] Visual hallucinations tend to worsen with dopamine agonist treatment[51] because of their effect on dopaminergic transmission in the brain.

Depression, anxiety, and apathy are also quite common in individuals with DLB and symptoms are frequently more severe in these patients than in those with Alzheimer disease.[52] There is limited evidence regarding selective serotonin uptake inhibitor (SSRI) use in DLB, but a trial is likely warranted, and SSRIs may improve depressive symptoms. One study showed that citalopram actually worsened neuropsychiatric symptoms and provided no benefit,[53] but more studies are needed comparing the efficacy of individual SSRIs to one another or to placebo.

PROGNOSIS

Unfortunately, DLB is a progressive neurodegenerative disease in which there is no cure or disease-modifying treatments. One epidemiologic study assessing risk factors and overall prognosis of α-synucleinopathies found a survival median of 4.7 years in those with DLB and 3.8 years in those diagnosed with PDD after the time of diagnosis.[5] There is thought to be an accelerated cognitive decline in patients with DLB in comparison with those with Alzheimer disease. Kramberger and colleagues[54] found that the mean annual cognitive decline as determined by the Mini-Mental Status Examination was −2.1 points in DLB, −1.6 points in Alzheimer disease, and −1.8 points in PDD. The rate of cognitive decline is even more accelerated in those with mixed disease of DLB and Alzheimer disease.[55] This, in combination with the often debilitating and difficult to treat visual hallucinations and sleep disturbances, yield a higher caregiver burden for those caring for these patients[56] and also a lower quality of life for the patients themselves.[57] In fact, one study found the median time from the diagnosis of DLB until entry into residential care to be 1.8 years, which is nearly 2 years shorter than in patients with Alzheimer disease,[58] and another study found that 24% of patients with DLB rated their health state to be worse than death versus 6% of patients with Alzheimer disease. Admission to the hospital has also been found to be higher in DLB and is mostly commonly due to falls, delirium, and pneumonia.[59] Fluctuating mental status in addition to hallucinations, both of which are frequently seen in DLB, can be misinterpreted as "delirium"[60] and can lead to increased health care utilization for workup and management. Considering earlier placement in residential care, increased hospitalization, and higher caregiver burden, it should not be surprising then that DLB has been found to have a higher economic burden than Alzheimer disease.[57]

SUMMARY

In conclusion, DLB is the second most common neurodegenerative dementia following Alzheimer disease. It stems from the formation of Lewy bodies, which contain aggregates of the misfolded protein, α-synuclein. These begin depositing in areas of the nervous system and brain, leading to neuronal cell death and causing clinically apparent symptoms. Diagnosis requires the presence of dementia, plus 2 or more core clinical features of parkinsonian motor symptoms, visual hallucinations, RBD, and fluctuations in mental status. Because of its clinical overlap with other forms of dementia, DLB is often underdiagnosed and misdiagnosed. There are currently no disease-modifying treatments or cures, and treatments are aimed at ameliorating specific symptoms. DLB confers a high caregiver burden, decreased quality of life, and increased health care utilization and costs over and above other dementias (**Box 1**).

> **Box 1**
> **Fast facts about dementia with Lewy bodies**
>
> - Second most common neurodegenerative dementia after Alzheimer dementia
> - Term "Lewy body dementia" encompasses both Parkinson disease with dementia and dementia with Lewy bodies
> - Results from the accumulation of the overexpressed protein α-synuclein into Lewy bodies
> - Symptoms correlate with location of Lewy body deposition in the brain and nervous system
> - Diagnosis requires the presence of dementia plus 2 or more core clinical features of parkinsonism, visual hallucinations, REM sleep behavioral disorder, and fluctuation in cognition
> - Imaging modalities other than MRI are not widely used to aid in diagnosis
> - There are no cures for DLB and treatments are aimed at ameliorating specific symptoms
> - DLB has a high caregiver burden, decreased quality of life for the affected individual, and higher health care utilization and costs than other forms of dementia

REFERENCES

1. Lewy F. Paralysis agitans. I. Pathologische anatomie. In: Lewandowski M, Abelsdorff G, et al, editors. Handbuch der Neurologie, vol. 3. Berlin: Springer Verlag; 1912. p. 920–33.
2. Spillantini M, Schmidt M, Lee V, et al. α-Synuclein in Lewy bodies. Nature 1997; 388:839–40.
3. Varkey J, Isas J, Mizuno N, et al. Membrane curvature induction and tubulation are common features of α-synuclein inclusion formation during aging. J Biol Chem 2010;285:32486–93.
4. McCann H, Stevens C, Cartwright H, et al. α-Synucleinopathy phenotypes. Parkinsonism Relat Disord 2014;20(Suppl 1):S62–7.
5. Savica R, Grossardt B, Bower J, et al. Diagnosed synucleinopathies with parkinsonism: a population-based study. JAMA Neurol 2017;74(7):839–46.
6. Emre M, Aarsland D, Brown R. Clinical diagnostic criteria for dementia associated with Parkinson's disease. Mov Disord 2007;22:1689–707.
7. Palmqvist S, Hansson O, Minthon L, et al. Practical suggestions on how to differentiate dementia with Lewy bodies from Alzheimer's disease with common cognitive tests. Int J Geriatr Psychiatry 2009;24(12):1405–12.
8. Vann Jones S, O'Brien J. The prevalence and incidence of dementia with Lewy bodies: a systematic review of population and clinical studies. Psychol Med 2014;44(4):673–83.
9. Galasko D. Lewy body disorders. Neurol Clin 2017;35:325–38.
10. Lippa C, Fujiwara H, Mann D, et al. Lewy bodies contain altered alpha-synuclein in brains of many familiar Alzheimer's disease patients with mutations in presenilin and amyloid precursor protein genes. Am J Pathol 1998; 153:1365–70.
11. Uchikado H, Lin W, DeLucia M, et al. Alzheimer disease with amygdala Lewy bodies: a distinct form of α-synucleinopathy. J Neuropathol Exp Neurol 2006; 65(7):685–97.
12. Rabinovici G, Carrillo M, Forman M, et al. Multiple comorbid neuropathologies in the setting of Alzheimer's disease neuropathology and implications for drug development. Alzheimers Dement 2016;3(1):83–91.

13. Bras J, Guerreiro R, Darwent L, et al. Genetic analysis implicates APOE, SNCA and suggests lysosomal dysfunction in the etiology of dementia with Lewy bodies. Hum Mol Genet 2014;23:6139–46.
14. Tsuang D, Leverenz J, Lopez O, et al. APOE ε4 increases risk for dementia in pure synucleinopathies. JAMA Neurol 2013;70:727–35.
15. Stefanis L. α-Synuclein in Parkinson's disease. Cold Spring Harb Perspect Med 2012;2(2):a009399.
16. Goedert M, Jakes R, Spillantini M. The synucleinopathies: twenty years on. J Parkinsons Dis 2017;7(9):S53–71.
17. Braak H, Del Tredici K, Rub U, et al. Staging of brain pathology related to sporadic Parkinson's disease. Neurobiol Aging 2003;24:197–211.
18. Dickson D, Fujishiro H, DelleDonne A, et al. Evidence that incidental Lewy body disease is pre-symptomatic Parkinson's disease. Acta Neuropathol 2008;115(4): 436–44.
19. Schneider J, Arvanitakis Z, Yu L, et al. Cognitive impairment, decline and fluctuations in older community-dwelling subjects with Lewy bodies. Brain 2012;135(Pt 10):3005–14.
20. Nelson PT, Jicha GA, Kryscio RJ, et al. Low sensitivity in clinical diagnosis of dementia with Lewy bodies. J Neurol 2010;257:359–66.
21. McKeith I, Dickson D, Lowe J, et al. Diagnosis and management of dementia with Lewy bodies. Neurology 2005;65:1863–72.
22. Postuma R, Berg D, Stern M, et al. Abolishing the 1-year rule: how much evidence will be enough? Mov Disord 2016;31:1623–7.
23. Whitwell J, Weigand S, Shiung M, et al. Focal atrophy in dementia with Lewy bodies on MRI: a distinct pattern from Alzheimer's disease. Brain 2007;l30(pt 3):708–19.
24. Tiraboschi P, Salmon D, Hansen L, et al. What best differentiates Lewy body from Alzheimer's disease in early-stage dementia? Brain 2006;129:729–35.
25. Petrova M, Mehrabian-Spasova A, Aarsland D, et al. Clinical and neuropsychological differences between mild Parkinson's disease dementia and dementia with Lewy bodies. Dement Geriatr Cogn Dis Extra 2015;5(2):212–20.
26. Bodis-Wollner I. Retinopathy in Parkinson disease. J Neural Transm (Vienna) 2009;116(11):1493–501.
27. Boeve B. REM sleep behavior disorder: updated review of the core features, the RBD-neurodegenerative disease association, evolving concepts, controversies, and future directions. Ann N Y Acad Sci 2010;1184:15–54.
28. Genier Marchand D, Montplaisir J, Postuma R, et al. Detecting the cognitive prodrome of dementia with Lewy bodies: a prospective study of REM sleep behavior disorder 2017;40(1). https://doi.org/10.1093/dleep/zsw014.
29. Mak E, Su L, Williams G. Longitudinal assessment of global and regional atrophy rates in Alzheimer's disease and dementia with Lewy bodies. Neuroimage Clin 2015;7:456–62.
30. Watson R, O'Brien J. Differentiating dementia with Lewy bodies and Alzheimer's disease using MRI. Neurodegener Dis Manag 2012;2:411–20.
31. Klein J, Eggers C, Kalbe E, et al. Neurotransmitter changes in dementia with Lewy bodies and Parkinson disease dementia in vivo. Neurology 2010;74: 885–92.
32. Graff-Radford J, Murray M, Lowe V, et al. Dementia with Lewy bodies: basis of cingulate island sign. Neurology 2014;83:801–9.
33. Piggot M, Marshall E, Thomas N, et al. Striatal dopaminergic markers in dementia with Lewy bodies, Alzheimer's and Parkinson's diseases: rostrocaudal distribution. Brain 1999;122:1449–68.

34. Lobotesis K, Fenwick J, Phipps A, et al. Occipital hypoperfusion on SPECT in dementia with Lewy bodies but not AD. Neurology 2001;56:643–9.

35. Rossi C, Volterrani D, Nicoletti V, et al. 'Parkinson-dementia' diseases: a comparison by double tracer SPECT studies. Parkinsonism Relat Disord 2009;15:762–6.

36. Hall S, Ohrfelt A, Constantinescu R, et al. Accuracy of a panel of 5 cerebrospinal fluid biomarkers in the differential diagnosis of patients with dementia and/or parkinsonian disorders. Arch Neurol 2012;69(11):1445–52.

37. Vanderstichele H, De Vreese K, Blennow K, et al. Analytical performance and clinical utility of the INNOTESTVR PHOSPHO-TAU (181P) assay for discrimination between Alzheimer's disease and dementia with Lewy bodies. Clin Chem Lab Med 2006;44:1472–80.

38. Abdelnour C, van Steenoven I, Londos E, et al. Alzheimer's disease cerebrospinal fluid biomarkers predict cognitive decline in Lewy body dementia. Mov Disord 2016;31:1203–8.

39. Kraybill M, Larson E, Tsuang D, et al. Cognitive differences in dementia patients with autopsy-verified AD, Lewy body pathology, or both. Neurology 2005;64:2069–73.

40. Stinton C, McKeith I, Taylor J, et al. Pharmacological management of Lewy body dementia: a systematic review and meta-analysis. Am J Psychiatry 2015;172:731–42.

41. Takahashi H, Yoshida K, Sugita T, et al. Quetiapine treatment of psychotic symptoms and aggressive behavior in patients with dementia with Lewy bodies: a case series. Prog Neuropsychopharmacol Biol Psychiatry 2003;27(3):549–53.

42. Cummings J, Street J, Masterman D, et al. Efficacy of olanzapine in the treatment of psychosis in dementia with Lewy bodies. Dement Geriatr Cogn Disord 2002;13(2):67–73.

43. Walker Z, Grace J, Overshot R, et al. Olanzapine in dementia with Lewy bodies: a clinical study. Int J Geriatr Psychiatry 1999;14(6):459–66.

44. Workman R, Orengo C, Bakey A, et al. The use of risperidone for psychosis and agitation in demented patients with Parkinson's disease. J Neuropsychiatry Clin Neurosci 1997;9:594–7.

45. Matsunaga S, Kishi T, Yasue I, et al. Cholinesterase inhibitors for Lewy body disorders: a meta-analysis. Int J Neuropsychopharmacol 2015;19(2) [pii:pyv086].

46. Wesnes K, Aarsland D, Ballard C, et al. Memantine improves attention and episodic memory in Parkinson's disease dementia and dementia with Lewy bodies. Int J Geriatr Psychiatry 2015;30(1):46–54.

47. Matsunaga S, Kishi T, Iwata N. Memantine for Lewy body disorders: systematic review and meta-analysis. Am J Geriatr Psychiatry 2015;23(4):373–83.

48. Molloy S, McKeith I, O'Brien J, et al. The role of levodopa in the management of dementia with Lewy bodies. J Neurol Neurosurg Psychiatry 2005;76(9):1200–3.

49. Bonelli S, Ransmayr G, Steffelbauer M, et al. L-dopa responsiveness in dementia with Lewy bodies, Parkinson disease with and without dementia. Neurology 2004;63:376–8.

50. Goldman J, Goetz C, Brandabur M, et al. Effects of dopaminergic medications on psychosis and motor function in dementia with Lewy bodies. Mov Disord 2008;23:2248–50.

51. Baker W, Silver D, White C, et al. Dopamine agonists in the treatment of early Parkinson's disease: a meta-analysis. Parkinsonism Relat Disord 2009;15(4):287–94.

52. Chiu P, Wang C, Tsai C, et al. Depression in dementia with Lewy bodies; a comparison with Alzheimer's disease. PLoS One 2017;12(6):e0179399.

53. Culo S, Mulsant B, Rosen J, et al. Treating neuropsychiatric symptoms in dementia with Lewy bodies: a randomized controlled-trial. Alzheimer Dis Assoc Disord 2010;24(4):360–4.

54. Kramberger M, Auestad B, Garcia-Ptacek S, et al. Long-term cognitive decline in dementia with Lewy bodies in a large multicenter, international cohort. J Alzheimers Dis 2017;57(3):787–95.

55. Blanc F, Mahmoudi R, Jonveaux T, et al. Long-term cognitive outcome of Alzheimer's disease and dementia with Lewy bodies: dual disease is worse. Alzheimers Res Ther 2017;9(1):47.

56. Ricci M, Guidoni S, Sepe-Monti M, et al. Clinical findings, functional abilities and caregiver distress in the early stage of dementia with Lewy bodies (DLB) and Alzheimer's disease (AD). Arch Gerontol Geriatr 2009;49:e101–4.

57. Bostrom F, Jonsson L, Minthon L, et al. Patients with dementia with Lewy bodies have more impaired quality of life than patients with Alzheimer disease. Alzheimer Dis Assoc Disord 2007;21:150–4.

58. Rongve A, Vossius C, Norse S, et al. Time until nursing home admission in people with mild dementia: comparison of dementia with Lewy bodies and Alzheimer's dementia. Int J Geriatr Psychiatry 2014;29:392–8.

59. Murman D, Juo S, Powel M, et al. The impact of parkinsonism on costs of care in patients with AD and dementia with Lewy bodies. Neurology 2003;61:944–9.

60. Vardy E, Holt R, Gerhard A. History of a suspected delirium is more common in dementia with Lewy bodies than Alzheimer's disease: a retrospective study. Int J Geriatr Psychiatry 2014;29(2):178–81.

Traumatic Brain Injury, Chronic Traumatic Encephalopathy, and Alzheimer Disease

Roula al-Dahhak, MD[a],*, Rita Khoury, MD[b], Erum Qazi, MD[b],
George T. Grossberg, MD[b]

KEYWORDS

- Traumatic brain injury • Concussion • Neurodegenerative disorders • Dementia
- Chronic traumatic encephalopathy

KEY POINTS

- Traumatic brain injury (TBI) has a relation with cognitive changes later on, but this relationship is likely related to several contributing factors as not all subjects with TBI develop dementia.
- Prevention of TBI is essential in reducing the risk of developing dementia later on in life.
- As aging population is increasing, and their risk of fall increase; we need to establish measures to address their exposure to TBI as the history of loss of consciousness is not always clear to them without a witnessed fall.

INTRODUCTION

Traumatic brain injury (TBI) is an acquired brain injury that is defined by an alteration in brain function, or other evidence of brain pathology, caused by an external force (bump, blow, jolt to the head, or a penetrating head injury). Alteration in brain function may involve one of the following: any period of loss or decreased level of consciousness, any loss of memory for events immediately before or after the injury, any alteration in the mental state at the time of injury. or the occurrence of any neurologic deficit.[1] TBIs affect more than 50 million individuals worldwide each year, and the annual incidence of TBI in the United States is approximately 3.5 million.[2] These numbers are probably an underestimation of the true prevalence of TBIs, as many

Disclosure Statement: The authors have no financial disclosure or conflicts.
[a] Department of Neurology, Saint Louis University, 1438 South Grand Boulevard, Suite 105, St Louis, MO 63104, USA; [b] Department of Psychiatry and Behavioral Neuroscience, Saint Louis University, 1438 South Grand Boulevard, St Louis, MO 63104, USA
* Corresponding author.
E-mail address: roula.aldahhak@health.slu.edu

Clin Geriatr Med 34 (2018) 617–635
https://doi.org/10.1016/j.cger.2018.06.008
0749-0690/18/© 2018 Elsevier Inc. All rights reserved.

geriatric.theclinics.com

cases go undetected by surveillance databases. For instance, a population-based study in Colorado has demonstrated that nearly one-third of those who reported a history of TBI did not seek any medical care in an emergency department or hospital settings and thus were not formally diagnosed.[3] TBI has a huge public health impact. The overall rate of TBI-related deaths was estimated to be 18.4 per 100,000 Americans, according to Centers for Disease Control and Prevention (CDC) data between 1997 and 2007.[4] The increased risk of death associated with severe TBI was shown to persist for at least 7 years following the initial injury.[5] Survivors of TBI have been shown to develop long-term disability that adversely impacts not only their lives, but their caregivers' lives and the entire society.[6] In a 1-year prospective study, 50% of TBI survivors were found to be moderately to severely disabled, regardless of TBI severity.[7] It is estimated that 3.2 to 5.3 million Americans are currently living with a TBI-related disability.[8] Those patients present higher rates of chronic pain and fatigue, major depressive disorder, posttraumatic stress disorder and other psychiatric disorders, social isolation, and neurodegenerative disorders, lasting for more than a decade after the initial injury.[9,10] The economic burden is also substantial: in 2013, the direct and indirect costs related to productivity loss have been estimated to reach $13.1 billion and $64.7 billion, respectively; medical costs ranged between $63.4 and $79.1 billion in the United States.[11]

More recently, TBI has been increasingly recognized as a risk factor for cognitive impairment: it was found to be associated with an increased risk of developing any dementia (Relative Risk [RR] = 1.63), and particularly Alzheimer disease (AD) (RR = 1.51).[12,13] Chronic traumatic encephalopathy (CTE) is another type of neurocognitive disorder associated with TBI, resulting from exposure to repetitive mild head injuries occurring for instance in contact sports (eg, boxing, American football, hockey) or in the military service, and found to be clinically and pathologically distinct from AD.[14]

EPIDEMIOLOGY

TBI contributes to approximately 30% of all deaths related to injuries in the United States.[8] According to the latest CDC estimates, TBIs accounted for 300,000 hospitalizations, 2.1 million emergency department visits, and 1.1 million physician office visits, yearly in the United States.[3] The leading causes of nonfatal TBIs in the general American population are falls (35%), followed by motor vehicle accidents (17%) and strikes to the head from or against an object such as in sports injuries (17%).[8] The rates may vary according to the age category. Recent epidemiologic studies have shown an increasing incidence of TBIs in the elderly population (65 years and older), especially in the high-income countries that have witnessed an improvement in traffic safety measures and an increase in life expectancy.[15] Moreover, the number of older Americans is projected to more than double, from 46 million today to more than 98 million by 2060, and the 65 and older age group's share of the total population will rise to nearly 24% from 15%.[16] Unintentional falls remain the most common cause of TBIs and TBI-related hospitalizations among older adults, especially the oldest old (85 years and older).[17,18] With aging, the risk of TBIs increases as the rate of falls increases due to multiple medical comorbidities, physical deterioration, including unsteadiness and reduced visual perception, in addition to medication-induced orthostatic hypotension.[19] Increasing severity of TBI and poorer outcomes may be partly linked to significantly higher prescription rates of anticoagulants in this vulnerable aging population.[20] The annual rate per 100,000 of TBI-related deaths caused by a fall increases from 1.0 in the age group 35 to 44 years to 6.8 in the age group 65 to 74 and 53.7 for those older than 85 years.[4]

CLASSIFICATION OF TRAUMATIC BRAIN INJURY

TBI is a heterogeneous disease. It has been traditionally classified using injury severity scores. The most commonly used scoring system is the Glasgow Coma Scale (GCS), which consists of 3 categories (eye opening response, verbal response, and motor response), assessing for impaired consciousness and coma, when administered in the first 24 hours following the injury. Scores range between 3 and 15, where higher scores indicate better function[21] (**Table 1**). A score of 13 to 15 represents a mild TBI (mTBI) also referred to as "concussion" injury, whereas a score <9 corresponds to a severe TBI. Besides the GCS, other severity measures include measures of loss of consciousness (LOC) and posttraumatic amnesia (PTA) durations.[22] PTA is defined as the interval from injury until the patient is oriented and able to recall newly formed memories.[23] A mild TBI can be considered if LOC is ≤ 30 minutes or PTA is ≤1 day; a severe TBI corresponds to a LOC longer than 24 hours and/or a PTA longer than 7 days.[22] Although the predictive value of these single indicators is well established, each may be influenced by other factors unrelated or indirectly related to the severity of TBI. Hence, the Mayo classification system that combines the afore-mentioned clinical indicators with neuroimaging abnormalities was developed to improve the reliability and accuracy of TBI severity assessment. It classifies TBI into 3 categories: moderate-severe (definite) TBI, mild (probable) TBI, and symptomatic (possible) TBI.[24]

The GCS is the accepted classification tool for TBI due to its simplicity and predictive value relative to overall prognosis.[25]

According to the World Health Organization (WHO) Task Force and the CDC, mTBI is defined as "An acute brain injury resulting from mechanical energy to the head from external physical forces." Operational criteria for clinical identification include (1) 1 or more of the following: confusion or disorientation, LOC for 30 minutes or less, PTA for less than 24 hours, and/or other transient neurologic abnormalities, such as focal signs, seizure, and intracranial lesion not requiring surgery; and (2) GCS score of 13–15, 30 minutes postinjury or later on presentation for health care. (c) These

Table 1 Glasgow Coma Scale		
Response	**Scale**	**Score (Points)**
Eye opening response	Eyes open spontaneously	4
	Eyes open to verbal command	3
	Eyes open to pain	2
	No eye opening	1
Verbal response	Oriented	5
	Confused conversation, but able to answer questions	4
	Inappropriate responses, but discernible words	3
	Incomprehensible sounds/speech	2
	No verbal response	1
Motor response	Obeys commands for movements	6
	Purposeful movements to painful stimuli	5
	Withdraws from pain	4
	Abnormal flexion; decortication	3
	Extensor response; decerebration	2
	No motor response	1

Data from Teasdale G, Jennett B. Assessment of coma and impaired consciousness. Lancet 1974;304(7872):81–4.

manifestations must not be due to drugs, alcohol, or medications; caused by other injuries or treatment for other injuries (eg, systemic injuries, facial injuries, or intubation); caused by other problems (eg, psychological trauma, language barrier, or coexisting medical conditions); or caused by penetrating cranio-cerebral injury.[26] The American Congress of Rehabilitation Medicine defines a patient with mTBI as someone having traumatically induced physiologic disruption of brain function, as manifested by at least 1 of the following: (1) any period of LOC; (2) any loss of memory for events immediately before or after the accident; (3) any alteration in mental state at the time of the accident (eg, feeling dazed, disoriented, or confused); and (4) focal neurologic deficit(s) that may or may not be transient, but where the severity of the injury does not exceed the following: LOC of approximately 30 minutes or less; after 30 minutes, an initial GCS score of 13 to 15; and a PTA not greater than 24 hours. One drawback shared by both classifications is their exclusion of more severe TBIs, such as penetrating head injuries.[2]

Other systems used to assess the severity of the head injury include the Abbreviated Injury Scale, the Trauma Score, and the Abbreviated Trauma Score. These systems need additional validation, are not as easily administered, and the results may not be as reproducible as the GCS system, which remains the optimal system in use to date.[27–29]

Regardless of the definition or classification used to categorize head injuries, mTBI constitutes most (70%–90%) of all diagnosed/treated TBIs.[30]

PATHOPHYSIOLOGY

Pathophysiological changes related to TBI are dynamic, since the initial/primary injury is followed over time by a continuum of molecular and cellular processes, also known as secondary injuries, thought to be the most important determinant of the final outcome and the extent of recovery.[31,32] Excitotoxicity mediated by an overproduction of excitatory neurotransmitters, such as glutamate in the extracellular space, is hypothesized to be the sentinel event after trauma occurrence. Glutamate's binding to the N-methyl-D-aspartate receptors is associated with an increase in calcium influx intracellularly, which leads to mitochondrial damage and release of oxygen radicals and other oxidative stress mediators, resulting in neuronal death.[31] Another pathway activated in response to TBI is neuroinflammation, which has both beneficial and deleterious consequences, manifested by the release of proinflammatory cytokines (interleukin [IL]-1, IL-6, and tumor necrosis factor α), anti-inflammatory cytokines (IL-10 and transforming growth factor- β) and chemokines like Chemokine Ligand-2 (CCL-2), along with microglial activation to promote tissue repair and neurogenesis.[33,34] Chronic and uncontrolled inflammation may lead to neurodegeneration: neuropathological evidence has shown that neuroinflammation may still be ongoing, up to 18 years following a single moderate/severe TBI.[33,35] Proinflammatory cytokines stimulate secretases and amyloid protein precursor (APP) processing, generating Aβ plaque deposits in the brain and contributing in some to the development of AD.[34] After TBI, several brain areas have been shown to suffer from hypoxic damage and secondary ischemia,[36] which have been implicated in the pathogenesis of AD by accelerating the accumulation of amyloid β and increasing the hyper-phosphorylation of tau, leading to the chronic process of neurodegeneration.[37] Moreover, there has been increasing evidence of widespread, diffuse, multifocal disruption of the blood-brain barrier (BBB), soon after the brain injury and even many years later.[38] BBB damage has been implicated in the slower clearance of senile plaques, also contributing to the pathophysiology of AD.[39] Findings from postmortem examination of brains of individuals with CTE have also improved our understanding of the heterogeneous neuropathological features associated with brain trauma. A common white-matter pathologic finding is diffuse axonal injury that can progress over months and even years after the injury,[35] evolving from impairment in axonal transport to axonal swelling, leading ultimately to Wallerian degeneration/demyelization.[40] Studies in individuals with repetitive concussive injuries (boxers, American football players, wrestlers, ice hockey players, and former veterans) have shown macroscopic changes including generalized or focal brain atrophy even after a single TBI, and the development of a cavum septum pellucidum coupled with ventricular enlargement.[41] Microscopically, accumulation of multiple proteins, such as neurofibrillary tangles (Tau), TAR DNA-binding protein (TDP-43), and β amyloid plaques have been reported.[41,42] TBI-induced encephalopathy can thus be considered a "polypathology," as it shares common neuropathological hallmarks found in other neurodegenerative disorders, including AD, fronto-temporal dementia, Lewy-body dementia and Parkinson disease (PD).[43] The 2 neuropathological hallmarks of AD consist of extracellular deposits of amyloid senile plaques and intracellular deposits of neurofibrillary tangles in the brain.[44] Amyloid β deposits have been found shortly after a TBI, in addition to an overexpression of β and γ-secretases and their substrate the APP, generating senile plaque deposits de novo.[34,45] In a cohort of 114 autopsied brains with CTE, Aβ deposits were found in 52% of the cases, with a significantly greater burden of Aβ1–40 plaques in the sulcal depths compared with the gyral crests.[46] In addition to the accelerated accumulation of Aβ deposits in the CTE brain, it is currently well established that the pathognomonic lesion of CTE consists of the accumulation of abnormal hyperphosphorylated tau tangles in a distinct pattern that involves preferentially the depth of the sulci in the neocortex, with perivascular accentuation.[42] Findings from the case series by McKee and colleagues[47] of 68 brains of individuals with a clinical history of repetitive TBI and histopathological evidence of CTE have revealed a spectrum of tauopathy ranging from perivascular accumulation of neurofibrillary tangles in the frontal cortex in the mild stages to a widespread brain distribution, including the medial temporal lobe in the most severe stages. The McKee criteria are hence used to grade the severity of CTE by categorizing it into the 4 stages presented in **Table 2**.

In 2016, the National Institute of Neurological Disorders and Stroke criteria for the pathologic diagnosis of CTE were published. In this consensus meeting, researchers agreed that the pathognomonic lesion required for CTE diagnosis consists of p-Tau aggregates in neurons, astrocytes, and cell processes around small vessels in an irregular pattern at the depths of the cortical sulci. **Fig. 1** shows stained slides of cerebral cortex in 3 cases of CTE showing irregular patches of p-Tau pathology most dense at the depth of the sulci, previously published by McKee and colleagues.[48] Some of the supportive neuropathological features of CTE include the preferential accumulation of abnormal p-Tau pretangles and NFTs (neurofibrillary tangles) in superficial layers (layers II–III), in contrast to layers III and V as in AD; accumulation of pretangles, NFTs, or extracellular tangles in the hippocampus preferentially affecting CA2 and CA4 in contrast with CA1 and subiculum involvement in AD; accumulation of abnormal p-Tau immunoreactive neuronal and astrocytic aggregates in subcortical nuclei, including the mammillary bodies and other hypothalamic nuclei, amygdala, nucleus accumbens, thalamus, midbrain tegmentum, and isodendritic core (nucleus basalis of Meynert, raphe nuclei, substantia nigra and locus coeruleus); and accumulation of p-Tau immunoreactive large grainlike and dotlike structures (in addition to some threadlike neurites).[48]

Current epidemiologic evidence indicates that nearly 1 in every 3 people who die as a consequence of TBI have β amyloid plaque deposits in their brains and that this is detectable within hours of the injury.[49] Widespread neurofibrillary tangles were also

Table 2	
The 4 neuropathological stages of chronic traumatic encephalopathy (CTE)	
Stage I CTE	p-Tau pathology restricted to discrete foci in the cerebral cortex most commonly in the superior, dorsolateral or lateral frontal cortex, typically around small vessels, at the depth of the sulci.
Stage II CTE	Multiple epicenters at the depths of the cerebral sulci and localized spread of neurofibrillary pathology from these epicenters to the superficial layers of adjacent cortex. The medial temporal lobe is spared.
Stage III CTE	p-Tau pathology is widespread englobing the frontal and temporal lobes, concentrated at the depth of the sulci. The amygdala, hippocampus, and entorhinal cortex show neurofibrillary pathology
Stage IV CTE	Severe p-Tau pathology affecting most regions of the cerebral cortex and the medial temporal lobe, sparing calcarine cortex in all but the most severe cases

Adapted from McKee AC, Stein TD, Nowinski CJ, et al. The spectrum of disease in chronic traumatic encephalopathy. Brain 2013;136(1):46; with permission.

present in up to one-third of patients many years after a single moderate to severe TBI.[50] However, these findings should be interpreted with caution, as these changes also may be found in cognitively intact individuals,[51] and their frequency increases with age.[52]

SYMPTOMATOLOGY

Symptoms associated with mTBI/concussion are usually broad and nonspecific. They are classified into 3 categories that include the following: (1) physical: headaches, reported by up to 90% of patients, dizziness, blurred vision, fatigue and photo/phonosensitivity; (2) psychiatric symptoms involving personality change, anxiety, depression, irritability, sleep disturbances, as well as psychosis in rare instances; and (3) Cognitive symptoms including mostly impairments in verbal/nonverbal memory, but also in attention, concentration, and executive functioning.[53] Postconcussion syndrome (PCS) is defined by the WHO International Classification of Diseases, 10th revision (ICD-10) as a syndrome that occurs following head trauma, that includes 3 or more of the following 8 symptoms: headache, dizziness, fatigue, irritability, insomnia,

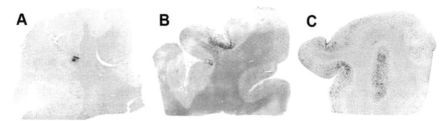

Fig. 1. Low-magnification inspection of p-Tau–stained slides often revealed the irregular spatial pattern of CTE pathology. AT8-stained slides of cerebral cortex in 3 cases of CTE showing irregular patches of p-Tau pathology most dense at the depths of the sulci. (*From* McKee AC, Cairns NJ, Dickson DW, et al. The first NINDS/NIBIB consensus meeting to define neuropathological criteria for the diagnosis of chronic traumatic encephalopathy. Acta Neuropathol 2016;131(1):79. Distributed under the terms of the Creative Commons Attribution 4.0 International License Available at: https://creativecommons.org/licenses/by/4.0/.)

concentration or memory difficulty, and intolerance of stress, emotion, or alcohol.[54] It occurs in 38% to 80% of patients after mTBI. The vast majority of individuals fully recover within 3 to 6 months, but up to 15% may have symptoms lasting for a year after the injury, and are thus considered suffering from persistent or long-term PCS.[53] Chronic PCS is thought to be a clinical entity distinct from CTE, as the onset of symptoms begins rapidly after the head trauma and persists but rarely progresses in PCS.[55] Recovery is very common after TBI: some studies observed continued recovery up to 2 years postinjury, but most noted a plateau beyond 1 year.[56] With respect to cognitive symptoms, a more accelerated recovery was found during the first 5 months rather than the last 7 months of the year postinjury, in those undergoing rehabilitation therapy.[56] Decreasing age was found to significantly impact the trajectory of cognitive recovery, by enhancing simple and complex speed of processing[57,58] and executive functioning,[58] up to a year postinjury. No effect of age was found on memory or attention. Premorbid intellectual functioning influenced outcome, with respect to level of functioning.[57]

On the other hand, concussions can be associated with a progressive neurologic dysfunction that was described for the first time in 1928 by Harrison S. Martland in his seminal paper about "Punch-Drunk" syndrome in boxers who had progressively developed parkinsonian symptoms, ataxia, and "mental deterioration" leading to institutionalization.[59] This syndrome became then known as "Dementia pugilistica," and involved dysarthria, ataxia, pyramidal signs, extrapyramidal signs, memory impairment, and personality changes.[60] With increasing neuropathogical evidence, the term CTE was later introduced,[61] and recognized not only in boxers, but also in other athletes, particularly American football players.[62] McKee and colleagues[47] demonstrated a clinicopathological correlation across the 4 stages of CTE: the superior, dorsolateral, and lateral frontal affected areas in stage I may underlie the clinical features of disinhibition, lack of insight, and poor executive functioning in these patients. Pathologic involvement of the inferior temporal lobe and amygdala might contribute to the frontal symptoms and to the irritability, impulsivity, and outbursts of aggression so commonly experienced as early manifestations of CTE. Pathology of the nucleus basalis of Meynert and septal nuclei might contribute to the cognitive symptoms. Mammillary body, anterior thalamic, and hippocampal pathology found in stage IV are the most important contributor to progressive cognitive impairment.

Traumatic Brain Injury and Dementia

To date, the mechanisms by which TBI leads to cognitive impairment are not completely understood. It is believed that TBI may either trigger a progressive neurodegenerative cascade, accelerate an established neurodegenerative cascade, or reduce cognitive reserve.[63]

The association between TBI and AD has been inconsistent throughout the literature: many studies reported an increased risk for AD after TBI,[12,64–66] and threefold higher risk of AD-related mortality among football players with TBI history,[67] whereas other studies reported no increased risk for AD.[68–71] In a large 33-year Swedish cohort of individuals previously enrolled in the military service, exposure to TBI with different severities (1 mTBI, more than 2 mTBIs or 1 severe TBI) was particularly associated with an increased likelihood of developing dementia of the non-AD type at a younger age (<65 year old). Surprisingly, none of these TBIs was significantly associated with an increased likelihood of developing young-onset AD.[72]

Several factors related to trauma severity, patient characteristics (genetics, age at the time of injury, gender, premorbid functioning, cognitive reserve), and management following the trauma are thought to influence the development of a neurocognitive disorder. For instance, moderate to severe TBI was found to be associated with an increased likelihood of developing dementia in individuals aged 55 years or older, whereas mild TBI was associated with increased dementia risk in those aged 65 years or older.[63] TBIs occurring in younger ages were associated with increased risk of dementia and AD in later life.[73,74] Compared with mTBI, both moderate and severe TBIs were found to be associated with a significantly higher risk of developing AD among veterans.[74] TBI with LOC, compared to without LOC, was associated with a significantly higher risk of subjective cognitive impairment, increasingly recognized as a risk factor for AD,[75] even after adjustment for depression.[76] In addition, the Apolipoprotein E4 (ApoE4) genotype is known to be the major genetic risk factor for AD.[77] Data from animal and human studies have consistently demonstrated the negative impact of the ApoE4 allele on the reparative capacity of the brain following a TBI.[78] Carriers of the apolipoprotein ApoE4 genotype were found to be overrepresented in victims of fatal TBIs with amyloid plaque deposits.[79] Studies also have demonstrated that possession of this genetic susceptibility may poorly impact the cognitive outcome, especially in the case of repetitive or more severe TBI exposure in professional athletes.[80,81] Moreover, male gender was particularly associated with a higher likelihood of developing AD after a TBI.[12,64,74] In a 9-year population-based study, fall-related moderate TBI (MTBI) was associated with an earlier onset of dementia, especially in APOE4 allele carriers.[82] In a retrospective study, TBI with LOC was also related to an earlier onset of AD by 2.5 years, regardless of gender or APOE4 genotype status. However, participants with both a history of TBI and ApoE4 genotype had the earliest age of onset compared with those with a history of TBI, or carrying the APOE4 allele alone.[83]

Dementia with Lewy bodies (DLB) is a neurodegenerative disorder associated with diffuse accumulation of Lewy bodies and alpha-synuclein protein in the brain. Its core clinical features involve fluctuating cognitive impairment, spontaneous features of parkinsonism, and early psychotic symptoms, usually recurrent visual hallucinations.[84] The association between TBI and DLB is not well established. Boot and colleagues[85] reported no association between TBI and risk of DLB when compared with controls or with patients with AD. Crane and colleagues[71] on the other hand found that TBI with a history of LOC was associated with pathologic findings of Lewy bodies in the frontal and temporal cortex on autopsy.

Frontotemporal dementia (FTD) is a leading cause of early-onset dementia. It is characterized by progressive deficits in behavior, executive function, and language.[86] There has been increasing evidence linking TBI to FTD. In a retrospective case-control study, patients who reported a history of TBI had 3.3-fold higher risk of being diagnosed with FTD.[87] In another case-control study conducted among veterans, the prevalence of TBI was shown to be significantly higher in patients with FTD compared with those with non-FTD dementias. Moreover, those with a history of TBI were 4.4-fold at higher risk of being diagnosed with FTD, compared with those who did not report a previous TBI history.[88] A retrospective study comparing a large sample of patients with FTD with controls has found that a lifetime history of TBI with more than 5 minutes LOC was associated with a 1.6 higher risk for FTD.[89]

Furthermore, a history of TBI with LOC was associated with an earlier age of symptom onset and age of diagnosis of FTD (2.8 and 3.2 years, respectively), and these effects were independent of family history of dementia and education.[90]

TBI and parkinsonian symptoms are well established vis à vis CTE; however, the relationship of TBI to the later development of PD is not well established. Both TBI and PD share similar mechanisms, including inflammation,[91,92] mitochondrial dysfunction,[93,94] and most importantly, the accumulation of alpha-synuclein protein.[95]

Small studies have reported parkinsonian symptoms following severe TBI that is sometimes responsive to dopaminergic medication.[96] The risk of PD following MTBI is less clear.[97] A recent meta-analysis has shown that TBI in general was associated with 1.57-fold higher risk for developing PD.[98] In a case-control study, an earlier age at first TBI with LOC was found to be significantly associated with a higher risk of PD.[99]

APPROACH TO DIAGNOSIS OF TRAUMATIC BRAIN INJURY
History and Examination

Detailed and careful history taking, including caretaker accounts related to the patient's symptoms, remains the cornerstone for diagnosis of TBI. It is especially important to inquire about history of falls. History of MTBI may not be obtained, as LOC may not be present in the history. History of posttraumatic amnesia is more reliable than LOC, so a thorough interview about the details of the patient's recall of the events preceding and following the trauma is important. History of unsteadiness, frequent falls, previous TBIs (as the recurrence in higher in the presence of previous fall or previous TBI, as mentioned earlier) and a review of medications list should be performed, carefully searching for common medications that are known for causing dizziness/orthostasis or altered LOC with secondary falls. Comorbidities, such as cardiac disease with syncopal risks, diabetes with orthostatic hypotension, and other contributing history, is essential information to obtain in the history. A detailed neurologic examination is critical. Mental status examination with cognitive functions, as well as eye movements, balance, gait, and coordination can be affected.[100] Carefully searching for extrapyramidal signs, such as tremors, rigidity, and bradykinesia, are helpful in determining parkinsonian symptoms that may predispose the patient to falls. Mood disorders are common, and an underlying structural/metabolic etiology should not be overlooked in patients with depression. Although definitive diagnosis of CTE is made via postmortem autopsy, Montenigro and colleagues[101] recently proposed the following criteria for the clinical diagnosis of traumatic encephalopathy syndrome: a history of multiple impacts including mTBI (minimum of 4) or moderate to severe TBI (minimum of 2), acquired in the course of contact sports, military service or any other setting of repetitive head injuries, present for at least 12 months, with no other neurologic disorder that could account for the clinical presentation, such as chronic residual symptoms from a single TBI or persistent postconcussion syndrome, and requiring at least 1 core feature and 2 supportive features to be present. Core features involve cognitive, behavioral, and mood changes, whereas some of the supportive features are suicidality, apathy, paranoia, and headaches.

Neuropsychological Testing

Neuropsychological testing is a comprehensive clinical tool, administered by a neuropsychologist, that aims to objectively assess different cognitive domains that may have been affected in TBIs, such as sensory-motor functions, language, visuospatial abilities, learning and memory, attention, executive functions, functional abilities, and emotional functioning/personality. It also provides information about the new baseline of cognitive abilities post-TBI, allowing for future measures of changes over time.[102]

More recently, computer-generated neuropsychological test programs have been developed and are currently being validated in the sports setting (but not yet available for clinical use). They offer the advantages of rapid scoring, ease of administration, and greater accessibility. They include the following: Immediate Post-Concussion Assessment and Cognitive Testing, Computerized Cognitive Assessment Tool,

Concussion Resolution Index, Automated Neuropsychological Assessment Metrics system and Concussion Vital Signs.[103]

Neuroimaging

Despite the potential usefulness of conventional imaging techniques, such as computed tomography (CT) scans and MRI in moderate to severe TBIs, these modalities have been shown to lack sensitivity for identifying diffuse axonal injuries typically found in mTBIs/concussions.[104]

More sensitive modalities involve (1) diffusion tensor imaging, an MRI-based technique, measuring white-matter integrity and detecting mTBI-related axonal injuries[105]; (2) functional MRI, measuring brain activity by detecting changes associated with blood flow and providing insight into various functional abnormalities, even in subconcussive injuries[106]; (3) magnetic resonance spectroscopy, a noninvasive technique measuring metabolic changes in N-acetyl aspartate/creatine ratio, as an indicator of neuronal damage following mTBI[107]; (4) positron emission tomography (PET) scan, measuring patterns of 2-fluro-2-deoxy-D-glucose uptake and its utilization in the brain after an injury, showing a broad pattern of hypometabolism in brain regions affected by the injury[108]; (5) single photon emission computer tomography, measuring cerebral perfusion and identifying hypoperfusion of brain regions affected by mTBI[109]; (6) susceptibility weighted imaging, sensitive for detection of micro-hemorrhages, venous thrombosis, and ischemia, commonly found after mTBI, but also mapping the extent of BBB disruption and perivascular tau deposition during the progression of CTE.[110]

Biomarkers of Brain Injury

The clinical and neuroimaging approaches to classify TBIs have been shown to be insufficient due to the challenging aspect of the brain and injury response.[111] Furthermore, despite recent development of specific diagnostic criteria,[48] CTE shares common neuropathological findings with other neurodegenerative disorders. Identifying reliable biomarkers for mTBI and CTE may improve diagnosis, disease characterization, and monitoring of severity, progression, and recovery.[2] Data from a Swedish cohort of professional ice hockey players have shown that total tau and S-100 calcium-binding protein B significantly increase in the blood after a concussion, and decrease after rehabilitation.[112] The calpain-derived all-spectrin N-terminal fragment (SNTF) is usually absent from healthy neurons, but accumulates in damaged axons after an mTBI. In this same cohort, serum concentrations of SNTF were shown to increase, along with total tau levels, as early as 1 hour after concussion, and remain significantly elevated for up to 6 days, before returning to baseline at the time of return to play. SNTF can thus be considered a promising marker of diffuse axonal injury, found in concussions.[113] The Glial neuronal ratio, which is the ratio between serum glial fibrillary acidic protein and ubiquitin carboxy-terminal hydrolase-L1, was found to be associated with the severity of head injury, in correlation with CT scan findings.[114] Serum concentrations of neuron-specific enolase (NSE) have been postulated to increase in patients with mTBI compared with controls, and to serve as a marker of neuronal death. However, the use of this marker is limited by the fact that NSE is found in many other tissues beside the brain, such as erythrocytes, platelets, neuroendocrine cells, and oligodendrocytes; yielding a lot of false-positive measures.[111]

Promising markers for CTE include cerebrospinal fluid measures of chemokine CCL-11, as increased levels were shown to discriminate between American football players with CTE and subjects with AD and controls.[115] Novel diagnostic approaches for CTE involve PET imaging using recently developed tau-ligands, such as [18F] T807.[116]

PREVENTION AND TREATMENT

No disease-modifying treatment is available for CTE and other neurocognitive disorders associated with TBIs. However, improving prevention strategies is vital to reducing the global burden of TBIs. Implementing safety measures to decrease road traffic accidents, mostly in low to middle-income countries, include changes in legislation and vehicle safety designs, improvements in infrastructure, promotion of seatbelt use, as well as other awareness campaigns focusing on speeding and driving under the influence.[2] Prevention of falls is a substantial intervention to reduce TBIs, especially in the elderly. Older adults who have fallen in the past, or with gait and balance problems are at higher risk of future falls.[117] Prevention strategies include promoting the use and acceptability of mobility assistive devices, such as walkers and canes[118]; implementing regular screenings for vision, balance, and gait problems; and rational de-prescribing of medication incriminated in orthostasis and falls.[119,120]

Furthermore, strict regulations need to be applied in contact sports. A player with a suspicion of a concussion needs to be immediately removed from play, and examined by a physician. Education with respect to concussions and CTE needs to be provided to players, parents, referees, coaches, and sports organization committees.[2] Protective equipment, such as headgear, helmets, and mouth guards, may reduce the risk of severe head injuries, but have not been shown to reduce the risk of concussions. In fact, their use can lead to a false sense of security, resulting in a more dangerous style of play, such as using the helmet to initiate contact[121]; although counterintuitive, a helmetless tackling training among American football players resulted in 28% reduction in head impacts for an entire season, in comparison with controls (players tackling with their helmets).[122]

Pharmacologic interventions are usually targeted toward neuropsychiatric symptoms post-TBI. Prescriptions should be personalized (on a case-by-case basis), favor monotherapy, and "start low and go slow." Caution is necessary regarding the patient's cardiovascular status and epileptogenic threshold, affected by the trauma.[123] Selective serotonin reuptake inhibitors (SSRIs) have been associated with improvements in severity of depressive symptoms, but not cognitive symptoms.[124] In one randomized controlled study, sertraline was shown to prevent the occurrence of a depressive episode at 24 weeks, when given at the dosage of 100 mg daily, within 4 weeks of a TBI.[125]

Beta-blockers (eg, propranolol, pindolol) and antiepileptics carry the most compelling evidence for the management of agitation, aggression, and irritability post-TBI.[126] Other options include antipsychotics, preferably second-generation, antidepressants (eg, trazodone, SSRIs), buspirone, and rarely, benzodiazepines.[123,126–128]

Limited evidence has shown a potential role of amantadine in improving cognition and apathy and reducing agitation.[129] However, a recent randomized controlled trial demonstrated its efficacy in accelerating the pace of recovery and promoting arousal from a vegetative state or minimally conscious state, when administered early after a severe TBI.[130]

Research in animal models with TBI has also shown a promising role of beta and gamma secretase inhibitors in reducing posttraumatic cell loss and improving motor and cognitive recovery after a TBI, probably through a reduction of Aβ amyloid production.[131]

Cognitive rehabilitation therapy is another approach to TBI treatment. It may help patients overcome their cognitive impairments and regain an optimal level of functionality. It begins with complete neuropsychological testing to identify strengths and weaknesses in the different cognitive arenas, followed by establishing a plan to retrain the brain to overcome these deficits.[132] Ultimate goals of rehabilitation include enhancing the independence of TBI survivors, retraining them for activities of daily living, facilitating return to work and community reintegration, and improving their quality of life. Unfortunately, most patients are confronted with lack of availability of these services, especially in underserved areas.[2]

SUMMARY

There is growing evidence linking TBI to the development of some neurocognitive disorders such as AD, DLB, FTD, and the challenging entity of CTE. However, the estimation of individualized risk is still very challenging. In addition to the methodological limitations of the current studies in the literature, both TBIs and neurocognitive disorders are very heterogeneous disorders, which currently limit our ability to accurately predict the risk of developing progressive cognitive impairment in TBI-exposed individuals.[133] Moreover, it is impossible to objectively assess for brain neuroplasticity and its capacity to recuperate over time, especially with rehabilitation. Future studies should aim at agreeing on a common classification system for TBI, to be used for research purposes, and developing objective blood or imaging biomarkers for TBI. In the meantime, prevention of TBI, including prevention of falls in the elderly and concussions among athletes remains the optimal approach to decreasing the impact of TBI in our society.

REFERENCES

1. Menon DK, Schwab K, Wright DW, et al. Position statement: definition of traumatic brain injury. Arch Phys Med Rehabil 2010;91(11):1637–40.
2. Maas AIR, Menon DK, Adelson PD, et al. Traumatic brain injury: integrated approaches to improve prevention, clinical care, and research. Lancet Neurol 2017;16(12):987–1048.
3. Whiteneck GG, Cuthbert JP, Corrigan JD, et al. Prevalence of self-reported lifetime history of traumatic brain injury and associated disability: a statewide population-based survey. J Head Trauma Rehabil 2016;31(1):E55–62.
4. Coronado VG, Xu L, Basavaraju SV, et al. Surveillance for traumatic brain injury-related deaths–United States, 1997-2007. MMWR Surveill Summ 2011;60(5):1–32.
5. McMillan TM, Teasdale GM. Death rate is increased for at least 7 years after head injury: a prospective study. Brain 2007;130(Pt 10):2520–7.
6. Selassie AW, Zaloshnja E, Langlois JA, et al. Incidence of long-term disability following traumatic brain injury hospitalization, United States, 2003. J Head Trauma Rehabil 2008;23(2):123–31.
7. Thornhill S, Teasdale GM, Murray GD, et al. Disability in young people and adults one year after head injury: prospective cohort study. BMJ 2000; 320(7250):1631–5.
8. Centers for Disease Control and Prevention. Report to congress on traumatic brain injury in the United States: epidemiology and rehabilitation. Atlanta (GA): National Center for Injury Prevention and Control; Division of Unintentional Injury Prevention; 2015. Available at: https://www-cdc-gov.ezp.slu.edu/traumaticbraininjury/pdf/tbi_report_to_congress_epi_and_rehab-a.pdf. Accessed January 14, 2018.
9. Jourdan C, Azouvi P, Genet F, et al. Disability and health consequences of traumatic brain injury: national prevalence. Am J Phys Med Rehabil 2018. https://doi.org/10.1097/PHM.0000000000000848.
10. Hoofien D, Gilboa A, Vakil E, et al. Traumatic brain injury (TBI) 10-20 years later: a comprehensive outcome study of psychiatric symptomatology, cognitive abilities and psychosocial functioning. Brain Inj 2001;15(3):189–209.

11. Ma VY, Chan L, Carruthers KJ. The incidence, prevalence, costs and impact on disability of common conditions requiring rehabilitation in the US: stroke, spinal cord injury, traumatic brain injury, multiple sclerosis, osteoarthritis, rheumatoid arthritis, limb loss, and back pain. Arch Phys Med Rehabil 2014;95(5):986–95.e1.

12. Fleminger S, Oliver DL, Lovestone S, et al. Head injury as a risk factor for Alzheimer's disease: the evidence 10 years on; a partial replication. J Neurol Neurosurg Psychiatry 2003;74(7):857–62.

13. Li Y, Li Y, Li X, et al. Head injury as a risk factor for dementia and Alzheimer's disease: a systematic review and meta-analysis of 32 observational studies. PLoS One 2017;12(1):e0169650.

14. Stern RA, Riley DO, Daneshvar DH, et al. Long-term consequences of repetitive brain trauma: chronic traumatic encephalopathy. PM R 2011;3(10, Supplement 2):S460–7.

15. Roozenbeek B, Maas AI, Menon DK. Changing patterns in the epidemiology of traumatic brain injury. Nat Rev Neurol 2013;9(4):231–6.

16. Mather M, Jacobsen L, Pollard K. Aging in the United States." Population Bulletin 70. no. 2. 2015. Available at: http://www.prb.org/pdf16/aging-us-population-bulletin.pdf. Accessed January 16, 2017.

17. Coronado VG, Thomas KE, Sattin RW, et al. The CDC traumatic brain injury surveillance system: characteristics of persons aged 65 years and older hospitalized with a TBI. J Head Trauma Rehabil 2005;20(3):215–28.

18. Harvey LA, Close JC. Traumatic brain injury in older adults: characteristics, causes and consequences. Injury 2012;43(11):1821–6.

19. Karibe H, Hayashi T, Narisawa A, et al. Clinical characteristics and outcome in elderly patients with traumatic brain injury: for establishment of management strategy. Neurol Med Chir (Tokyo) 2017;57(8):418–25.

20. Smith K, Weeks S. The impact of pre-injury anticoagulation therapy in the older adult patient experiencing a traumatic brain injury: a systematic review. JBI Libr Syst Rev 2012;10(58):4610–21.

21. Teasdale G, Jennett B. Assessment of coma and impaired consciousness. Lancet 1974;304(7872):81–4.

22. O'Neil ME, Carlson K, Storzbach D, et al. Classification of TBI severity. complications of mild traumatic brain injury in veterans and military personnel: a systematic review [Internet]. 2013. Available at: https://www-ncbi-nlm-nih-gov.ezp.slu.edu/books/NBK189784/table/appc.t1/. Accessed January 13, 2018.

23. Nakase-Richardson R, Sherer M, Seel RT, et al. Utility of post-traumatic amnesia in predicting 1-year productivity following traumatic brain injury: comparison of the Russell and Mississippi PTA classification intervals. J Neurol Neurosurg Psychiatry 2011;82(5):494–9.

24. Malec JF, Brown AW, Leibson CL, et al. The Mayo classification system for traumatic brain injury severity. J Neurotrauma 2007;24(9):1417–24.

25. Saatman KE, Duhaime AC, Bullock R, et al. Classification of traumatic brain injury for targeted therapies. J Neurotrauma 2008;25(7):719–38.

26. Carroll LJ, Cassidy JD, Holm L, et al. Methodological issues and research recommendations for mild traumatic brain injury: the WHO Collaborating Centre Task Force on mild traumatic brain injury. J Rehabil Med 2004;43(Suppl):113–25.

27. Champion HR, Copes WS, Sacco WJ, et al. The major trauma outcome study: establishing national norms for trauma care. J Trauma 1990;30(11):1356–65.

28. Champion HR, Sacco WJ, Copes WS, et al. A revision of the trauma score. J Trauma 1989;29(5):623–9.

29. Baker SP, O'Neill B. The injury severity score: an update. J Trauma 1976;16(11): 882–5.

30. Cassidy JD, Carroll LJ, Peloso PM, et al. Incidence, risk factors and prevention of mild traumatic brain injury: results of the WHO Collaborating Centre Task Force on mild traumatic brain injury. J Rehabil Med 2004;43(Suppl):28–60.

31. Greve MW, Zink BJ. Pathophysiology of traumatic brain injury. Mt Sinai J Med 2009;76(2):97–104.

32. Stocchetti N, Zanier ER. Chronic impact of traumatic brain injury on outcome and quality of life: a narrative review. Crit Care 2016;20(1):148.

33. Ziebell JM, Morganti-Kossmann MC. Involvement of pro- and anti-inflammatory cytokines and chemokines in the pathophysiology of traumatic brain injury. Neurotherapeutics 2010;7(1):22–30.

34. Breunig J, Guillot-Sestier M-V, Town T. Brain injury, neuroinflammation and Alzheimer's disease. Front Aging Neurosci 2013;5:26.

35. Johnson VE, Stewart JE, Begbie FD, et al. Inflammation and white matter degeneration persist for years after a single traumatic brain injury. Brain 2013;136(Pt 1):28–42.

36. Huang RQ, Cheng HL, Zhao XD, et al. Preliminary study on the effect of trauma-induced secondary cellular hypoxia in brain injury. Neurosci Lett 2010;473(1): 22–7.

37. Zhang X, Le W. Pathological role of hypoxia in Alzheimer's disease. Exp Neurol 2010;223(2):299–303.

38. Hay JR, Johnson VE, Young AM, et al. Blood-brain barrier disruption is an early event that may persist for many years after traumatic brain injury in humans. J Neuropathol Exp Neurol 2015;74(12):1147–57.

39. Shibata M, Yamada S, Kumar SR, et al. Clearance of Alzheimer's amyloid-β(1-40) peptide from brain by LDL receptor–related protein-1 at the blood-brain barrier. J Clin Invest 2000;106(12):1489–99.

40. Johnson VE, Stewart W, Smith DH. Axonal pathology in traumatic brain injury. Exp Neurol 2013;246(Supplement C):35–43.

41. Smith DH, Johnson VE, Stewart W. Chronic neuropathologies of single and repetitive TBI: substrates of dementia? Nat Rev Neurol 2013;9(4):211–21.

42. Hay J, Johnson VE, Smith DH, et al. Chronic traumatic encephalopathy: the neuropathological legacy of traumatic brain injury. Annu Rev Pathol 2016;11: 21–45.

43. Washington PM, Villapol S, Burns MP. Polypathology and dementia after brain trauma: does brain injury trigger distinct neurodegenerative diseases, or should they be classified together as traumatic encephalopathy? Exp Neurol 2016; 275(Pt 3):381–8.

44. Bloom GS. Amyloid-beta and tau: the trigger and bullet in Alzheimer disease pathogenesis. JAMA Neurol 2014;71(4):505–8.

45. Uryu K, Chen X-H, Martinez D, et al. Multiple proteins implicated in neurodegenerative diseases accumulate in axons after brain trauma in humans. Exp Neurol 2007;208(2):185–92.

46. Stein TD, Montenigro PH, Alvarez VE, et al. Beta-amyloid deposition in chronic traumatic encephalopathy. Acta Neuropathol 2015;130(1):21–34.

47. McKee AC, Stein TD, Nowinski CJ, et al. The spectrum of disease in chronic traumatic encephalopathy. Brain 2013;136(1):43–64.

48. McKee AC, Cairns NJ, Dickson DW, et al. The first NINDS/NIBIB consensus meeting to define neuropathological criteria for the diagnosis of chronic traumatic encephalopathy. Acta Neuropathol 2016;131(1):75–86.

49. Johnson VE, Stewart W, Smith DH. Traumatic brain injury and amyloid-β pathology: a link to Alzheimer's disease? Nat Rev Neurosci 2010;11(5):361–70.
50. Johnson VE, Stewart W, Smith DH. Widespread tau and amyloid-beta pathology many years after a single traumatic brain injury in humans. Brain Pathol 2012; 22(2):142–9.
51. Gu Y, Razlighi QR, Zahodne LB, et al. Brain amyloid deposition and longitudinal cognitive decline in nondemented older subjects: results from a multi-ethnic population. PLOS One 2015;10(7):e0123743.
52. Braak H, Thal DR, Ghebremedhin E, et al. Stages of the pathologic process in Alzheimer disease: age categories from 1 to 100 years. J Neuropathol Exp Neurol 2011;70(11):960–9.
53. Hall RC, Hall RC, Chapman MJ. Definition, diagnosis, and forensic implications of postconcussional syndrome. Psychosomatics 2005;46(3):195–202.
54. ICD-10. Postconcussional syndrome. 2016. Available at: http://apps.who.int/classifications/icd10/browse/2016/en#/F07.2. Accessed January 18, 2018.
55. Ling H, Hardy J, Zetterberg H. Neurological consequences of traumatic brain injuries in sports. Mol Cell Neurosci 2015;66(Pt B):114–22.
56. Christensen BK, Colella B, Inness E, et al. Recovery of cognitive function after traumatic brain injury: a multilevel modeling analysis of Canadian outcomes. Arch Phys Med Rehabil 2008;89(12, Supplement):S3–15.
57. Green RE, Colella B, Christensen B, et al. Examining moderators of cognitive recovery trajectories after moderate to severe traumatic brain injury. Arch Phys Med Rehabil 2008;89(12 Suppl):S16–24.
58. Rabinowitz AR, Hart T, Whyte J, et al. Neuropsychological recovery trajectories in moderate to severe traumatic brain injury: influence of patient characteristics and diffuse axonal injury. J Int Neuropsychol Soc 2018. https://doi.org/10.1017/S1355617717000996.
59. Martland HS. Punch drunk. J Am Med Assoc 1928;91(15):1103–7.
60. Castellani RJ, Perry G. Dementia pugilistica revisited. J Alzheimers Dis 2017; 60(4):1209–21.
61. Miller H. Mental after-effects of head injury. Proc R Soc Med 1966;59(3): 257–61.
62. Omalu BI, DeKosky ST, Minster RL, et al. Chronic traumatic encephalopathy in a national football league player. Neurosurgery 2005;57(1):128–34 [discussion: 128–34].
63. Gardner RC, Burke JF, Nettiksimmons J, et al. Dementia risk after traumatic brain injury vs nonbrain trauma: the role of age and severity. JAMA Neurol 2014;71(12):1490–7.
64. Mortimer JA, van Duijn CM, Chandra V, et al. Head trauma as a risk factor for Alzheimer's disease: a collaborative re-analysis of case-control studies. EURODEM risk factors research group. Int J Epidemiol 1991;20(Suppl 2):S28–35.
65. Suhanov AV, Pilipenko PI, Korczyn AD, et al. Risk factors for Alzheimer's disease in Russia: a case-control study. Eur J Neurol 2006;13(9):990–5.
66. Lee YK, Hou SW, Lee CC, et al. Increased risk of dementia in patients with mild traumatic brain injury: a nationwide cohort study. PLoS One 2013;8(5):e62422.
67. Lehman EJ, Hein MJ, Baron SL, et al. Neurodegenerative causes of death among retired National Football League players. Neurology 2012;79(19):1970–4.
68. Launer LJ, Andersen K, Dewey ME, et al. Rates and risk factors for dementia and Alzheimer's disease: results from EURODEM pooled analyses. EURODEM incidence research group and work groups. European studies of dementia. Neurology 1999;52(1):78–84.

69. Mehta KM, Ott A, Kalmijn S, et al. Head trauma and risk of dementia and Alzheimer's disease: the Rotterdam study. Neurology 1999;53(9):1959–62.

70. Dams-O'Connor K, Gibbons LE, Bowen JD, et al. Risk for late-life re-injury, dementia and death among individuals with traumatic brain injury: a population-based study. J Neurol Neurosurg Psychiatry 2013;84(2):177–82.

71. Crane PK, Gibbons LE, Dams-O'Connor K, et al. Association of traumatic brain injury with late-life neurodegenerative conditions and neuropathologic findings. JAMA Neurol 2016;73(9):1062–9.

72. Nordstrom P, Michaelsson K, Gustafson Y, et al. Traumatic brain injury and young onset dementia: a nationwide cohort study. Ann Neurol 2014;75(3):374–81.

73. Schofield PW, Tang M, Marder K, et al. Alzheimer's disease after remote head injury: an incidence study. J Neurol Neurosurg Psychiatry 1997;62(2):119–24.

74. Plassman BL, Havlik RJ, Steffens DC, et al. Documented head injury in early adulthood and risk of Alzheimer's disease and other dementias. Neurology 2000;55(8):1158–66.

75. Rabin LA, Smart CM, Amariglio RE. Subjective cognitive decline in preclinical Alzheimer's disease. Annu Rev Clin Psychol 2017;13(1):369–96.

76. Gardner RC, Langa KM, Yaffe K. Subjective and objective cognitive function among older adults with a history of traumatic brain injury: a population-based cohort study. PLoS Med 2017;14(3):e1002246.

77. Kim J, Basak JM, Holtzman DM. The role of apolipoprotein E in Alzheimer's disease. Neuron 2009;63(3):287–303.

78. Crawford F, Wood M, Ferguson S, et al. Apolipoprotein E-genotype dependent hippocampal and cortical responses to traumatic brain injury. Neuroscience 2009;159(4):1349–62.

79. Nicoll JA, Roberts GW, Graham DI. Apolipoprotein E epsilon 4 allele is associated with deposition of amyloid beta-protein following head injury. Nat Med 1995;1(2):135–7.

80. Jordan BD, Relkin NR, Ravdin LD, et al. Apolipoprotein E epsilon4 associated with chronic traumatic brain injury in boxing. JAMA 1997;278(2):136–40.

81. Kutner KC, Erlanger DM, Tsai J, et al. Lower cognitive performance of older football players possessing apolipoprotein E epsilon4. Neurosurgery 2000;47(3):651–7 [discussion: 657–8].

82. Luukinen H, Viramo P, Herala M, et al. Fall-related brain injuries and the risk of dementia in elderly people: a population-based study. Eur J Neurol 2005;12(2):86–92.

83. LoBue C, Wadsworth H, Wilmoth K, et al. Traumatic brain injury history is associated with earlier age of onset of Alzheimer disease. Clin Neuropsychol 2017;31(1):85–98.

84. McKeith IG, Dickson DW, Lowe J, et al. Diagnosis and management of dementia with Lewy bodies: third report of the DLB consortium. Neurology 2005;65(12):1863–72.

85. Boot BP, Orr CF, Ahlskog JE, et al. Risk factors for dementia with Lewy bodies: a case-control study. Neurology 2013;81(9):833–40.

86. Bang J, Spina S, Miller BL. Frontotemporal dementia. Lancet 2015;386(10004):1672–82.

87. Rosso SM, Landweer EJ, Houterman M, et al. Medical and environmental risk factors for sporadic frontotemporal dementia: a retrospective case–control study. J Neurol Neurosurg Psychiatry 2003;74(11):1574.

88. Kalkonde YV, Jawaid A, Qureshi SU, et al. Medical and environmental risk factors associated with frontotemporal dementia: a case-control study in a veteran population. Alzheimers Dement 2012;8(3):204–10.

89. Deutsch MB, Mendez MF, Teng E. Interactions between traumatic brain injury and frontotemporal degeneration. Dement Geriatr Cogn Disord 2015;39(0):143–53.

90. LoBue C, Wilmoth K, Cullum CM, et al. Traumatic brain injury history is associated with earlier age of onset of frontotemporal dementia. J Neurol Neurosurg Psychiatry 2016;87(8):817–20.

91. McGeer PL, McGeer EG. Inflammation and the degenerative diseases of aging. Ann N Y Acad Sci 2004;1035:104–16.

92. Gentleman SM, Leclercq PD, Moyes L, et al. Long-term intracerebral inflammatory response after traumatic brain injury. Forensic Sci Int 2004;146(2–3):97–104.

93. Arundine M, Tymianski M. Molecular mechanisms of glutamate-dependent neurodegeneration in ischemia and traumatic brain injury. Cell Mol Life Sci 2004; 61(6):657–68.

94. Winklhofer KF, Haass C. Mitochondrial dysfunction in Parkinson's disease. Biochim Biophys Acta 2010;1802(1):29–44.

95. Smith DH, Uryu K, Saatman KE, et al. Protein accumulation in traumatic brain injury. Neuromolecular Med 2003;4(1–2):59–72.

96. Formisano R, Zasler ND. Posttraumatic parkinsonism. J Head Trauma Rehabil 2014;29(4):387–90.

97. Marras C, Hincapie CA, Kristman VL, et al. Systematic review of the risk of Parkinson's disease after mild traumatic brain injury: results of the international collaboration on mild traumatic brain injury prognosis. Arch Phys Med Rehabil 2014;95(3 Suppl):S238–44.

98. Jafari S, Etminan M, Aminzadeh F, et al. Head injury and risk of Parkinson disease: a systematic review and meta-analysis. Mov Disord 2013;28(9):1222–9.

99. Taylor KM, Saint-Hilaire MH, Sudarsky L, et al. Head injury at early ages is associated with risk of Parkinson's disease. Parkinsonism Relat Disord 2016;23: 57–61.

100. Arciniegas DB, Anderson CA, Topkoff J, et al. Mild traumatic brain injury: a neuropsychiatric approach to diagnosis, evaluation, and treatment. Neuropsychiatr Dis Treat 2005;1(4):311–27.

101. Montenigro PH, Baugh CM, Daneshvar DH, et al. Clinical subtypes of chronic traumatic encephalopathy: literature review and proposed research diagnostic criteria for traumatic encephalopathy syndrome. Alzheimers Res Ther 2014; 6(5):68.

102. Soble JR, Critchfield EA, O'Rourke JJ. Neuropsychological evaluation in traumatic brain injury. Phys Med Rehabil Clin N Am 2017;28(2):339–50.

103. Straus LB. Neurocognitive testing for concussions: computerized neuropsychological tests. 2013. Available at: http://www.momsteam.com/health-safety/concussion-safety/recognition-evaluation/neuropsychological-testing-for-concussions?page=0%2C1. Accessed January 20, 2018.

104. Shenton ME, Hamoda HM, Schneiderman JS, et al. A review of magnetic resonance imaging and diffusion tensor imaging findings in mild traumatic brain injury. Brain Imaging Behav 2012;6(2):137–92.

105. Basser PJ, Mattiello J, LeBihan D. MR diffusion tensor spectroscopy and imaging. Biophys J 1994;66(1):259–67.

106. McDonald BC, Saykin AJ, McAllister TW. Functional MRI of mild traumatic brain injury (mTBI): progress and perspectives from the first decade of studies. Brain Imaging Behav 2012;6(2):193–207.

107. Tshibanda L, Vanhaudenhuyse A, Galanaud D, et al. Magnetic resonance spectroscopy and diffusion tensor imaging in coma survivors: promises and pitfalls. Prog Brain Res 2009;177:215–29.

108. Byrnes KR, Wilson CM, Brabazon F, et al. FDG-PET imaging in mild traumatic brain injury: a critical review. Front Neuroenergetics 2013;5:13.

109. Raji CA, Tarzwell R, Pavel D, et al. Clinical utility of SPECT neuroimaging in the diagnosis and treatment of traumatic brain injury: a systematic review. PLoS One 2014;9(3):e91088.

110. Turner RC, Lucke-Wold BP, Robson MJ, et al. Repetitive traumatic brain injury and development of chronic traumatic encephalopathy: a potential role for biomarkers in diagnosis, prognosis, and treatment? Front Neurol 2012;3:186.

111. Mondello S, Schmid K, Berger RP, et al. The challenge of mild traumatic brain injury: role of biochemical markers in diagnosis of brain damage. Med Res Rev 2014;34(3):503–31.

112. Shahim P, Tegner Y, Wilson DH, et al. Blood biomarkers for brain injury in concussed professional ice hockey players. JAMA Neurol 2014;71(6):684–92.

113. Siman R, Shahim P, Tegner Y, et al. Serum SNTF increases in concussed professional ice hockey players and relates to the severity of postconcussion symptoms. J Neurotrauma 2015;32(17):1294–300.

114. Mondello S, Jeromin A, Buki A, et al. Glial neuronal ratio: a novel index for differentiating injury type in patients with severe traumatic brain injury. J Neurotrauma 2012;29(6):1096–104.

115. Cherry JD, Stein TD, Tripodis Y, et al. CCL11 is increased in the CNS in chronic traumatic encephalopathy but not in Alzheimer's disease. PLoS One 2017;12(9): e0185541.

116. Gandy S, Ikonomovic MD, Mitsis E, et al. Chronic traumatic encephalopathy: clinical-biomarker correlations and current concepts in pathogenesis. Mol Neurodegener 2014;9:37.

117. Ganz DA, Bao Y, Shekelle PG, et al. Will my patient fall? JAMA 2007;297(1): 77–86.

118. Luz C, Bush T, Shen X. Do canes or walkers make any difference? Nonuse and fall injuries. Gerontologist 2017;57(2):211–8.

119. Tinetti ME. Preventing falls in elderly persons. N Engl J Med 2003;348(1): 42–9.

120. Frank C, Weir E. Deprescribing for older patients. CMAJ 2014;186(18):1369–76.

121. Daneshvar DH, Baugh CM, Nowinski CJ, et al. Helmets and mouth guards: the role of personal equipment in preventing sport-related concussions. Clin Sports Med 2011;30(1):145–63.

122. Swartz EE, Broglio SP, Cook SB, et al. Early results of a helmetless-tackling intervention to decrease head impacts in football players. J Athl Train 2015;50(12): 1219–22.

123. Plantier D, Luauté J. Drugs for behavior disorders after traumatic brain injury: systematic review and expert consensus leading to French recommendations for good practice. Ann Phys Rehabil Med 2016;59(1):42–57.

124. Yue JK, Burke JF, Upadhyayula PS, et al. Selective serotonin reuptake inhibitors for treating neurocognitive and neuropsychiatric disorders following traumatic brain injury: an evaluation of current evidence. Brain Sci 2017; 7(8) [pii:E93].

125. Jorge RE, Acion L, Burin DI, et al. Sertraline for preventing mood disorders following traumatic brain injury: a randomized clinical trial. JAMA Psychiatry 2016;73(10):1041–7.

126. Luaute J, Plantier D, Wiart L, et al. Care management of the agitation or aggressiveness crisis in patients with TBI. Systematic review of the literature and practice recommendations. Ann Phys Rehabil Med 2016;59(1):58–67.

127. Fleminger S, Greenwood RJ, Oliver DL. Pharmacological management for agitation and aggression in people with acquired brain injury. Cochrane Database Syst Rev 2006;(4):CD003299.

128. Lombard LA, Zafonte RD. Agitation after traumatic brain injury: considerations and treatment options. Am J Phys Med Rehabil 2005;84(10):797–812.

129. Leone H, Polsonetti BW. Amantadine for traumatic brain injury: does it improve cognition and reduce agitation? J Clin Pharm Ther 2005;30(2):101–4.

130. Giacino JT, Whyte J, Bagiella E, et al. Placebo-controlled trial of amantadine for severe traumatic brain injury. N Engl J Med 2012;366(9):819–26.

131. Loane DJ, Pocivavsek A, Moussa CEH, et al. Amyloid precursor protein secretases as therapeutic targets for traumatic brain injury. Nat Med 2009;15(4): 377–9.

132. Tsaousides T, Gordon WA. Cognitive rehabilitation following traumatic brain injury: assessment to treatment. Mt Sinai J Med 2009;76(2):173–81.

133. LoBue C, Cullum CM, Didehbani N, et al. Neurodegenerative dementias after traumatic brain injury. J Neuropsychiatry Clin Neurosci 2018. https://doi.org/10.1176/appi.neuropsych.17070145.

Behavioral Problems and Dementia

Ladislav Volicer, MD, PhD*

KEYWORDS

- Dementia • Behavior • Agitation • Apathy • Rejection of care • Depression
- Psychosis

KEY POINTS

- Main consequences of dementia are functional impairment and in some cases also mood disorders and psychosis.
- Main behavioral problems in people with dementia are apathy, agitation, and rejection of care/aggression.
- Agitation and rejection of care/aggression are 2 different syndromes requiring different symptom management.
- Physical causes of behavioral symptoms, for example, pain, should be investigated and eliminated before concluding that they are caused by dementia.
- Nonpharmacologic interventions should be the first strategy used in the management of behavioral symptoms of dementia.

INTRODUCTION

Behavioral and psychological symptoms of dementia are common, and a recent study found that they occur in up to 90% of people living in residential care facilities.[1] These symptoms are often more disturbing than cognitive impairment and are associated with increased health care use, earlier institutionalization,[2] excess morbidity and mortality, greater caregiver distress, and depression.[3] Behavioral symptoms caused by dementia have 3 main consequences: functional impairment, which is necessary to be present for diagnosis of dementia, and in some people also mood disorders and psychosis (**Fig. 1**). The 3 main consequences, alone or in combination, lead to secondary and peripheral symptoms. It is a mistake to treat peripheral symptoms instead of addressing the primary dementia consequences. For instance, treating insomnia with hypnotics, instead of providing meaningful activity that keeps the person with dementia awake during the day, or using benzodiazepines for treatment of anxiety instead of treating depression.

Disclosure: The author has nothing to disclose.
University of South Florida, Tampa, FL, USA
* 2337 Dekan Lane, Land O'Lakes, FL 34639.
E-mail address: lvolicer@usf.edu

Clin Geriatr Med 34 (2018) 637–651
https://doi.org/10.1016/j.cger.2018.06.009
0749-0690/18/© 2018 Elsevier Inc. All rights reserved.

geriatric.theclinics.com

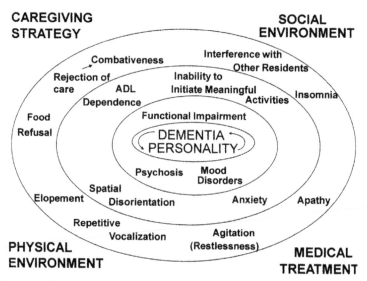

Fig. 1. Hierarchy of behavioral symptoms of dementia. ADL, activities of daily living. (*Modified from* Mahoney E, Volicer L, Hurley AC. Management of challenging behaviors in dementia. Baltimore (MD): Health Profession Press; 2000; with permission.)

Behavioral symptoms may be modified by changes in a person's personality. Personality changes may occur before dementia diagnosis and differ according to type of dementia.[4] In Alzheimer disease, there is an increase of neuroticism, decline in extraversion, and decline in conscientiousness scores. In fronto-temporal dementia, personality changes include loss of empathy, inappropriateness of affect, and behavioral disinhibition. In addition, in contrast to Alzheimer disease, they may have stereotypic behavior, change in food preference, and loss of social awareness. Persons who have dementia with Lewy bodies have frequently apathy, diminished emotional responsiveness, and purposeless hyperactivity, and they relinquish hobbies. Personality changes in vascular dementia include apathy, disinhibition, and accentuation of previous traits, such as egocentricity, paranoid attitudes, and irritability.

Behavioral symptoms of dementia also depend on environmental influences. Caregiving strategy may precipitate or prevent rejection of care, and social environment may precipitate or prevent problematic interaction with other residents. There is an advantage of having on a unit only residents with dementia, because they are less bothered by another resident entering their room than would residents who are cognitively intact. Physical environment should be safe for residents to wander and prevent elopement. Finally, medical treatment may precipitate behavioral problems because persons with dementia may not understand their need and purpose and may resist care providers.

There are many problematic behaviors in persons with dementia, as shown in **Box 1**, which lists behaviors evaluated by one of the most commonly used scale: Cohen-Mansfield Agitation Inventory.[5] However, most of these behaviors could be considered part of 2 behavioral syndromes: agitation and rejection of care, which are most common in nursing home residents.[6] Another most common behavioral syndrome, occurring in most persons with dementia, is apathy. Therefore, this article concentrates on description and suggestions for treatment of apathy, agitation, and rejection of care.

Box 1
Cohen-Mansfield Agitation Inventory (CMAI)

Physical/Aggressive
1. Hitting (including self)
2. Kicking
3. Grabbing onto people
4. Pushing
5. Throwing things
6. Biting
7. Scratching
8. Spitting
9. Hurting self or others
10. Tearing things or destroying property
11. Making physical sexual advances

Physical/Nonaggressive
12. Pace, aimless wandering
13. Inappropriate dress or disrobing
14. Trying to get to a different place
15. Intentional falling
16. Eating/drinking inappropriate substance
17. Handling things inappropriately
18. Hiding things
19. Hoarding things
20. Performing repetitive mannerisms
21. General restlessness

Verbal/Aggressive
22. Screaming
23. Making verbal sexual advances
24. Cursing or verbal aggression

Verbal/Nonaggressive
25. Repetitive sentences or questions
26. Strange noises (weird laughter or crying)
27. Complaining
28. Negativism
29. Constant unwarranted request for attention or help

From Cohen-Mansfield J. Instruction Manual for Jiska Cohen-Mansfield Agitation Inventory (CMAI). 1991. Available at: https://shine-dementia.wikispaces.com/file/view/Cohen-Mansfield+Agitation+Inventory+(CMAI).pdf; with permission. © Cohen-Mansfield.

APATHY

Management of apathy is a very important issue, because many residents suffer from this syndrome that decreases quality of life.[7] In Alzheimer disease, apathy is the most common behavioral syndrome.[8] It may occur already in people with mild cognitive impairment (MCI)[9] and it occurs in 27% of individuals with dementia living in the community.[10] The prevalence of apathy increases with progression of dementia,[11,12] and it is present in up to 92% of patients with advanced dementia.[13]

Apathy may be a behavioral marker of a more aggressive dementia, characterized by a faster progression of cognitive, functional, and emotional impairment[14] and could indicate elevated risk of progression of MCI into dementia, especially in people with Apolipoprotein E4.[12] Apathy is related to neurofibrillary tangles in the anterior cingulate[15] and to reduced perfusion in the left anterior cingulate, right inferior and medial gyrus frontalis, and left orbitofrontal gyrus and right gyrus lingualis.[16]

Apathy also occurs in dementia with Lewy bodies[11] and in Parkinson disease without dementia.[17] Caregivers' reports of apathy may predict progression to dementia.[18] Apathy is a common feature of Huntington disease, in almost 25% of presymptomatic individuals, and the prevalence increases to approximately 50% in the late stage of the disease.[19] In amyotrophic lateral sclerosis, apathy is characterized by decreased initiation apathy and less emotional apathy.[20] Apathy is also a significant syndrome in alcohol-related dementia.[21]

Apathy in vascular dementia depends on the site of the lesion. Lesions in the anterior thalamic radiation were related to apathy in MCI.[22] Deep white matter lesions cause apathetic behavior even in community-dwelling elderly subjects without dementia,[23] and in a behavioral variant of frontotemporal dementia.[24] Vascular lesions also may be responsible for occurrence of apathy in persons with type 2 diabetes.[25]

People with apathy are sometimes considered to be depressed. However, it is now well recognized that apathy is a separate syndrome from depression, although these 2 conditions often occur simultaneously.[26] Depression may cause loss of interest and diminished activity, but is perceived as sadness. In contrast, apathy is a neutral experience for the apathetic person because it is an emotional deficit state (**Table 1**).

Table 1
Criteria for diagnosis of apathy
For a Diagnosis of Apathy, the Patient Should Fulfill the Criteria A, B, C, and D
A	Loss of or diminished motivation in comparison with the patient's previous level of functioning and that is not consistent with his or her age or culture. These changes in motivation may be reported by the patient himself or herself, or by the observations of others.
B	Presence of at least 1 symptom in at least 2 of the 3 following domains for a period of at least 4 wk and present most of the time. *Domain B1:* Loss of, or diminished, goal-directed behavior as evidenced by at least 1 of the following: loss of self-initiated behavior (for example, starting conversation, doing basic tasks of day-to-day living, seeking social activities, communicating choices), loss of environment-stimulated behavior (for example, responding to conversation, participating in social activities). *Domain B2:* Loss of, or diminished, goal-directed cognitive activity as evidenced by at least 1 of the following: loss of spontaneous ideas and curiosity for routine and new events (ie, challenging tasks, recent news, social opportunities, personal/family and social affairs), loss of environment-stimulated ideas and curiosity for routine and new events (ie, in the person's residence, neighborhood, or community). *Domain B3:* Loss of, or diminished, emotion as evidenced by at least 1 of the following: loss of spontaneous emotion, observed or self-reported (for example, subjective feeling of weak or absent emotions, or observation by others of a blunted affect), loss of emotional responsiveness to positive or negative stimuli or events (for example, observer-reports of unchanging affect, or of little emotional reaction to exciting events, personal loss, serious illness, emotional-laden news).
C	These symptoms (A–B) cause clinically significant impairment in personal, social, occupational, or other important areas of functioning.
D	The symptoms (A–B) are not exclusively explained or due to physical disabilities (eg, blindness and loss of hearing), to motor disabilities, to diminished level of consciousness, or to the direct physiologic effects of a substance (eg, drug of abuse, a medication).

From Robert P, Onyike CU, Leentjens AF, et al. Proposed diagnostic criteria for apathy in Alzheimer's disease and other neuropsychiatric disorders. Eur Psychiatry 2009;24:101; with permission.

Apathy influences daily functioning more than depression and may, therefore, require increased need for help from the caregivers.[9] In addition to different symptomatology and their independent effects on quality of life, there is also evidence from neuropathological studies indicating that apathy is associated with brain small blood vessel disease, whereas depression is not associated with this condition.[27] In addition, another study with patients after stroke showed that apathy, but not depression, was correlated negatively with functional improvement after rehabilitation.[28]

Apathy also has been shown to be associated with increased caregiver burden in patients with Alzheimer disease and other patients with dementia.[28] Apathy is significantly related to reduced independent activities of daily living, survival duration after nursing home admission, and poor outcomes in rehabilitation.[29] It has strong association with mortality, negative impact on disability, management of other diseases,[30] and may cause increased weight loss.[31]

TREATMENT OF APATHY

Apathy is a common disorder, but can be easily overlooked because the apathetic person does not cause problems for his or her care providers. Research has indicated that apathy is associated with various adverse outcomes but seems to be treatable. Because there no medications that are specifically approved for treatment of apathy, nonpharmacologic interventions should be used.

Nonpharmacologic strategies do not have to be specific for apathy, and various therapeutic activities are effective.[29] The type of activities is not as important as quality and duration. Ideally, activities should be tailored to the severity of dementia and provided as a continuous activity programming, 7 days a week.[32] Therapeutic activities should be person-centered and benefit all residents. Presence of apathy in a resident population could indicate insufficient activity programming in this setting. Providing activity for residents with advanced dementia is especially important because they are often isolated in their rooms, placed by a nursing station, or placed on the periphery of an activity in which they cannot participate. Specialized programs, for example, Namaste Care, which takes place in a pleasant environment and provides activities with loving touch approach, may decrease apathy in residents with advanced dementia.[33] This program is described in more detail in the section on rejection of care.

Additional programs that decreased apathy include the lifestyle engagement activity program (LEAP),[34] environmental modifications,[35] and the use of social robots.[36] The LEAP program trains case managers to set meaningful social and/or recreational goals, and trains care workers in good communication, and promotion of residents' independence and choice. The program significantly decreased apathy and increased engagement.[34] An environment modification study found that clarity and strength of environmental stimulation were significantly associated with lower apathy levels.[35] A study investigating social robots used humanoid and pet robots. This study found that both robots decreased apathy but also increased delusions in the group treated with the humanoid robot and increased irritability in both robot groups.[36]

Pharmacologic Treatment

There is no medication that is specifically approved for treatment of apathy. Early studies reported some effectiveness of cholinesterase inhibitors[28] and memantine[37] for treatment of apathy, but later studies could not replicate these results.[38] However, one study found the combination of donepezil with a cholinergic precursor (choline alphoscerate) decreased apathy scores.[39,40] Two studies reported beneficial effect of methyphenidate.[41,42] Discontinuation of antipsychotics may decrease apathy, but low doses of atypical antipsychotics may actually decrease apathy.[37] Although discontinuation of antipsychotics may decrease apathy, low doses of atypical antipsychotics may also decrease apathy.[43]

AGITATION

Development of strategies for management of behavioral symptoms of dementia is hindered by confusing terminology. Many investigators consider behavioral and psychological symptoms of dementia to be a singular phenomenon, using the abbreviation BPSD. This approach assumes that all of these symptoms may be improved by the same strategy.

Other investigators call all behavioral symptoms of dementia agitation[44] (see **Box 1**). Using factor analysis, they divided these symptoms into physically aggressive symptoms, verbally aggressive symptoms, physically nonaggressive symptoms, and verbally nonaggressive symptoms. The main problem of this system is that it labels people with dementia aggressive. This "aggressive" behavior is in most cases caused by rejection of care, when the person with dementia does not understand the need for care or misinterprets the carer's intention. If the carer insists on providing care, the person with dementia defends himself or herself from this unwanted attention and may become combative. This could be called reactive aggression, as is described in more detail later in this article.

The confusing terminology is further complicated by the Neuropsychiatric Inventory scale, which labels one domain Agitation/Aggression. The probing questions for this domain are "Does the resident have periods when he/she refuses to let people help him/her? Is he/she hard to handle? Is he/she noisy or uncooperative? Does the resident attempt to hurt or hit others?" indicating that the domain is actually asking about rejection of care that may sometimes escalate into reactive aggression. Behaviors that represent actual agitation are measured in this scale by domains called Disinhibition and Aberrant Motor Behavior.

The distinction between rejection of care and agitation is supported by different relationships of these syndromes to dementia severity. Agitation may occur in the early stages of dementia, and the prevalence remains the same, whereas rejection of care starts in moderate dementia and increases as the dementia progresses (**Fig. 2**). This increase is parallel with a decrease of the ability of persons with dementia to understand their care providers. This indicates that lack of understanding is a major factor in rejection of care.[45] The distinction between rejection of care and agitation is very important, because nonpharmacologic management strategies differ in these 2 conditions, as is described later in this article.

There are several definitions of agitation in the literature,[46] and the best is considered to be "motor restlessness, heightened responsivity to stimuli, irritability, inappropriate and/or purposeless verbal or motor activity, decreased sleep, and fluctuation of symptoms over time."[47] Agitation may be caused or enhanced by physical, environmental, or psychiatric conditions.

Physical Conditions

Several physical conditions may trigger agitation. They include hunger, thirst, physical illnesses (congestive heart failure, chronic obstructive pulmonary disease, brain tumors, infection, anemia), and metabolic disorders (renal failure, dehydration, hyponatremia, acid-base disturbance, hypoglycemia or hyperglycemia, hepatic failure,

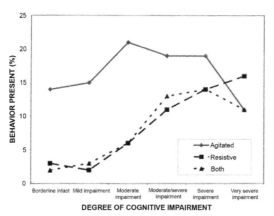

Fig. 2. Relationships between cognitive impairment and behavioral symptoms of dementia. (*From* Volicer L, Bass EA, Luther SL. Agitation and resistiveness to care are two separate behavioral syndromes of dementia. J Am Med Dir Assoc 2007;8:529; with permission.)

thyroid dysfunction, hypercalcemia), but the most prevalent is pain. Pain is very common in nursing home residents with dementia. A survey of 181 nursing home residents with dementia in Norway found that pain intensity greater than 0 on a 10-cm visual analog scale[48] was observed in 141 (78%) patients, and 3 or higher in 98 (54%) patients. Approximately 37% of mentally healthy controls received opioid analgesics, compared with 24% of the patients with severe dementia.[49] Another recent study found that 58% of residents with dementia had persistent pain.[50]

Treatment of pain was reported to decrease agitation[51] but recent meta-analysis of studies concerning pain, neuropsychiatric symptoms, and physical function found that the relationship of pain and agitation may be more complicated. The studies found association between pain and depression and longitudinal studies suggested that the effect of pain on neuropsychiatric symptoms is mediated by depression.[52] These results support the important role depression plays in development of agitation as is further described later in this article.

Environmental Factors

Environmental factors may precipitate development of agitation, but may also decrease or prevent agitated behavior. Factors that may precipitate agitation include exit control, which residents with dementia do not understand and try to overcome, sound levels,[53] restraints and lack of an individual space, and uncomfortable temperatures. Factors that decrease or prevent agitation include small-scale, homelike facilities,[54] and availability of outdoor spaces with safe walking paths.[55]

A recent review of articles discussing environmental design for dementia care concluded that there are 6 areas that need to be addressed: (1) organization of space (allowing residents to use the space according to their norm and values), (2) space-induced social cohesion (facilitation of social relationships and caring for residents), (3) residential or institutional ambiance, (4) privacy (space allowing use according to intimate and personal characteristics of the residents), (5) display of care (space allowing balance of relationship between residents and staff, including assistance, authority, collaboration, and empathy), and (6) control-attention (supervision of residents ensuring their safety, attention of staff toward residents overseeing their relationship with each other and the environment).[56]

Psychiatric Conditions

Two important conditions in persons with dementia are depression and delusions/hallucinations. Depression is very common, in up to 50% of residents with dementia, whereas delusions/hallucinations are present in 15% of them.[57] The importance of depression for the development of agitation was documented in a longitudinal study (**Fig. 3**). Using the Minimum Data Set (MDS), the subjects were divided into 4 groups according to the changes of agitation during the analysis period. The first group had agitation scores lower on the first assessment than on the last assessment (agitation increased), the second group had higher agitation score on the first assessment than on the last assessment (agitation decreased), the third group exhibited agitation on both the first and last assessments (stable problem), and the fourth group did not exhibit agitation on either the first or the last assessment (no problem). In all groups, the agitation scores for the second and third assessment were intermediate between the first and last assessment. Depression scores were significantly higher in the stable problem group than in no problem group. In addition, depression scores increased in the agitation increased group and decreased in the agitation decreased group.[57]

The relationship between agitation and psychotic symptoms (delusions + hallucinations) was similar to the relationship between depression and agitation. In contrast, the pain scores plots did not differ significantly among the 4 agitation groups.[57] Although pain may play a role in agitation in some residents, it was not highly related to agitation in this study. The close relationship of depression and agitation is not surprising, because agitated depression is one of the clinical forms even in cognitively intact individuals.[58]

TREATMENT OF AGITATION

The first step in treatment of agitation should be careful attention to physical and environmental factors. When these factors were excluded, or agitation continued after correction of these factors, the next step should be initiation of meaningful activities because agitation may be precipitated by boredom. Various types of activities are effective, including occupational therapy[59] and individual music,[60] but the most effective are live human stimuli.[61] It is important to provide these activities as continuous

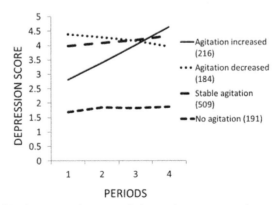

Fig. 3. Relationship between changes of depression scores and severity of agitation. (*From* Volicer L, Frijters DH, Van der Steen JT. Relationship between symptoms of depression and agitation in nursing home residents with dementia. Int J Geriatr Psychiatry 2012;27:751; with permission.)

activity programming instead of isolated sessions. In the interval between sessions, the residents wander, have undesirable interaction with each other, and are prone to falls.[32]

If activity programs are unable to improve agitation, pharmacologic treatments should be considered. Because of the important relationship between agitation and depression, antidepressant treatment should be considered. If there is evidence that the resident is bothered by unpleasant delusions or hallucinations, antipsychotics may be indicated. Atypical antipsychotics, for example, aripiprazole, also may be useful to augment antidepressant treatment effects. However, antipsychotics should not be the first line medication without evidence of delusion and hallucinations because of significant side effects.[62] Benzodiazepines are not recommended for treatment of agitation because there is no good evidence for their effectiveness and they may increase confusion and falls.[63]

AGGRESSION

Aggression is overt behavior of animals or humans involving intent to harm another organism or inanimate object.[64] It is possible to distinguish 2 types of aggression based on motivation: proactive and reactive aggression. Proactive aggression is defined as behavior that anticipates a reward and involves planning and premeditation, whereas reactive aggression is an impulsive aggressive response to a perceived threat, loss, danger, or provocation.[65,66] Persons with dementia rarely exhibit proactive aggression, because their executive function is impaired. However, they may exhibit reactive aggression as a response to care approaches that they do not understand or that are causing discomfort or pain. This behavior may be a consequence of rejection of care (resistiveness to care in the MDS 2.0), which may escalate into combative behavior if the carer insists in providing care despite defensive behavior of the care recipient.

In agreement with this concept, we have found by analysis of MDS 2.0 data that lack of understanding was one of the most important factors leading to resistiveness to care that leads to abusive behavior (or behavior directed toward others, in the MDS 3.0) (**Fig. 4**).[67] The second important factor was depression, which in addition to increasing resistiveness to care may also lead to physical and verbal abuse in residents who are not resistive to care. Resistiveness to care is also increased by delusions and hallucinations, but their relationship with resistiveness to care is less significant. In this study, we did not find significant relationship between pain and resistiveness to care, but another study found that pain was associated with verbal and physical aggression in residents who could not articulate their pain.[68] This finding stresses the importance of communication in rejection of care and abusive behavior.

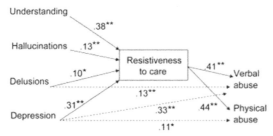

Fig. 4. Factors leading to abusive behavior in residents with dementia. * P <.05; ** P <.01. (*From* Volicer L, Van der Steen JT, Frijters DH. Modifiable factors related to abusive behaviors in nursing home residents with dementia. J Am Med Dir Assoc 2009;10:619; with permission.)

Table 2
Communication tips for Alzheimer disease (AD)

Mild AD	Moderate AD	Severe AD
• Don't make assumptions about a person's ability to communicate because of an Alzheimer diagnosis. The disease affects each person differently.	• Allow time for response so the person can think about what he or she wants to say.	• Treat the person with dignity and respect. Avoid talking down to the person or as if he or she isn't there.
• Don't exclude the person with the disease from conversations with others.	• Engage the person in one-on-one conversation in a quiet space that has minimal distractions.	• Approach the person from the front and identify yourself.
• Speak directly to the person if you want to know how he or she is doing.	• Be patient and supportive. Offering comfort and reassurance can encourage the person to explain his or her thoughts.	• Encourage nonverbal communication. If you don't understand what is being said, ask the person to point or gesture.
• Take time to listen to how the person is feeling, what he or she is thinking or may need.	• Maintain eye contact. It shows you care about what he or she is saying.	• Sometimes the emotions being expressed are more important than what is being said. Look for the feelings behind words or sounds.
• Give the person time to respond. Don't interrupt or finish sentences unless he or she asks for help finding a word or finishing a sentence.	• Avoid criticizing or correcting. Instead, listen and try to find the meaning in what is being said. Repeat what was said to clarify.	• Use touch, sights, sounds, smells, and tastes as a form of communication with the person.
• Talk with the person about what he or she is still comfortable doing and what he or she may need help with.	• Avoid arguing. If the person says something you don't agree with, let it be.	• It's OK if you don't know what to do or say; your presence and friendship are most important to the person.
• Explore which method of communication is most comfortable for the person. This could include face-to-face conversations, e-mail, or phone calls.	• Don't overwhelm the person with lengthy requests. Offer clear, step-by-step instructions for tasks.	
• It's OK to laugh. Sometimes humor lightens the mood and makes communication easier.	• Speak slowly and clearly.	
• Be honest and frank about your feelings. Don't pull away; your friendship and support are important to the person.	• Ask "yes" or "no" questions. For example, "Would you like some coffee?" rather than "What would you like to drink?"	
	• Ask one question at a time.	
	• Give visual cues. To help demonstrate the task, point or touch the item you want the individual to use. Or, begin the task for the person.	
	• Written notes can be helpful when a spoken word seems confusing.	

From Alzheimer's Association. Communication and Alzheimer's. Available at: https://www.alz.org/help-support/caregiving/daily-care/communications. Accessed July 26, 2018; with permission.

This was also supported by a longitudinal study that found that lack of understanding and depression are important factors in development of rejection of care and behaviors directed toward others.[69]

TREATMENT OF AGGRESSION

The first strategy for management of aggression should be nonpharmacologic approaches, which should concentrate on efforts to improve communication. Communication style should consider the severity of dementia (**Table 2**). Communication with people who have dementia may be improved by training the caregiving staff,[70] but this strategy is not always effective.[71] Communication also could be improved by using cognitive-linguistic stimulation in people with dementia.[72] Another strategy for management of rejection of care is changing the type of caregiving intervention. For instance, substituting bed bath for shower that the resident did not like.[73]

Nonverbal communication could be improved by massage therapy. Although there is only limited evidence for effectiveness of massage in general,[74] there is some evidence that frequent limited massage could decrease significantly rejection of care and combative behavior.[75] A program called Namaste Care[76] combined massage of hands, feet, and scalp with a pleasant environment, and significantly decreased rejection of care. Caregivers reported that the residents became more tactile and the pleasant touch during Namaste Care sessions made them more accepting of touch during bathing and other activities of daily living.

If nonpharmacologic interventions are not effective, pharmacologic treatment may be necessary. There is some evidence that cholinesterase inhibitors and memantine may help in addressing communication difficulties,[72] but in view of the strong relationship between abusive behavior and depression, described previously, antidepressant treatment should be considered. If the resident exhibits delusions and/or hallucinations that are troublesome for her or him, antipsychotic treatment is indicated. Second-generation antipsychotics may be also indicated to augment the effect of antidepressants.[77]

SUMMARY

Management of behavioral symptoms of dementia is important to preserve quality of life of persons with dementia and their care providers. Although there are several kinds of behavioral symptoms, the most common are agitation and aggression. It is important to distinguish these 2 syndromes because nonpharmacologic strategy for their management differs. Depression is related to both syndromes and, therefore, antidepressant therapy may be considered.

REFERENCES

1. Loi SM, Lautenschlager NT. Investigating the current methods of assessing behavioral and psychological symptoms in residential aged care facilities in a metropolitan city. Int Psychogeriatr 2017;29:855–8.

2. Phillips VL, Diwan S. The incremental effect of dementia-related problem behaviors on the time to nursing home placement in poor, frail, demented older people. J Am Geriatr Soc 2003;51:188–93.

3. Kales HC, Gitlin LN, Lyketsos CG, et al. Management of neuropsychiatric symptoms of dementia in clinical settings: recommendations from a multidisciplinary expert panel. J Am Geriatr Soc 2014;62:762–9.

4. Cipriani G, Borin G, Del Debbio A, et al. Personality and dementia. J Nerv Ment Dis 2015;203:210–4.

5. Cohen-Mansfield J. Instruction manual for Jiska Cohen-Mansfield agitation inventory (CMAI). 1991. Available at: https://shine-dementia.wikispaces.com/file/view/Cohen-Mansfield+Agitation+Inventory+(CMAI).pdf. Accessed July 24, 2018.

6. Cohen-Mansfield J, Jensen B. Physicians' perceptions of their role in treating dementia-related behavior problems in the nursing home: actual practice and the ideal. J Am Med Dir Assoc 2008;9:552–7.

7. Mjorud M, Kirkevold M, Rosvik J, et al. Variables associated to quality of life among nursing home patients with dementia. Aging Ment Health 2014;18: 1013–21.

8. Landes AM, Sperry SD, Strauss ME, et al. Apathy in Alzheimer's disease. J Am Geriatr Soc 2001;49:1700–7.

9. Zahodne LB, Tremont G. Unique effects of apathy and depression signs on cognition and function in amnestic mild cognitive impairment. Int J Geriatr Psychiatry 2013;28:50–6.

10. Lyketsos CG, Steinberg M, Tschanz JT, et al. Mental and behavioral disturbances in dementia: findings from the Cache County study on memory in aging. Am J Psychiatry 2000;157:708–14.

11. Brodaty H, Connors MH, Xu J, et al. Prime study group. The course of neuropsychiatric symptoms in dementia: a 3-year longitudinal study. J Am Med Dir Assoc 2015;16:380–7.

12. Stella F, Laks J, Govone JS, et al. Association of neuropsychiatric syndromes with global clinical deterioration in Alzheimer's disease patients. Int Psychogeriatr 2016;28:786.

13. Mega MS, Cummings JL, Fiorello T, et al. The spectrum of behavioral changes in Alzheimer's disease. Neurology 1996;46:130–5.

14. Starkstein SE, Jorge R, Mizrahi R, et al. A prospective longitudinal study of apathy in Alzheimer's disease. J Neurol Neurosurg Psychiatry 2006;77:8–11.

15. Tekin S, Mega MS, Masterman DM, et al. Orbitofrontal and anterior cingulate cortex neurofibrillary tangle burden is associated with agitation in Alzheimer disease. Ann Neurol 2001;49:355–61.

16. Benoit M, Koulibaly PM, Migneco O, et al. Brain perfusion in Alzheimer's disease with and without apathy: a SPECT study with statistical parametric mapping analysis. Psychiatry Res Neuroimaging 2002;114:103–11.

17. Wang F, Yu SY, Zuo LJ, et al. Excessive iron and a-synuclein oligomer in brain are relevant to pure apathy in Parkinson disease. J Geriatr Psychiatry Neurol 2016; 29(4):187–94.

18. Fitts W, Weintraub D, Massimo L, et al. Caregiver report of apathy predicts dementia in Parkinson's disease. Parkinsonism Relat Disord 2015;21:992–5.

19. Mason S, Barker RA. Rating apathy in Huntington's disease: patients and companions agree. J Huntingtons Dis 2015;4:49–59.

20. Radakovic R, Stephenson L, Colville S, et al. Multidimensional apathy in ALS: validation of the dimensional apathy scale. J Neurol Neurosurg Psychiatry 2016. https://doi.org/10.1136/jnnp-2015-310772.

21. Mulders AJ, Fick IW, Bor H, et al. Prevalence and correlates of neuropsychiatric symptoms in nursing home patients with young-onset dementia: the BEYOnD study. J Am Med Dir Assoc 2016;17(6):495–500.

22. Torso M, Serra L, Giulietti G, et al. Strategic lesions in the anterior thalamic radiation and apathy in early Alzheimer's disease. PLoS One 2015;10:e0124998.

23. Yao H, Takashima Y, Araki Y, et al. Leisure-time physical inactivity associated with vascular depression or apathy in community-dwelling elderly subjects: the Sefuri study. J Stroke Cerebrovasc Dis 2015;24:2625–31.

24. Powers JP, Massimo L, McMillan CT, et al. White matter disease contributes to apathy and disinhibition in behavioral variant frontotemporal dementia. Cogn Behav Neurol 2014;27:206–14.

25. Bruce DG, Nelson ME, Mace JL, et al. Apathy in older patients with type 2 diabetes. Am J Geriatr Psychiatry 2015;23:615–21.

26. Mortby ME, Maercker A, Forstmeier S. Apathy: a separate syndrome from depression in dementia? A critical review. Aging Clin Exp Res 2012;24:305–16.

27. Hollocks MJ, Lawrence AJ, Brookes RL, et al. Differential relationships between apathy and depression with white matter microstructural changes and functional outcomes. Brain 2015;138:3803–15.

28. Ishii S, Weintraub N, Mervis JR. Apathy: a common psychiatric syndrome in the elderly. J Am Med Dir Assoc 2009;10:381–93.

29. Brodaty H, Burns K. Nonpharmacological management of apathy in dementia: a systematic review. Am J Geriatr Psychiatry 2012;20:549–64.

30. van der Linde RM, Matthews FE, Dening T, et al. Patterns and persistence of behavioural and psychological symptoms in those with cognitive impairment: the importance of apathy. Int J Geriatr Psychiatry 2016;32(3):306–15.

31. Volicer L, Frijters DH, Van der Steen JT. Apathy and weight loss in nursing home residents: longitudinal study. J Am Med Dir Assoc 2013;14:417–20.

32. Volicer L, Simard J, Pupa JH, et al. Effects of continuous activity programming on behavioral symptoms of dementia. J Am Med Dir Assoc 2006;7:426–31.

33. Simard J. The end-of-life Namaste Care program for people with dementia. Baltimore (MD): Health Professions Press; 2007.

34. Low LF, Baker JR, Harrison F, et al. The lifestyle engagement activity program (LEAP): implementing social and recreational activity into case-managed home care. J Am Med Dir Assoc 2015;16:1069–76.

35. Jao YL, Algase DL, Specht JK, et al. The association between characteristics of care environments and apathy in residents with dementia in long-term care facilities. Gerontologist 2015;55:S27–39.

36. Valenti Soler M, Aguera-Ortiz L, Olazaran Rodriquez J, et al. Social robots in advanced dementia. Front Aging Neurosci 2015;7:133.

37. Berman K, Brodaty H, Withall A, et al. Pharmacologic treatment of apathy in dementia. Am J Geriatr Psychiatry 2012;20:104–22.

38. Harrison F, Aerts L, Brodaty H. Apathy in dementia: systematic review of recent evidence on pharmacological treatments. Curr Psychiatry Rep 2016;18:103.

39. Peters ME, Vaidya V, Drye LT, et al. Citalopram for the treatment of agitation in Alzheimer dementia: genetic influences. J Geriatr Psychiatry Neurol 2016;29:59–64.

40. Rea R, Carotenuto A, Traini E, et al. Apathy treatment in Alzheimer's disease: interim results of the ASCOMALVA trial. J Alzheimers Dis 2015;48:377–83.

41. Rosenberg PB, Lanctot KL, Drye LT, et al. Safety and efficacy of methylphenidate for apathy in Alzheimer's disease: a randomized, placebo-controlled trial. J Clin Psychiatry 2013;74:810–6.

42. Lancot KL, Chau SA, Herrmann N, et al. Effect of methylphenidate on attention in apathetic AD patients in a randomized, placebo-controlled trial. Int Psychogeriatr 2014;26:239–46.

43. Padala PR, Padala KP, Monga V, et al. Reversal of SSRI-associated apathy syndrome by discontinuation of therapy. Ann Pharmacother 2012;46:e8.

44. Cohen-Mansfield J, Marx MS, Rosenthal AS. A description of agitation in a nursing home. J Gerontol 1989;44:M77–84.

45. Volicer L, Bass EA, Luther SL. Agitation and resistiveness to care are two separate behavioral syndromes of dementia. J Am Med Dir Assoc 2007;8:527–32.

46. Volicer L, Citrome L, Volavka J. Measurement of agitation and aggression in adult and aged neuropsychiatric patients: review of definitions and frequently used measurement scales. CNS Spectr 2017;22:407–14.

47. Lindenmayer JP. The pathophysiology of agitation. J Clin Psychiatry 2000;61: 5–10.

48. Husebo BS, Strand LI, Moe-Nilssen R, et al. Mobilization-observation-behavior-intensity-dementia pain scale (MOBID): development and validation of a nurse-administered pain assessment tool for use in dementia. J Pain Symptom Manage 2007;34:67–80.

49. Husebo BS, Strand LI, Moe-Nilssen R, et al. Who suffers most? Dementia and pain in nursing home patients: a cross-sectional study. J Am Med Dir Assoc 2008;9:427–43.

50. van Kooten J, Smalbrugge M, van der Wouden JC, et al. Evaluation of a pain assessment procedure in long-term care residents with pain and dementia. J Pain Symptom Manage 2017;54:727–31.

51. Husebo BS, Ballard C, Cohen-Mansfield J, et al. The response of agitated behavior to pain management in persons with dementia. Am J Geriatr Psychiatry 2014;22:708–17.

52. van Dalen-Kok AH, Pieper MJ, de Waal MW, et al. Association between pain, neuropsychiatric symptoms, and physical function in dementia: a systematic review and meta-analysis. BMC Geriatr 2015;19:49.

53. Joosse LL. Do sound levels and space contribute to agitation in nursing home residents with dementia? Res Gerontol Nurs 2012;5:174–84.

54. Verbeek H, Zwakhalen SM, Van Rossum E, et al. Effects of small-scale, home-like facilities in dementia care on residents' behavior, and use of physical restraints and psychotropic drugs: a quasi-experimental study. Int Psychogeriatr 2014; 26:657–68.

55. Whear R, Coon JT, Bethel A, et al. What is the impact of using outdoor spaces such as gardens on the physical and mental well-being of those with dementia? A systematic review of quantitative and qualitative evidence. J Am Med Dir Assoc 2014;15:697–705.

56. Charras K, Eynard C, Viatour G. Use of space and human rights: planning dementia friendly settings. J Gerontol Soc Work 2016;59:181–204.

57. Volicer L, Frijters DH, Van der Steen JT. Relationship between symptoms of depression and agitation in nursing home residents with dementia. Int J Geriatr Psychiatry 2012;27:749–54.

58. Maj M, Pirozzi R, Magliano L, et al. Agitated "unipolar" major depression: prevalence, phenomenology, and outcome. J Clin Psychiatry 2006;67:712–9.

59. Gitlin LN, Arthur P, Piersol C, et al. Targeting behavioral symptoms and functional decline in dementia: a randomized clinical trial. J Am Geriatr Soc 2017. https://doi.org/10.1111/jgs.15194.

60. Sancheza A, Masedaa A, Marante-Moarb MP, et al. Comparing the effects of multisensory stimulation and individualized music sessions on elderly people with severe dementia: a randomized controlled trial. J Alzheimers Dis 2016;52: 303–15.

61. Cohen-Mansfield J, Thein K, Marx MS, et al. The relationships of environment and personal characteristics to agitated behaviors in nursing home residents with dementia. J Clin Psychiatry 2012;73:392–9.

62. Sturm AS, Trinkley KE, Porter K, et al. Efficacy and safety of atypical antipsychotics for behavioral symptoms of dementia among patients residing in long-term care. Int J Clin Pharm 2017. https://doi.org/10.1007/s11096-017-0555-y.

63. Zaman H, Sampson SJ, Beck AL, et al. Benzodiazepines for psychosis-induced aggression or agitation. Cochrane Database Syst Rev 2017;(12):CD003079.

64. Volavka J. Neurobiology of violence. 2nd edition. Washington (DC): American Psychiatric Publishing; 2002.

65. Gardner KJ, Archer J, Jackson S. Does maladaptive coping mediate the relationship between borderline personality traits and reactive and proactive aggression? Aggress Behav 2012;38:403–13.

66. Miller JD, Lynam DR. Reactive and proactive aggression: similarities and difference. Personality and Individual Differences 2006;41:1469–80.

67. Volicer L, Van der Steen JT, Frijters DH. Modifiable factors related to abusive behaviors in nursing home residents with dementia. J Am Med Dir Assoc 2009;10: 617–22.

68. Ahn H, Garvan C, Lyon D. Pain and aggression in nursing home residents with dementia: Minimum Data Set 3.0 analysis. Nurs Res 2015;64:256–63.

69. Galindo-Garre F, Volicer L, Van der Steen JT. Factors related to rejection of care and behaviors directed towards others: a longitudinal study in nursing home residents with dementia. Dement Geriatr Cogn Dis Extra 2015;5:123–34.

70. Bourgeois MS, Dijkstra K, Burgio LD, et al. Communication skills training for nursing aides of residents with dementia. Clin Gerontol 2004;27:119–38.

71. Machiels M, Metzelthin SF, Hamers JP, et al. Interventions to improve communication between people with dementia and nursing staff during daily nursing care: a systematic review. Int J Nurs Stud 2017;66:37–46.

72. Woodward M. Aspects of communication in Alzheimer's disease: clinical features and treatment options. Int Psychogeriatr 2013;25:877–85.

73. Sloane PD, Rader J, Barrick A-L, et al. Bathing person with dementia. Gerontologist 1995;35:672–8.

74. Moyle W, Murfield JE, O'Dwyer S, et al. The effect of massage on agitated behaviours in older people with dementia: a literature review. J Clin Nurs 2013;22: 601–10.

75. Manzar BA, Volicer L. Effects of Namaste Care: pilot study. Am J Alzheim Dis 2015;2:24–37.

76. Simard J. The end-of-life Namaste program for people with dementia. 2nd edition. Baltimore (MD): Health Professions Press; 2013.

77. Papakostas GI, Shelton RC, Smith J, et al. Augmentation of antidepressants with atypical antipsychotic medications for treatment-resistant major depressive disorder: a meta-analysis. J Clin Psychiatry 2007;68:826–31.

Cognitive Stimulation Therapy for Dementia

Harleen Rai, MSc[a],*, Lauren Yates, BSc, PhD[b], Martin Orrell, PhD, FRCPsych[c]

KEYWORDS

- Dementia • Cognitive Stimulation Therapy • CST • Psychological treatment
- Psychosocial intervention • Cognition • Quality of life • Well-being

KEY POINTS

- Cognitive Stimulation Therapy is a psychological treatment for people with mild and moderate dementia.
- It is offered in both a group and individual format showing various benefits on cognitive functioning, quality of life, and quality of the caregiving relationship.
- The intervention provides a fun and meaningful approach toward staying mentally stimulated and engaged.
- The World Alzheimer's Report 2014 recommends Cognitive Stimulation Therapy to be offered routinely to people with dementia around the world.
- In the future, Cognitive Stimulation Therapy based approaches will hopefully grow and be made available to people who want and need it the most.

INTRODUCTION

Cognitive Stimulation Therapy (CST) is a brief psychological treatment for people with mild to moderate dementia. It offers a person-based approach to help people with dementia to stay mentally stimulated and engaged while providing an optimal learning environment. Over the course of 20 years, CST has grown to be widely used with 3 CST manuals published to date. Currently, CST is the only nonpharmacologic therapy

Disclosure Statement: Royalties from the sale of the Making a Difference manuals go to the support of the international CST center at UCL run by Dr Aimee Spector. H. Rai is working with Eumedianet on the development of a web app version of CST as part of her PhD.
[a] Division of Psychiatry and Applied Psychology, Institute of Mental Health, School of Medicine, University of Nottingham, Jubilee Campus, Triumph Road, Nottingham NG7 2TU, UK; [b] Division of Psychiatry and Applied Psychology, Institute of Mental Health, School of Medicine, University of Nottingham, Jubilee Campus, University of Nottingham Innovation Park, Triumph Road, Nottingham NG7 2TU, UK; [c] Division of Psychiatry and Applied Psychology, Faculty of Medicine and Health Sciences, Institute of Mental Health, University of Nottingham, Jubilee Campus, University of Nottingham Innovation Park, Triumph Road, Nottingham NG7 2TU, UK
* Corresponding author.
E-mail address: Harleen.Rai@nottingham.ac.uk

Clin Geriatr Med 34 (2018) 653–665
https://doi.org/10.1016/j.cger.2018.06.010
0749-0690/18/© 2018 Elsevier Inc. All rights reserved.

geriatric.theclinics.com

recommended by the National Institute for Health & Clinical Excellence guidelines (2006) for treating cognitive symptoms of dementia in the UK. These guidelines advise that CST should be available to people with dementia regardless of medication received. In addition, nearly all memory services in the UK currently offer CST in regular groups with people with dementia.[1] On a global level, CST is now recommended to be offered routinely to people with dementia around the world in the World Alzheimer's Report produced by Alzheimer Disease International in 2011. The International CST Center at University College London (UCL) has supported the adaptation and/or implementation of CST in more than 25 countries. Furthermore, the first 2 international CST conferences brought together researchers, clinicians, and other stakeholders from around the world to discuss past work and to exchange new and exciting ideas regarding CST. In Hong Kong, delegates learned about the concept of a virtual feature for CST groups where people would be able to attend CST groups from the comfort of their homes, connecting with others via a video/audio channel on a technological device. CST shows measurable benefits on cognition and quality of life (QoL) comparable with the effects of some antidementia mediation. In addition, it is cost effective[2] and very much enjoyed by people with dementia. All of these factors have undoubtedly supported the national and international uptake of the intervention.

The field of CST remains ever evolving and further to what has been achieved so far, there is much to look forward to in terms of innovations.

BACKGROUND

CST was developed 20 years ago at a time when there were few psychological therapies available for people with dementia and the potential for engagement in mentally stimulating, enjoyable activities in everyday life to preserve cognitive health and protect against decline had not been realized. From the perspective of the population, there was a clear need to have something available that would provide people with dementia with a meaningful way to spend their time. Clinicians and policymakers anticipated the development of new antidementia medication because the benefits of tacrine, the only pharmacologic therapy available, were modest and the risks of adverse events made the drug unsuitable for some people with dementia. Therefore, the field of psychological treatments remained unexplored and trials for psychological interventions were often small in scale and methodologically unsound. From a research perspective, the need for more rigorous investigation of new and/or existing psychological therapies for people with dementia was evident. Considering both the gaps in research and the needs of people with dementia, a research team in the UK set out to develop a novel, psychological therapy whose evaluation would be built on a strong methodological foundation comparable with that of pharmacologic treatments.[3]

The first steps toward developing CST included the review of evidence from existing psychological therapies which could serve as a strong foundation. This review included 2 systematic literature reviews on reality orientation (RO) and reminiscence therapy (RT), 2 widely used psychological approaches. In addition, the work on CST was influenced by Breuil's approach to cognitive stimulation.[4] Whereas RO is described as the presentation and repetition of orientation-based information, Breuil's approach differed from traditional RO by setting out to engage people in enjoyable cognitive tasks provided in a group format. Breuil and colleagues (1994)[4] conducted a randomized, controlled trial among 56 people with dementia and found their cognitive stimulation approach had positive effects on cognitive functioning. The workgroup went on to combine the effective techniques from key therapies (RO, RT and, Breuil and colleagues's work) and multisensory stimulation to form the CST program.

CST consists of 14 twice-weekly group sessions (**Table 1**) that take place over the course of 7 weeks.[5] All sessions are diverse in nature and the program offers a wide array of topics to ensure it meets the group's interests and cognitive abilities. Every CST group has personalized elements to it, such as choice of a group name and song. These are displayed on an RO board during the session. Sessions last 45 minutes including a 10-minute noncognitive warmup and a 10-minute closing activity (summary and/or the group song). CST is typically delivered by a trained health care professional or care assistant to groups of 5 to 8 people. The facilitators are encouraged to adhere to the key principles of CST, which helps to create the most optimal environment for mental stimulation and enjoyment. Examples of the 18 key principles are mental stimulation, using reminiscence as an aid to the here and now, implicit learning, fun, choice, building/strengthening relationships, and focusing on opinions, rather than facts. These features are unique to CST.

EVIDENCE

The development of CST followed the guidance of the Medical Research Council framework for developing complex interventions.[6] This framework includes a development–evaluation–implementation process in which all the phases interact with each other.

The first draft version of CST was taken forward in a pilot study.[7] A total of 27 people with dementia, recruited from a day center and 3 residential homes, were included. Seventeen were randomized to the treatment group receiving CST and 10 were allocated to a treatment as usual control group. The results were promising and indicated that for the CST treatment group there were positive signs regarding cognition, and depression and anxiety seemed to be reduced compared with the control group.

Table 1 Cognitive Stimulation Therapy sessions	
Session	**Content**
1	Physical games
2	Sound
3	Childhood
4	Food
5	Current affairs
6	Faces/scenes
7	Associated words
8	Being creative
9	Categorizing objects
10	Orientation
11	Using money
12	Number games
13	Word games
14	Team games

Data from Spector A. Introduction. In: Yates LA, Yates J, Orrell M, et al, editors. Cognitive stimulation therapy for dementia: history, evolution and internationalism. 1st edition. Oxford (England): Routledge; 2017. p. 177–93.

No negative effects were observed as a result of the treatment. The positive findings from this pilot study formed a strong argument for investigating the effects of CST in a large randomized, controlled trial.

After a few adjustments to the CST program according to the findings from the pilot study, a single-blind, multicenter randomized, controlled trial was conducted that included 201 people with dementia.[8] The participants were distributed over 23 CST groups and were recruited from 5 day centers and 18 care homes. The following inclusion criteria applied to all participants:

- *Diagnostic and Statistical Manual of Mental Disorders, fourth edition,* criteria for dementia[9];
- Score of between 10 and 24 on the Mini Mental State Examination[10];
- Some ability to communicate and understand (eg, ability to give informed consent);
- Able to see and hear well enough to participate in the group and make use of most of the material in the program; and
- No major physical illness, learning disability, or other disability that could affect participation.

These inclusion criteria have been commonly applied in CST studies since, and are now referred to as the Spector and colleagues (2003) standardized criteria.

Participants were randomized to either a CST group (n = 115) or a treatment as usual control group (n = 86). Researchers aimed to assess benefits across several outcomes measures with primary outcomes of cognitive functioning and QoL. The trial results were positive: participants in the CST group showed significant improvements in cognitive functioning as measured by the Mini Mental State Examination[10] and the Alzheimer's Disease Assessment Scale Cognitive Subscale (ADAS-Cog)[11] compared with the treatment as usual group. Self-rated QoL was higher in the CST group as measured by the Quality of Life-AD.[12] Last, there was a positive trend for communication (Holden Communication Scale).[13] No significant differences were found for the secondary outcomes such as functional ability, anxiety, and depression.

The trial met some challenges and the research team made key observations that helped them to better understand the results.[14] One of the limitations was the short follow-up period, which consisted of 8 weeks and did not allow for any evidence regarding long-term effects of CST. In addition, none of the staff-rated scales showed any significant benefits (behavior, mood, communication). The researchers did observe a considerable amount of variation between centers in terms of the effects on the outcome measures. This finding could be due to the role of staff members and the quality of the environment, but also to the level of impairment of participants. At times, if people with dementia were functioning quite well already, there was little room for significant improvement. It could also be difficult to run groups with people with different stages of dementia because those with mild impairment sometimes grew frustrated with participants with a greater degree of impairment. To maximize the effectiveness of the intervention, it is crucial to create an optimal learning environment, including pitching the sessions to an appropriate level according to the needs of the group participants. Despite these challenges, the significant improvements on the primary outcome measures and the fact that people with dementia really enjoyed CST encouraged the research team to publish the CST training manual and to make it more widely available.

A few years later, the CST findings from the trial were supported with qualitative data when researchers investigated the experiences of people with dementia, carers, and group facilitators who attended CST groups.[15] This study included 38 participants recruited from 3 existing CST groups. Two main themes (along with 7 subthemes) emerged from the focus groups and interviews: positive experiences of being in the group and changes experienced in everyday life. Participants shared many reflections, some of which are highlighted herein. Regarding changes in everyday life, participants reported noticing some benefits in their memory:

Yes, remembering the recent events have been a lot more simple and a lot more logical than it was certainly.
                                                                    —Person with dementia

Cognitive benefits in other areas such as communication were also observed by carers.

She's clearer on the telephone. Clearer I suppose in the way she holds the conversation it's not that she speaks differently. It's just that the flow of the conversation is a little easier.
                                                                    —Carer

Personal experiences reported by participants support the notion of CST being a positive and mentally stimulating experience, which is in line with previous quantitative findings.[15]

MAINTENANCE COGNITIVE STIMULATION THERAPY

The first CST trial showed positive results. However, the need for more research regarding potential longer term outcomes and more CST content for people with dementia in general, led to the development of an extended version of CST called maintenance CST (MCST).[16] The MCST program includes the regular 7-week CST program with an extension of an additional 24 weekly maintenance sessions. **Box 1** gives an overview of all the MCST themes in the published MCST manual.

Before finalizing the MCST program, an exploratory pilot study was conducted in 4 residential homes.[17] After completion of the standard CST program, 2 residential homes were offered 16 once weekly MCST sessions and the 2 remaining homes served as treatment as usual control groups. Thirty-five participants were recruited for the study which were allocated to 1 of the 3 groups: (1) MCST and CST (n = 8), (2) CST only (n = 12), and (3) no CST (n = 15). Results indicated a continuous, significant improvement at follow-up on cognitive functioning as measured by the Mini Mental State Examination among participants receiving MCST (CST plus MCST) compared with the CST only or the no CST groups. No significant effects were found for QoL, communication, or behavior after MCST. It was evident that a fully developed MCST program was needed to formally investigate the effects of CST delivered over a longer term basis.[17]

The researchers considered the theory behind the original CST program and the findings from the exploratory pilot study while finalizing the MCST program. In line with CST, MCST was developed according to the Medical Research Council framework and used a mixed methods approach.[16] Evidence from the following sources were combined: (1) a Cochrane review of cognitive stimulation for people with dementia,[18] (2) a Delphi consensus process (involving key stakeholders), (3) focus groups with key stakeholders, and (4) a Delphi survey. This process led to the development of the MCST manual, which includes themed sessions and resembles the consistent structure of CST (eg, group name/song, noncognitive warmup).[19] The finalized MCST program was evaluated in a large-scale randomized, controlled trial.

Box 1
Maintenance Cognitive Stimulation Therapy sessions themes

My life

Current affairs

Food

Being creative

Number game

Team games, quiz

Sound

Physical games

Categorizing objects

Household treasures (new)

Useful tips (new)

Thinking cards (new)

Visual clips (new)

Art discussion (new)

Faces/scenes

Word game

Associated words, discussion

Orientation

Using money

Data from Orrell M, Forrester L. Group cognitive stimulation therapy: clinical trials. In: Yates LA, Yates J, Orrell M, et al, editors. Cognitive stimulation therapy for dementia: history, evolution and internationalism. 1st edition. Oxford (England): Routledge; 2017. p. 49–67.

The MCST trial was a single-blind, multicenter, pragmatic randomized, controlled trial of the effects of MCST groups after the completion of the standard CST program versus CST followed by treatment as usual.[20] A total of 236 participants were recruited from 9 care homes and 9 community services (eg, day centers). After completion of the original CST program, participants were randomly allocated to either the additional MCST program (n = 123) or the treatment as usual control group (n = 113). Participants were assessed at baseline before randomization had taken place, at 3 months, and after 6 months. Similarly, with the previous CST trial, the primary outcomes measures were the ADAS-Cog[11] and QoL-AD.[12]

Trial results indicated that, at the 6-month follow-up, the MCST treatment group showed significant improvements in self-rated QoL-AD compared with the treatment as usual control group.[21] At the 3-month follow-up, results showed positive effects for people with dementia on the proxy-rated QoL (Dementia Quality of Life questionnaire)[22] by carers and care staff, and daily activities (Alzheimer's Disease Cooperative Study Activities of Daily Living Inventory).[23] No significant effects were found on the ADAS-Cog or other secondary outcomes at either follow-up.

The most notable difference between the findings from the MCST trial and the first CST trial was the absence of improvements on cognition after MCST.[21] Because dementia is associated with a progressive decline in cognition, participants in both the

MCST and the control group were likely to have shown cognitive deterioration at the 6 month follow-up. This decline might have limited further cognitive improvement with MCST after the standard CST program. Another key finding came from a substudy of the MCST trial that investigated the use of acetylcholinesterase inhibitor medication in combination with MCST. The substudy found that less cognitive decline occurred in the MCST group taking acetylcholinesterase inhibitor medication compared with the MCST group without medication and the treatment as usual group. This finding indicates that better results might be obtained if pharmacologic treatments are combined with CST. The research team concluded that more research is needed regarding continued CST because this was the first rigorous trial of MCST and the results did not seem to be conclusive. However, because the significant improvements on QoL owing to MCST were an encouraging finding, the research team published the MCST manual.

INDIVIDUAL COGNITIVE STIMULATION THERAPY

With the increasing evidence for the benefits of CST and its uptake in routine services, the need to offer CST through different avenues became apparent. It was acknowledged that CST is not always accessible for those who are either unwilling or unable to attend groups. Taking their needs and wishes in consideration, the individual version of CST (iCST) was developed. Unlike CST and MCST, iCST is home based and is facilitated by an informal carer (eg, a family member, friend, or anyone who is close to the person with dementia) or a paid carer (eg, home support worker).

The development of iCST followed the Medical Research Council framework and included several research activities.[24] In the first stages of development, people with dementia, carers, and care staff were asked to share their feedback and thoughts on the idea of iCST in an informal survey. The research team then reviewed existing literature of CST, MCST, one-to-one programs of cognitive stimulation, and RO. The evidence collated from the literature was then reviewed by a small group of key stakeholders such as carers and health care professionals who provided their advice on important considerations for the adaptation of CST to iCST. These activities led to the first draft of sessions 1 to 12 of the iCST manual, which were appraised in focus groups and interviews with people with dementia and carers. Participants were generally positive about the iCST materials and also shared their views on mentally stimulating activities and the feasibility of iCST. The research team proceeded with a field testing phase of the full program, which included both informal carers and paid carers. Both quantitative (eg, questionnaires, rating of enjoyment, interest, communication, and level of interest) and qualitative data (eg, through telephone support) were collected. Last, a 2-stage modified Delphi consensus process (online survey and conference) was used to reach consensus on themes that participants of focus groups, interviews, and field testing could not agree on. The sample consisted of academic, health care professionals, researchers, and carers.[24,25]

The iCST intervention follows the same principles of group CST; however, a few adjustments had to be made to make it suitable for use at home. Instead of the introduction and closing element of group CST, iCST sessions begin with a discussion of orientation information and current affairs followed by a themed activity. Each iCST session lasts around 20 to 30 minutes and each CST and MCST session was split to create 2 iCST sessions, which resulted in a 75-session program lasting over 25 weeks. **Box 2** gives an overview of the iCST session themes; some themes occur more than once. The iCST omits the key principles geared toward the group process;

> **Box 2**
> **Individual Cognitive Stimulation Therapy session themes**
>
> My life
>
> Current affairs
>
> Food
>
> Being creative
>
> Number games
>
> Quiz games
>
> Sounds
>
> Physical games
>
> Categorizing objects
>
> Household treasures
>
> Useful tips
>
> Thinking cards
>
> Visual clips discussion
>
> Art discussion
>
> Faces/scenes
>
> Word games
>
> Slogans (new)
>
> Associated words discussion
>
> Orientation
>
> Using money
>
> Childhood (new)
>
> *Data from* Yates LA. Individual cognitive stimulation therapy (iCST). Group cognitive stimulation therapy: clinical trials. In: Yates LA, Yates J, Orrell M, et al, editors. Cognitive stimulation therapy for dementia: history, evolution and internationalism. 1st edition. Oxford (England): Routledge; 2017. p. 69–88.

rather, it stimulates discussion between the person with dementia and the carer and encourages them to enjoy the time they spend together.

The final iCST program was tested in a multicenter, single-blind, large-scale randomized, controlled trial.[26] A total of 356 participants were recruited from a variety of community settings and allocated to either the iCST intervention group (n = 180) or the treatment as usual control group (n = 176). All participants met the Spector and colleagues (2003) standardized criteria with the addition of the following 2 criteria: living in the community and the availability of an informal carer. The main outcome measures were cognition (ADAS-Cog)[11] and QoL for the person with dementia (QoL-AD),[12] and QoL of the carer (Short Form-12).[27] The primary and secondary outcomes measures were completed at 3 time points: baseline, first follow-up at 13 weeks, and second follow-up at 26 weeks. Throughout the trial, participants received support from the research team in the form of regular telephone support and monitoring visits. The trial results demonstrated no differences between the iCST and treatment as usual control group on any of the primary outcome measures at both follow-up time points. However, for one of the secondary outcome measures, significant improvements in the quality of the caregiving relationship from the person with dementia's perspective were found. For the carers, scores on a secondary QoL measure (EQ-5D)[28] were significantly better in the iCST group at the second follow-up.[26]

The results of this trial are not consistent with previous CST findings and the following reflections may help us to better understand the iCST evidence. Because iCST is a longer intervention, the findings might indicate that a short-term, more intense dose of CST could be more beneficial or effective. The social setting provided during the group CST might also be crucial to enhancing cognition and QoL; thus, lacking this feature, iCST may not elicit benefits. It is suggested, in previous research, that improvements in cognition from CST mediate improvements in QoL for people with dementia.[18] Hence, the lack of change in cognition experienced by iCST participants could explain the lack of results on QoL. The greatest challenge of the trial proved to be adherence to iCST. The research team observed that, on average, dyads completed just less than one-half of the recommended 75 sessions over 25 weeks. Although, before the trial, during the development phase, carers determined the current iCST format to be feasible, in reality carers identified several barriers to delivering the intervention after the trial, such as time constraints, physical health problems, and motivation.

Despite the lack of significant effects on cognition and QoL, this trial was innovative for several reasons. The iCST trial is the largest known piece of CST research to date and it is the first trial investigating a home-based, carer-led format of CST. This trial demonstrated that, in general, carers are able to deliver an intervention, which is a key finding supporting carer-led interventions. The observed improvements in the quality of the caregiving relationship are encouraging and could enhance the QoL of people with dementia. The results from this trial are not conclusive and there is a need for continued research on iCST to determine its exact effectiveness.

INTERNATIONAL COGNITIVE STIMULATION THERAPY

CST was initially developed and implemented in the UK and, after its success, began to attract international attention. Given the cultural differences in almost every country, in addition to the language barriers, it was deemed crucial to have some kind of framework in place that could facilitate the adaptation of CST. Therefore, the research team at UCL set out to create guidelines that could inform the process of adapting and translating the CST content and structure without compromising on its effectiveness.[29]

The research team reviewed existing frameworks and theoretic methods that have been developed to guide the cultural adaptation of existing interventions. Of the frameworks reviewed, the formative method for adapting psychotherapy (FMAP) was chosen to develop the CST guidelines owing to its community-based developmental approach.[30] This is a bottom-up approach in which people with dementia and other service users are consulted as a preliminary step to uncover their ideas and opinions (eg, how dementia is perceived in their culture). This step is essential because it provides an early understanding of how CST can be catered toward the needs of service users in that specific country. The FMAP approach together with evidence from existing international CST groups resulted in guidelines consisting of 5 phases, which are described in **Fig. 1**.

Currently, CST is used in all of the following developed and developing countries: Australia, Brazil, Canada, Chile, China, Denmark, Germany, Greece, Hong Kong, India, Israel, Italy, Ireland, Indonesia, Japan, Nepal, the Netherlands, New Zealand,

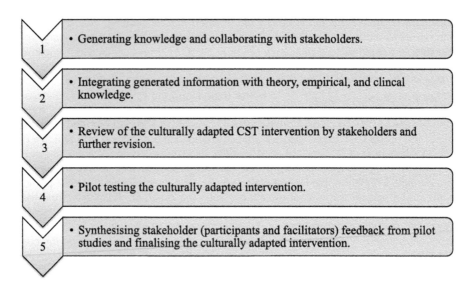

1 • Generating knowledge and collaborating with stakeholders.

2 • Integrating generated information with theory, empirical, and clincal knowledge.

3 • Review of the culturally adapted CST intervention by stakeholders and further revision.

4 • Pilot testing the culturally adapted intervention.

5 • Synthesising stakeholder (participants and facilitators) feedback from pilot studies and finalising the culturally adapted intervention.

Fig. 1. The 5 phases of Cognitive Stimulation Therapy adaptation guidelines.

Nigeria, Philippines, Portugal, Singapore, South Africa, South Korea, Tanzania, Turkey, and the United States.[31] CST is especially relevant for developing countries because it provides an effective low-cost intervention to help improve cognition and QoL. Establishing the international CST center at UCL has been a crucial step toward making CST more widely available because the center has been facilitating collaborations and knowledge exchange between the more than 25 countries currently offering CST.

COGNITIVE STIMULATION THERAPY IN THE UNITED STATES: A CASE STUDY

CST has been successfully adapted and implemented in the United States.[32] The first comprehensive CST program was developed at the Perry County Memorial Hospital, a small rural hospital in southeastern Missouri. Before its development, professionals received visits and CST training from members of the UCL research team. CST was found to be easily adaptable for the US population because the language barrier was minimal and sessions that focused on universal topics such as faces and scenes or food allowed for cultural adaptation.[32] After the adaptation of group CST, researchers compared pre-CST and post-CST data among both community-based and residential-dwelling people with dementia (n = 79) in which they found scores for cognition and QoL to be higher after the CST. These findings have been encouraging and allowed for the expansion of CST at Perry County Memorial Hospital from one, 6-member CST group to 10 CST groups currently running every week catering for 90 people with dementia. With regard to iCST, a family carer (daughter of a person with dementia) evaluated it quite positively as illustrated by the following quote:

> From discussion they had over architecture to deep thoughts on top news stories to exploring timeless paintings to simply relishing in discussing the glorious days of old, dad lover every moment. These weekly visits continued throughout dad's stay in the hospital and extended to his home post discharge. Dad would continue on in thought and articulate communication. Their session bled over into the everyday. And over time, dad became increasingly more fluent and lucid.

The US research team continues to provide CST training around the country and plans to establish a US CST National Training Center are underway. The team hopes to publish an adapted CST manual in the near future.

SUMMARY AND FUTURE DIRECTIONS

The CST journey has spanned for more than 20 years so far and innovations continue to be made in this field. When CST was developed, it helped to fill the existing gap in evidence-based psychological treatments for people with dementia. In this regard, it can be seen as a fundamental step toward shifting some of the focus from pharmacologic treatments to psychological ones. The positive effects of CST further amplified the importance of looking beyond antidementia medication and it fueled the realization that the two might actually provide the most optimal benefits to people with dementia when combined. Findings regarding experiences of people with dementia were just as encouraging; people have reported enjoyment and even increased confidence after CST. Therefore, CST has managed to provide both a meaningful and stimulating way for people with dementia to spend their time. The success of the original group CST made it possible to go even further and develop extensions of group CST ensuring that the intervention can be offered to people with different needs. In addition, the adaptation guidelines made it possible for CST to successfully be adapted and offered in a variety of countries around the world.

Still, there is more to be explored in the field of CST because some questions remain unanswered. The optimal dose for long-term CST is unknown and future research could help to give an indication of what the most beneficial duration and frequency of CST could be. Other work could focus on experimenting with iCST; for example, enhancing methods of support and training could help to improve adherence. In terms of exploring different platforms for CST, incorporating technology seems to be an attractive option; the use of technology can benefit the cognitive functioning of older people. A pilot study in Italy has investigated a tablet-based version of CST that can be delivered at home.[33] Results suggest the need for more research in this area.

For the future, we hope to maintain this growth of CST and explore different avenues for offering CST on both a national and international level. We aim to continue connecting stakeholders from around the world at our CST conferences and generate ideas and discussions on what works and what can be done even better. This would help to create an even better understanding of CST and encourage other researchers and clinicians to explore the field of CST so that CST will continue to be available to people with dementia who want and need it.

REFERENCES

1. Hodge S, Hailey E, Orrell M, editors. Memory services national accreditation programme - standards for memory services. 4th edition. London: Royal College of Psychiatrists; 2014.
2. Knapp M, Spector A, Thorgrimsen L, et al. Cognitive Stimulation Therapy for people with dementia: cost effectiveness analysis. Br J Psychiatry 2006;188:574–80.
3. Orrell M, Woods B. Editorial comment. Tacrine and psychological therapies in dementia – no contest? Int J Geriatr Psychiatry 1996;11(3):189–92.
4. Breuil V, De Rotrou J, Forette F, et al. Cognitive stimulation of patients with dementia. Int J Geriatr Psychiatry 1994;9(3):211–7.
5. Spector A, Thorgrimsen L, Woods B, et al. Making a difference: an evidence based group program to offer Cognitive Stimulation Therapy (CST) to people with dementia. London: Hawker Publications; 2006.

6. Craig P, Dieppe P, Macintyre S, et al. Developing and evaluating complex interventions: the new Medical Research Council guidance. BMJ 2008;29(337):a1655.

7. Spector A, Orrell M, Davies S, et al. Can reality orientation be rehabilitated? Development and piloting of an evidence-based programme of cognition-based therapies for people with dementia. Neuropsychol Rehabil 2001;11(3/4): 377–97.

8. Spector A, Thorgrimsen L, Woods B, et al. Efficacy of an evidence-based cognitive stimulation therapy programme for people with dementia: randomised controlled trial. Br J Psychiatry 2003;183:248–54.

9. American Psychiatric Association. Diagnostic and statistical manual of mental health disorders. 4th edition. Washington, DC: APA; 1994.

10. Folstein MF, Folstein SE, McHugh PR. "Mini mental state". A practical method for grading the cognitive state of patients for the clinician. J Psychiatr Res 1975; 12(3):189–98.

11. Rosen WG, Mohs RC, Davis KL. A new rating scale for Alzheimer's Disease. Am J Psychiatry 1984;141(11):1356–64.

12. Logsdon RG, Gibbons LE, McCurry SM, et al. Quality of life in Alzheimer's disease: patient and caregiver reports. J Ment Health Aging 1999;5:21–32.

13. Holden UP, Woods RT. Positive approaches to dementia care. 3rd edition. Edinburgh (Scotland): Churchill-Livingstone; 1995.

14. Orrell M, Forrester L. Group cognitive stimulation therapy: clinical trials. In: Yates LA, Yates J, Orrell M, et al, editors. Cognitive stimulation therapy for dementia: history, evolution and internationalism. 1st edition. Abingdon (England): Routledge; 2017. p. 49–67.

15. Spector A, Gardner C, Orrell M. The impact of Cognitive Stimulation Therapy groups on people with dementia: views from participants, their carers and group facilitators. Aging Ment Health 2011;15(8):945–9.

16. Aguirre E, Spector A, Hoe J, et al. Development of an evidence-based extended programme of maintenance Cognitive Stimulation Therapy (CST) for people with dementia. Non-pharmacological Therapies in Dementia Journal 2011;1:198–215.

17. Orrell M, Spector A, Thorgrimsen L, et al. A pilot study examining the effectiveness of Maintenance Cognitive Stimulation Therapy (Maintenance CST) for people with dementia. Int J Geriatr Psychiatry 2005;11:446–51.

18. Woods B, Aguirre E, Spector A, et al. Cognitive stimulation to improve cognitive functioning in people with dementia. Cochrane Database Syst Rev 2012;(2):CD005562.

19. Aguirre E, Spector A, Streater A, et al. Making a Difference 2: an evidence based group program to offer maintenance Cognitive Stimulation Therapy (CST) to people with dementia. London: Hawker Publications; 2006.

20. Aguirre E, Hoare Z, Streater A, et al. Cognitive Stimulation Therapy (CST) for people with dementia – who benefits most? Int J Geriatr Psychiatry 2013;28(3): 284–90.

21. Orrell M, Aguirre E, Spector A, et al. Maintenance Cognitive Stimulation Therapy (CST) for dementia: a single-blind, multi-centre, randomised controlled trial of Maintenance CST vs. CST for dementia. Br J Psychiatry 2014;204:454–61.

22. Smith SC, Lamping DL, Banerjee S, et al. Measurement of health-related quality of life for people with dementia: development of a new instrument (DEMQOL) and an evaluation of current methodology. Health Technol Assess 2005;9(10).

23. Galasko D, Bennet D, Sano M, et al. An inventory to assess activities of daily living for clinical trials in Alzheimer's disease: the Alzheimer Disease Cooperative Study. Alzheimer Dis Assoc Disord 1997;11:S33–9.

24. Yates LA, Leung P, Orgeta V, et al. The development of individual cognitive stimulation therapy (iCST) for dementia. Clin Interv Aging 2015;10:95–104.

25. Yates L, Orrell M, Leung P, et al. Making a difference 3 individual CST: a manual for carers. London: Hawker Publications; 2014.

26. Orrell M, Yates L, Leung P, et al. The impact of individual Cognitive Stimulation Therapy (iCST) on cognition, quality of life, caregiver health, and family relationships in dementia: a randomised controlled trial. PLoS Med 2017;14(3):1–22.

27. Ware J Jr, Kosinski M, Keller SD. A 12-Item short form health survey: construction of scales and preliminary tests of reliability and validity. Med Care 1996;34:220–33.

28. EuroQoL Group. EuroQoL–a new facility for the measurement of health-related quality of life. Health Policy 1990;16:199–208.

29. Aguirre E, Werheid K. Guidelines for adapting cognitive stimulation therapy to other cultures. In: Yates LA, Yates J, Orrell M, et al, editors. Cognitive stimulation therapy for dementia: history, evolution and internationalism. 1st edition. Abingdon (England): Routledge; 2017. p. 177–93.

30. Hwang WC. The formative method for adapting psychotherapy (FMAP): a community-based developmental approach to culturally adapting therapy. Prof Psychol Res Pr 2009;40(4):369.

31. International CST Groups. 2018. CST Dementia website Available at: http://www.cstdementia.com. Accessed January 24, 2018.

32. Lundy L, Hayden D, Berg-Weger M, et al. United States. In: Yates LA, Yates J, Orrell M, et al, editors. Cognitive stimulation therapy for dementia: history, evolution and internationalism. 1st edition. Abingdon (England): Routledge; 2017. p. 215–26.

33. Gardini S, Michelini G, Tirelli P, Morciano E, Caffarra P. The development of a home-based and computerized Cognitive Stimulation Therapy for people living with dementia: preliminary results. Proceedings from the Second International Meeting of the Milan Center for Neuroscience (Neuromi): Prediction and Prevention of Dementia: New Hope; July 6-8, 2016; Milan, Italy. S24.

Cognitive Frailty in Geriatrics

Hidenori Arai, MD, PhD[a],*, Shosuke Satake, MD, PhD[b,c], Koichi Kozaki, MD, PhD[d]

KEYWORDS

• Aging • Frailty • Mild cognitive impairment • Dementia • Disability • Exercise

KEY POINTS

- Cognitive frailty can be defined by the presence of physical frailty and cognitive impairment. However, the definition has not reached a consensus yet.
- Physical frailty and cognitive impairment have a close relationship. The deterioration of one component can affect the other and may form a vicious cycle.
- A multimodal intervention including the combination of different kinds exercise, nutritional support, and metabolic management is effective for cognitive frailty.

INTRODUCTION

Population aging is a global issue. Health care professionals need to deal with more and more older patients with multiple complex disorders with or without disability. Among several geriatric syndromes, dementia and frailty are common problems in people older than 75 and these 2 entities are considered to have a strong relationship. For example, we sometimes observe a rapid cognitive decline in a cognitively impaired older patient when he or she shows reduced activities due to physical limitations in geriatric care, which suggests a strong connection between cognitive function and physical fitness or physical activities. This indicates that both physical and cognitive assessment is required for elderly care. In this article, we reviewed clinical and epidemiologic studies related to "cognitive frailty" and tried to address the definition of cognitive frailty, its clinical and epidemiologic significance and pathogenesis, and the implication of interventions.

Disclosure: The authors have nothing to disclose.

[a] National Center for Geriatrics and Gerontology, 7-430, Morioka-cho, Obu, Aichi 474-8511, Japan; [b] Section of Frailty Prevention, Department of Frailty Research, Center for Gerontology and Social Science, 7-430, Morioka-cho, Obu, Aichi 474-8511, Japan; [c] Department of Geriatric Medicine, National Center for Geriatrics and Gerontology, 7-430, Morioka-cho, Obu, Aichi 474-8511, Japan; [d] Department of Geriatric Medicine, Kyorin University School of Medicine, 6-20-2 Shinkawa, Mitaka, Tokyo 181-8611, Japan
* Corresponding author.
E-mail address: harai@ncgg.go.jp

DEFINITION OF COGNITIVE FRAILTY

Frailty is characterized by the increased vulnerability of an individual to acute stressors caused by age-related cumulative decline of multiple physiologic systems and is a multidimensional syndrome that encompasses physical, social, and cognitive dimensions.[1–3] Cognitive impairment is one of the components of frailty; thus, the association between physical frailty and cognitive impairment has been widely investigated. Because of the close relationship between frailty and cognitive impairment, several lines of evidence have shown the link between physical frailty and cognitive impairment or dementia in cross-sectional and longitudinal studies.[4–6]

In terms of "cognitive frailty," Paganini-Hill and colleagues,[7] in 2001, were the first to use it in their study that examined the association of Clock Drawing Test with potential protective and risk factors for Alzheimer disease (AD). "Cognitive frailty" was then used by Panza and colleagues[8] as the title of the article. However, they did not define cognitive frailty, but rather focused on the possible role of vascular risk factors in modulating the risk of age-related cognitive decline. In fact, the concept and operational definition of "cognitive frailty" was first coined by the international consensus group composed of experts from the International Academy of Nutrition and Aging (IANA) and the International Association of Gerontology and Geriatrics (IAGG) in 2013,[9] based on the accumulation of extensive evidence of the significant association between physical frailty and cognitive impairment in older people. In their consensus paper, cognitive frailty was defined by the simultaneous presence of both physical frailty (phenotype model) and cognitive impairment (clinical dementia rating [CDR] = 0.5). Importantly, they excluded the presence of definite dementia and cognitive impairment due to neurodegenerative disorders when defining cognitive frailty.[9] As physical frailty, reversibility is supposed to be a characteristic feature of cognitive frailty, and cognitive frailty would be the reasonable target for the prevention of dependency and disability in older people. However, there are several issues that limit the clinical and research applications of this concept of cognitive frailty proposed by the international consensus group. For example, many researchers consider that it is difficult to reverse older people with cognitive frailty under the definition of IANA/IAGG, because those who satisfy the definition are few in the community and too frail to be reversed. In an attempt to refine the framework for the definition of cognitive frailty, Ruan and colleagues[10] proposed a new definition of cognitive frailty. The new operational definition includes 2 subtypes: "reversible" cognitive frailty and "potentially reversible" cognitive frailty. Reversible cognitive frailty is defined as the presence of physical frailty or prefrailty and subjective cognitive decline (SCD) and/or positive biomarkers; and absence of acute impairment, and clinical diagnosis of neurodegenerative and other mental conditions. Potentially reversible cognitive frailty is defined by the presence of physical frailty or prefrailty and cognitive impairment (CDR = 0.5), and absence of concurrent AD or other dementia. At this moment, the definition of cognitive frailty has not reached a consensus and needs further discussion.

RELATIONSHIP BETWEEN PHYSICAL FRAILTY AND COGNITIVE IMPAIRMENT

Many pathologic processes have been shown to contribute to cognitive impairment. Age is obviously the most important risk factor for cognitive impairment and frailty; therefore, age per se leads to cognitive decline and physical frailty in older people. The implication of cognitive impairment in a definition of frailty has been extensively discussed.[11] Some of the frailty measures include cognition, whereas the others do not. Among many frailty measures, the most widely used operational definition is proposed by Fried and colleagues,[12] in which unintentional weight loss, weakness, slowness, exhaustion, and low physical activity are the 5 components for frailty assessment, and the combination of 3 or more is considered frailty. Additionally, cognition does not correlate strongly with these components and may not be part of the frailty syndrome.[13,14] Therefore, physical frailty and cognitive impairment would be related, but distinct entities that frequently occur in a same older person.

Yuki and colleagues[15] have shown that physical activity and total energy expenditure are significant predictors of frontal lobe atrophy progression during an 8-year period, indicating the role of physical activity on the maintenance of brain function. Another Japanese study shows that subjects with exercise habits have larger subcortical gray matter volumes than those without exercise habits in community-dwelling older people.[16] Specifically, the volume of the nucleus accumbens correlates with both exercise habits and cognitive preservation.

In terms of the relationship between physical frailty and cognitive impairment, a Taiwanese group has shown that dynapenia is significantly associated with cognitive impairment in multiple dimensions and global cognitive function, indicating that reduced muscle strength and/or physical performance is strongly associated with cognitive impairment.[17] Bunce and colleagues[18] have shown that frailty is associated with poorer baseline performance in processing speed, verbal fluency, and so on. However, no significant effects of frailty on slopes of cognition are observed, suggesting that frailty-related cognitive deficits may exist independently of mechanisms that cause neurodegenerative disorders, such as AD. Buchman and colleagues[19] also showed that AD pathology, macroinfarcts, and nigral neuronal loss had independent associations with the progression of frailty. However, Gray and colleagues[20] found that frailty was associated with developing non-AD dementia, but not AD. Buracchio and colleagues[21] showed that gait speed starts to decrease 12 years before the development of mild cognitive impairment (MCI). Thus, they concluded that longitudinal changes in motor function may be useful in the early detection of cognitive decline, which is consistent with the Mayo Clinic Study of Aging.[22] Although brain plays an important role for both physical frailty and cognitive impairment, these data suggest that clinical manifestation might occur in a different timing.

In terms of the reversibility of frailty and cognitive impairment, a systematic review has shown that exercise and cognitive training improve specific factors associated with falls, such as gait speed, cognitive function, and balance in people with MCI.[23] As with the concept of physical frailty, cognitive frailty should be also characterized with the potential for reversibility.

EPIDEMIOLOGY OF COGNITIVE FRAILTY

Since the consensus conference by IANA/IAGG, several articles have evaluated the frequency of cognitive frailty on their own definitions; however, the definition and the frequency differ according to the report.

Cross-Sectional Study

First we describe the prevalence of cognitive frailty mainly in community-dwelling older people. In the earliest report by Shimada and colleagues,[24] 5104 people were evaluated for frailty using the Cardiovascular Health Study (CHS) criteria for community-dwelling older people, and MCI was evaluated using the National Center for Geriatrics and Gerontology-Functional Assessment Tool (NCGG-FAT). As a result, the prevalence of frailty, MCI, and cognitive frailty was 11.3%, 18.8%, and 2.7%, respectively. In this article, they did not use the term cognitive frailty, but physical frailty + MCI is regarded as cognitive frailty. In another study, the same group showed that the prevalence of frailty, cognitive dysfunction, and cognitive frailty was 7.2%, 5.2%, and 1.2%, respectively, in 8164 community-dwelling older people.[25] In a French cohort study (Multidomain Alzheimer Preventive Trial [MAPT] study, n = 1617) by Delrieu and colleagues,[26] cognitive frailty was defined by the presence of CDR0.5 + frailty or prefrailty based on the CHS criteria, and its prevalence was 22% (356 in 1617 people), whereas that of frailty and prefrailty was 24%. In this article, the prevalence of cognitive frailty was high because prefrailty was included in cognitive frailty. In 2017, Roppolo and colleagues[27] evaluated frailty by the modified CHS criteria and declined cognitive function as Mini-Mental State Examination (MMSE) ≤25 points and examined the prevalence of the 2 combinations. Among the 594 subjects, the prevalence of frailty and cognitive frailty was 14.0% and 4.4%, respectively. In a prospective study for older residents living in Italy, frailty was judged using the modified CHS criteria and cognitive impairment was judged by MCI instead of CDR 0.5 for 2373 people. As a result, the prevalence of nonfrailty + non-MCI, nonfrailty + MCI, frailty + non-MCI, and frailty + MCI (cognitive frailty) was 86.8%, 3.9%, 8.4%, and 1.0%, respectively. Regarding cognitive function, CDR 0.5 was proposed by the IANA/IAGG consensus conference, whereas other reports use MCI instead of CDR 0.5. There are also reports that use a subjective memory loss. On the other hand, for frailty, the CHS criteria are used in many cases, but there are some cases in which the evaluation method of the 5 domains is different from the original version, or prefrailty is included depending on the report. Based on the previous discussion, the prevalence of cognitive frailty is estimated to be 1% to 5% by the original definition (physical frailty + CDR 0.5 or MCI) in community-dwelling older adults, although it differs depending on the operational definitions and the study subjects.

Longitudinal Study

Next we describe the outcomes of cognitive frailty. Montero-Odasso and colleagues[28] followed 252 subjects from the Gait and Brain Study aged 65 years or older. The mean age was 77 years. The mean follow-up was 18 months. Frailty was defined by the CHS criteria and cognitive impairment defined as Montreal Cognitive Assessment (MoCA) <26 and CDR = 0.5. In their study, cognitive frailty increased the incident rate of dementia, but not risk for progression to dementia. Additionally, the combination of slow gait and cognitive impairment showed the highest risk for progression to dementia. Feng and colleagues[29] conducted a 3-year population-based longitudinal study with 2375 subjects aged 55 years or older in Singapore (mean age, 66 years). Frailty was defined with the modified CHS criteria and cognitive impairment defined as MMSE less than 26. They found that prefrailty and frailty with cognitive impairment were associated with an increased incidence of functional disability, poor quality of life, and mortality. In an Italian Longitudinal Study on Aging, Solfrizzi and colleagues[30] showed that cognitive frailty offered additional predictive value for the risk of disability during 3.5-year follow-up. The same group also investigated the association between reversible cognitive frailty and the incidence of dementia,[31] with reversible cognitive frailty defined by the presence of physical frailty and pre-MCI-SCD, and physical frailty operationalized by the CHS criteria, and pre-MCI-SCD assessed according to the positive response to the item of the Geriatric Depression Scale–30: "Do you feel you have more problems with memory than most?" The study found the prevalence of reversible cognitive frailty to be 2.5%, and that reversible cognitive frailty was a short-term (3.5 years) and long-term (7.0 years) predictor of all-cause mortality and overall dementia, particularly vascular dementia. In Japan, Shimada and colleagues[32] found significant relationships between incident dementia and cognitive frailty (hazard ratio 6.19, 95% confidence interval 2.7–13.99), but not with physical frailty without cognitive impairment. In contrast to the community settings, Jha and colleagues[33] studied cognitive frailty in 156 patients with advanced heart failure referred for heart transplantation. Their mean age was 53 years. Frailty was defined by the presence of 3 or more domains from 6 domains including the 5 physical domains of the modified CHS criteria and cognitive impairment defined as MoCA less than 26. Cognitive frailty was present in 39.7% of the patients and was shown to be a predictor of early mortality. Thus, in clinical settings dealing with patients with heart failure and other wasting disorders, for example, the prevalence of cognitive frailty was higher than community-dwelling older people with poorer outcomes. Although the consensus of major outcomes of cognitive frailty is not determined, major outcomes that should be taken into account are incident dementia, disability, and mortality.

PREVENTION OF COGNITIVE FRAILTY

For older people, we can propose the promotion of physical activities, exercise, and a healthy diet; the cessation of smoking; active social participation; avoidance of polypharmacy; and oral care and metabolic control as preventive measures for frailty. For those with potential cognitive frailty, we should provide a comprehensive geriatric assessment followed by individualized multimodal interventions, such as exercise and nutrition support. In fact, a multimodal intervention seems to be efficient in the prevention of cognitive frailty as described in the following studies.

It is well established that aerobic exercises, such as walking, may prevent cognitive decline in older adults.[34] In terms of other type of exercises, it has been observed that resistance training contributes positively and significantly to the improvement of executive function and response inhibition.[35,36] Additionally, a meta-analysis has shown that Tai Chi can positively affect cognitive performance in older adults.[37] In terms of the combination of exercise, Langlois and colleagues[38] conducted a study showing that an aerobic exercise and strength training program for frail older adults improved functional capacity and physical endurance, cognition, and quality of life. The significant improvements in cognition were due to increased scores in working memory, processing speed, and executive function. In terms of a multimodal approach, Ng and colleagues[39] have shown in a randomized control trial that physical, nutritional, and cognitive interventional approaches were effective in reversing frailty among community-living older persons. Suzuki and colleagues[40] examined the effects of a multicomponent exercise program on the cognitive function of older adults with amnestic MCI and found that a multicomponent exercise improved cognitive performance. Additionally, Bossers and colleagues[41] have shown that compared with a non-exercise control group, a combination of aerobic and strength training is more effective than aerobic training in slowing cognitive decline even in older adults with dementia. However, further research is needed on the role of exercise parameters, such as volume, types, and intensity on specific cognitive functions. Additionally, a question remains whether the same kind of multicomponent interventions are effective for physical frailty and cognitive frailty. Cognitive frailty might be more responsive to the interventions, including dual-task exercise, which is shown to be effective for older people with cognitive impairment.[40,42]

MOTORIC COGNITIVE RISK SYNDROME

As a similar pathologic entity to cognitive frailty, Verghese and colleagues[43] proposed motoric cognitive risk syndrome (MCR) as the presence of both slow gait speed and subjective cognitive complaints. They also excluded concurrent dementia or mobility disability as cognitive frailty. Slow gait speed is defined based on walking speed 1.0 SD or more below age and gender-specific means. Cognitive complaints do not require formal cognitive testing and are obtained based on responses to items on standardized questionnaires. In a recent multicenter study, the prevalence of MCR is estimated at 9.7% in 26,082 older adults from 17 countries.[44] Additionally, the overall age-adjusted and gender-adjusted incidence of MCR was 51 to approximately 80 per 1000 person-years.[44] MCR is associated with stroke, cerebral small vessel disease, depressive symptoms, inactivity, and obesity.[44] Additionally, MCR is associated with increased risk of dementia, especially vascular dementia.[43,45] Thus, MCR seems to be a similar entity, but may be milder than cognitive frailty.

SUMMARY

From the establishment of first operational definition of cognitive frailty in 2013, several population-based studies focused on this cognitive frailty model. In community settings, the prevalence of cognitive frailty was less than 5%, but higher in clinical settings when the definition is applied to the patients with wasting disorders, such as heart failure and renal failure. Cognitive frailty has a higher risk for adverse health outcomes, including disability, poor quality of life, dementia, and mortality.

In spite of the accumulated evidence, there still remain conceptual and methodological issues that we need to address. Pathoetiologically, it is difficult to determine whether cognitive impairment is caused by neurodegenerative disease or cardiovascular risk factors in most of the clinical and research settings.[46] Furthermore, cognitive frailty should have a potential for reversibility and would be a target for disability prevention; however, the lower prevalence of cognitive frailty suggests a limited clinical utility and a need for modification of the criteria. New definition of reversible cognitive frailty including elderly with physical prefrailty and SCD may resolve this issue.[10] Close association of physical frailty and cognitive impairment suggests the presence of a common underlying mechanisms shared by them, such as cardiovascular risk factors, chronic inflammation, nutritional problems, cerebral small vascular disease, and AD or other neurodegenerative pathology.[4,5] Identification of common modifiable factors of this concept combined physical dysfunction and cognitive impairment will help develop the successful strategies for prevention of disability and dementia progression among elderly.

In conclusion, there is still no consensus on the definition of cognitive frailty applicable in the clinical and community settings. Additionally, a consensus remains to be reached on which measures to be used for screening and diagnosing cognitive impairment. Further study is required to develop successful preventive strategies for older people with cognitive frailty to prevent the progression of dementia and disability for healthy aging.

REFERENCES

1. Rodriguez-Manas L, Feart C, Mann G, et al. Searching for an operational definition of frailty: a Delphi method based consensus statement: the frailty operative definition-consensus conference project. J Gerontol A Biol Sci Med Sci 2013; 68(1):62–7.

2. Cesari M, Prince M, Thiyagarajan JA, et al. Frailty: an emerging public health priority. J Am Med Dir Assoc 2016;17(3):188–92.

3. Clegg A, Young J, Iliffe S, et al. Frailty in elderly people. Lancet 2013;381(9868): 752–62.

4. Panza F, Seripa D, Solfrizzi V, et al. Targeting cognitive frailty: clinical and neuro-biological roadmap for a single complex phenotype. J Alzheimers Dis 2015;47(4): 793–813.

5. Panza F, Solfrizzi V, Barulli MR, et al. Cognitive frailty: a systematic review of epidemiological and neurobiological evidence of an age-related clinical condition. Rejuvenation Res 2015;18(5):389–412.

6. Robertson DA, Savva GM, Kenny RA. Frailty and cognitive impairment–a review of the evidence and causal mechanisms. Ageing Res Rev 2013;12(4):840–51.

7. Paganini-Hill A, Clark LJ, Henderson VW, et al. Clock drawing: analysis in a retirement community. J Am Geriatr Soc 2001;49(7):941–7.

8. Panza F, D'Introno A, Colacicco AM, et al. Cognitive frailty: predementia syndrome and vascular risk factors. Neurobiol Aging 2006;27(7):933–40.

9. Kelaiditi E, Cesari M, Canevelli M, et al. Cognitive frailty: rational and definition from an (I.A.N.A./I.A.G.G.) international consensus group. J Nutr Health Aging 2013;17(9):726–34.

10. Ruan Q, Yu Z, Chen M, et al. Cognitive frailty, a novel target for the prevention of elderly dependency. Ageing Res Rev 2015;20:1–10.

11. Aubertin-Leheudre M, Woods AJ, Anton S, et al. Frailty clinical phenotype: a physical and cognitive point of view. Nestle Nutr Inst Workshop Ser 2015;83: 55–63.

12. Fried LP, Tangen CM, Walston J, et al. Frailty in older adults: evidence for a phenotype. J Gerontol A Biol Sci Med Sci 2001;56(3):M146–56.

13. Sourial N, Bergman H, Karunananthan S, et al. Contribution of frailty markers in explaining differences among individuals in five samples of older persons. J Gerontol A Biol Sci Med Sci 2012;67(11):1197–204.

14. Sourial N, Wolfson C, Bergman H, et al. A correspondence analysis revealed frailty deficits aggregate and are multidimensional. J Clin Epidemiol 2010;63(6): 647–54.

15. Yuki A, Lee S, Kim H, et al. Relationship between physical activity and brain atrophy progression. Med Sci Sports Exerc 2012;44(12):2362–8.

16. Yamamoto M, Wada-Isoe K, Yamashita F, et al. Association between exercise habits and subcortical gray matter volumes in healthy elderly people: a population-based study in Japan. eNeurologicalSci 2017;7:1–6.

17. Huang CY, Hwang AC, Liu LK, et al. Association of dynapenia, sarcopenia, and cognitive impairment among community-dwelling older Taiwanese. Rejuvenation Res 2016;19(1):71–8.

18. Bunce D, Batterham PJ, Mackinnon AJ. Long-term associations between physical frailty and performance in specific cognitive domains. J Gerontol B Psychol Sci Soc Sci 2018. [Epub ahead of print].

19. Buchman AS, Yu L, Wilson RS, et al. Association of brain pathology with the progression of frailty in older adults. Neurology 2013;80(22):2055–61.

20. Gray SL, Anderson ML, Hubbard RA, et al. Frailty and incident dementia. J Gerontol A Biol Sci Med Sci 2013;68(9):1083–90.

21. Buracchio T, Dodge HH, Howieson D, et al. The trajectory of gait speed preceding mild cognitive impairment. Arch Neurol 2010;67(8):980–6.

22. Mielke MM, Roberts RO, Savica R, et al. Assessing the temporal relationship between cognition and gait: slow gait predicts cognitive decline in the Mayo Clinic study of aging. J Gerontol A Biol Sci Med Sci 2013;68(8):929–37.

23. Lipardo DS, Aseron AMC, Kwan MM, et al. Effect of exercise and cognitive training on falls and fall-related factors in older adults with mild cognitive impairment: a systematic review. Arch Phys Med Rehabil 2017;98(10):2079–96.

24. Shimada H, Makizako H, Doi T, et al. Combined prevalence of frailty and mild cognitive impairment in a population of elderly Japanese people. J Am Med Dir Assoc 2013;14(7):518–24.

25. Shimada H, Makizako H, Lee S, et al. Impact of cognitive frailty on daily activities in older persons. J Nutr Health Aging 2016;20(7):729–35.

26. Delrieu J, Andrieu S, Pahor M, et al. Neuropsychological profile of "cognitive frailty" subjects in MAPT study. J Prev Alzheimers Dis 2016;3(3):151–9.

27. Roppolo M, Mulasso A, Rabaglietti E. Cognitive frailty in Italian community-dwelling older adults: prevalence rate and its association with disability. J Nutr Health Aging 2017;21(6):631–6.

28. Montero-Odasso MM, Barnes B, Speechley M, et al. Disentangling cognitive-frailty: results from the gait and brain study. J Gerontol A Biol Sci Med Sci 2016;71(11):1476–82.

29. Feng L, Zin Nyunt MS, Gao Q, et al. Cognitive frailty and adverse health outcomes: findings from the Singapore longitudinal ageing studies (SLAS). J Am Med Dir Assoc 2017;18(3):252–8.

30. Solfrizzi V, Scafato E, Lozupone M, et al. Additive role of a potentially reversible cognitive frailty model and inflammatory state on the risk of disability: the Italian longitudinal study on aging. Am J Geriatr Psychiatry 2017;25(11):1236–48.

31. Solfrizzi V, Scafato E, Seripa D, et al. Reversible cognitive frailty, dementia, and all-cause mortality. The Italian longitudinal study on aging. J Am Med Dir Assoc 2017;18(1):89.e1–8.

32. Shimada H, Makizako H, Tsutsumimoto K, et al. Cognitive frailty and incidence of dementia in older persons. J Prev Alzheimers Dis 2018;5(1):42–8.

33. Jha SR, Hannu MK, Gore K, et al. Cognitive impairment improves the predictive validity of physical frailty for mortality in patients with advanced heart failure referred for heart transplantation. J Heart Lung Transplant 2016;35(9):1092–100.

34. Scherder E, Scherder R, Verburgh L, et al. Executive functions of sedentary elderly may benefit from walking: a systematic review and meta-analysis. Am J Geriatr Psychiatry 2014;22(8):782–91.

35. Chang YK, Tsai CL, Huang CC, et al. Effects of acute resistance exercise on cognition in late middle-aged adults: general or specific cognitive improvement? J Sci Med Sport 2014;17(1):51–5.

36. Dunsky A, Abu-Rukun M, Tsuk S, et al. The effects of a resistance vs. an aerobic single session on attention and executive functioning in adults. PLoS One 2017; 12(4):e0176092.

37. Wayne PM, Walsh JN, Taylor-Piliae RE, et al. Effect of tai chi on cognitive performance in older adults: systematic review and meta-analysis. J Am Geriatr Soc 2014;62(1):25–39.

38. Langlois F, Vu TT, Chasse K, et al. Benefits of physical exercise training on cognition and quality of life in frail older adults. J Gerontol B Psychol Sci Soc Sci 2013; 68(3):400–4.

39. Ng TP, Feng L, Nyunt MS, et al. Nutritional, physical, cognitive, and combination interventions and frailty reversal among older adults: a randomized controlled trial. Am J Med 2015;128(11):1225–36.e1.

40. Suzuki T, Shimada H, Makizako H, et al. Effects of multicomponent exercise on cognitive function in older adults with amnestic mild cognitive impairment: a randomized controlled trial. BMC Neurol 2012;12:128.

41. Bossers WJ, van der Woude LH, Boersma F, et al. A 9-week aerobic and strength training program improves cognitive and motor function in patients with dementia: a randomized, controlled trial. Am J Geriatr Psychiatry 2015;23(11):1106–16.

42. Doi T, Shimada H, Makizako H, et al. Cognitive function and gait speed under normal and dual-task walking among older adults with mild cognitive impairment. BMC Neurol 2014;14:67.
43. Verghese J, Wang C, Lipton RB, et al. Motoric cognitive risk syndrome and the risk of dementia. J Gerontol A Biol Sci Med Sci 2013;68(4):412–8.
44. Verghese J, Ayers E, Barzilai N, et al. Motoric cognitive risk syndrome: multi-center incidence study. Neurology 2014;83(24):2278–84.
45. Verghese J, Annweiler C, Ayers E, et al. Motoric cognitive risk syndrome: multi-country prevalence and dementia risk. Neurology 2014;83(8):718–26.
46. Kapasi A, DeCarli C, Schneider JA. Impact of multiple pathologies on the threshold for clinically overt dementia. Acta Neuropathol 2017;134(2):171–86.

Nutrition and Alzheimer Disease

Shirley Steffany Muñoz Fernández, MSc[a], Sandra Maria Lima Ribeiro, PhD[b],*

KEYWORDS

- Nutrients • Food • Dietary pattern • Alzheimer disease • Prevention • Management

KEY POINTS

- One of the most accepted hypothesis related to Alzheimer disease (AD) is the neuroinflammation cascade, which is correlated with systemic inflammation and can be originated by immunosenescence, adipose tissue, and/or the intestinal imbalance.
- There are several antioxidants and/or anti-inflammatory nutrients or food components with epigenetic properties, which certainly can help in attenuating or postponing the development of the disease.
- Inappropriate dietary patterns can facilitate the development of the disease, whereas a healthier style, such as the Mediterranean diet, can enhance body mechanisms to prevent AD.

INTRODUCTION

Pharmacologic therapies attempting to cure Alzheimer disease (AD) are, until now, only partial inhibitors rather than curative.[1] Thereby, nonpharmacologic interventions may be considered fundamental to prevent or postpone the development of the disease; there is strong evidence supporting nutrition in this context.[2] As such, this article intended to gather some theoretical and practical concepts related to the importance of nutrition in the prevention and management of AD.

DESCRIPTION OF ALZHEIMER DISEASE UNDER A NUTRITIONAL POINT OF VIEW

Histologically, the main hallmarks of AD are the extracellular neuritic plaques and the intracellular neurofibrillary tangle, composed mainly of 2 protein-derived molecules. The first one is the amyloid β peptide (Aβ), produced from the amyloid precursor protein (APP; from amyloidogenic pathway, under the action of β and γ-secretases). The

Disclosure Statement: The authors have nothing to disclose.
[a] Department of Nutrition, School of Public Health, University of São Paulo, Av. Dr. Arnaldo, 715, São Paulo CEP - 01246-904, São Paulo, SP, Brazil; [b] School of Public Health and School of Arts, Sciences and Humanities, University of São Paulo, Av. Dr. Arnaldo, 715, São Paulo CEP - 01246-904, Brazil and Av. Arlindo Bettio, 1000 CEP 03828-000, São Paulo, SP, Brazil
* Corresponding author.
E-mail address: smlribeiro@usp.br

Clin Geriatr Med 34 (2018) 677–697
https://doi.org/10.1016/j.cger.2018.06.012
0749-0690/18/© 2018 Elsevier Inc. All rights reserved.

geriatric.theclinics.com

second molecule is the hyperphosphorylated Tau protein, originated from different Tau pathologies.[3] The accumulation of plaques is associated with several events, such as mitochondrial dysfunction, impaired cell stress response, abnormal accumulation of transition metals, altered lipid metabolism, enzymatic dysregulation, neuroinflammation, and oxidative stress.[4]

The events associated with the Aβ deposition are considered an insult to the immune system, which activates the astrocytes and microglia nearby. These activated molecules are responsible for the production of inflammatory mediators, but this production generally is below the capacity of overcoming the Aβ deposition; consequently, the plaques become amyloid fibrils.[5–7] These neuroinflammatory processes generate many toxic products (reactive species, nitric oxide, proteolytic enzymes, and others).[8]

Some investigators have associated the neuroinflammation with low-grade systemic inflammation, a common picture in aging.[9] Systemic proinflammation-derived molecules cause a breach in the blood-brain barrier (BBB), allowing their entry into the brain, contributing to chronic neuroinflammation.[10]

The exact origin of such systemic inflammation remains unknown[11]; however, different hypotheses have been proposed.[12] **Box 1** and **Figs. 1** and **2** describe 3 of these hypotheses: the immunosenescence, intestinal imbalance, and adiposity.

From those hypotheses, the intestinal hypothesis does not have a relevant number of clinical and epidemiological studies to prove its association with AD so far.[6,20] Nevertheless, it is important to highlight that the diet and physical activity are factors capable of positively modifying the gut environment. Regarding adiposity, it is clear that the body composition (therefore, nutritional status) is associated with inflammatory status, which consequently increases the risk of AD. It is relatively well demonstrated that a high body weight, especially obesity, in middle adulthood is associated with impairment in cognitive functioning, dementias,[21,22] and white matter atrophy.[23]

Additionally, the epigenetic component, which is strongly associated with nutrition, should be highlighted.[24,25] Epigenetic mechanisms occur throughout life, due to environmental aspects, such as diet, toxin exposure, variations in maternal energy status, and others. They can activate or silence gene expression in specific gene loci of specific cells, yielding particular phenotypes; sometimes, the pathological manifestations occur only at late-life.[24] **Box 2** describes the categories of epigenetic modifications, and some examples of these changes in AD.

Box 1
The immunosenescence hypothesis to inflammaging

- With the continued exposure to antigens throughout life, antigen-presenting cells, especially macrophages, gradually become hyperstimulated, increasing their secretion of inflammatory cytokines. Although the immunosenescence in microglia is still poorly understood, it is believed to be one of the main features of Alzheimer disease.

- The microglial senescence means the loss of fundamental neuroprotective aspects: clearing of debris, production of neurotrophic factors, autoprotection from damage by synthesis of glutathione from glutamate, sequestration of free iron from ferritin, regulation of plasticity of neuronal circuits.

Data from Franceschi C, Bonafè M, Valensin S, et al. Inflamm-aging. An evolutionary perspective on immunosenescence. Ann N Y Acad Sci 2000;908:244–54; and Streit WJ, Xue QS. Alzheimer's disease, neuroprotection, and CNS immunosenescence. Front Pharmacol 2012;3:138.

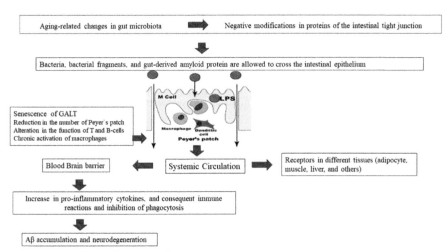

Fig. 1. Intestinal hypothesis to inflammaging. Senescence changes the GALT (gut-associated lymphoid tissue) functions, and modifies the balance between bacterial species, modifying trophic activity, defense, and barrier function. As a consequence, bacteria, bacterial fragments, and amyloid protein (produced by some gut bacteria) can then invade the systemic circulation, cross the BBB, and accumulate in the brain. LPS, lipopolysaccharide. (*Data from* Refs.[13–19])

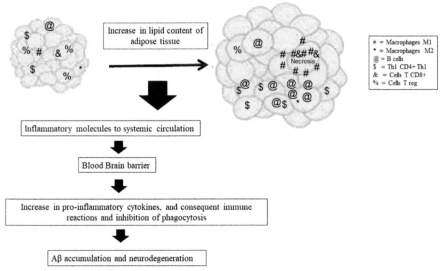

Fig. 2. Adipose tissue hypothesis to inflammaging. The increase in the lipid content of adipocytes increases the inflammatory status; immune cells infiltrate the adipocytes and release inflammatory molecules into circulation. (*Data from* Nishimura S, Manabe I, Nagasaki M, et al. CD8+ effector T cells contribute to macrophage recruitment and adipose tissue inflammation in obesity. Nat Med 2009;15(8):914–20; and Kalupahana NS, Moustaid-Moussa N, Claycombe KJ. Immunity as a link between obesity and insulin resistance. Mol Aspects Med 2012;33(1):26–34.)

Box 2

Different categories of epigenetic modifications, and some examples of these modifications with Alzheimer disease (AD)

DNA methylation

- Addition of a methyl group to the cytosine bases, by DNA methyltransferases (DNMTs), and with S-adenosyl-L-methionine (SAM) as methyl group donor. It causes silencing of gene transcription.

- Synaptic plasticity, learning, memory, modulation of neuronal gene expression, neuronal survival, and repair are dependent on DNA methylation.

- Hydroxymethylation of DNA is a result of oxidative stress, especially in neurons.

- *Some results of human and nonhuman studies:* Aging decreases the gene expression of specific DNMTs in different areas of human brain. Reductions or unusual methylation patterns have been associated with decline in learning and memory and have also been identified in patients with AD. Target genes primarily involved in AD pathogenesis have displayed changes in methylation patterns. Although with some controversies between different studies, there are possibly, with aging, hypomethylation and consequent changes in the expression of the promoter region of the amyloid precursor protein (APP) gene, as well as of other susceptible genes (encoding Apo E, methylenetetrahydrofolate reductase, PSEN1), leading to increased accumulation of Aβ.

Histone posttranslational modifications

- Histone posttranslational modifications include acetylation, methylation, phosphorylation, ubiquitination, and sumoylation.

- These reactions are catalyzed by different enzymes and can (1) activate gene transcription (histone acetyltransferases, HAT), (2) limit the accessibility and inactivation of gene for transcription (histone deacetylases, HDACs), (3) contribute to transcriptionally inactive chromatin (histone methyltransferases, HMTs, and histone demethylases).

- Chromatin remodeling consists of different histone/DNA conformations formed after interactions between DNA and histone proteins. Different forms of remodeling can either silence genes or allow gene expression. Histone H3 phosphorylation and acetylation are important in the formation of long-term memory.

- *Some results of human and nonhuman studies:* The balance between acetylation and deacetylation is greatly impaired in AD, mainly due to hyperphosphorylation of different histones in specific regions of the brain; these processes are associated with memory and learning and are frequent in AD brains. Different studies have associated different classes of HDAC, including sirtuins, with AD pathology.

MicroRNAs (miRNAs)

- Short RNA sequences that affect the transcriptional and translational processes by binding to their target in RNAs.

- miRNAs can control the expression of DNMTs and histone-modifying enzymes.

- miRNAs influence cellular processes, such as neuronal survival.

- *Some results of human and nonhuman studies:* Misregulation (upregulation or downregulation) of some members of the messenger RNA family have been shown in patients with AD; these misregulations may contribute to the alterations in gene expression and consequent neuronal degeneration. A number of miRNAs are associated with processes, such as control of oxidative stress, and expression of APP, BACE1, amyloidβ, BDNF, and SIRT1.

Abbreviations: BACE1, beta-secretase-1; BDNF, brain-derived neurotrophic factor; SIRT1, sirtuin 1.
Data from Sezgin Z, Dincer Y. Alzheimer's disease and epigenetic diet. Neurochem Int 2014;78:105–16.

NUTRIENTS AND PREVENTION OR ATTENUATION OF ALZHEIMER DISEASE

Evidence has established a strong association between diet and mental health, supporting the pivotal role of nutrients in brain functioning, which encompass cognitive function, memory, mood, and the overall mental health. In situations of nutritional deficits, particularly during senescence, brain functions may be altered, favoring the occurrence of neuropsychiatric disorders.[26] Hence, the appropriate brain function depends on the quality and quantity of dietary intake of nutrients, along with their absorption, biological utilization, and their ability to cross the BBB.

Energy Status, Nutrients, and Brain

Energy

Energy status is related to energy intake, which in turn, is controlled by hormones and growth factors. These molecules modulate gene expression related to brain development and functioning. The energy status of the body regulates epigenetic events associated with mental health, mainly the mitochondrial energy metabolism, regulation of the neurotrophic factor genes, and synaptic plasticity.[24] Aβ accumulation in AD is associated with impaired mitochondrial biogenesis, which entails mitochondrial dysfunction and consequent disruption in energy metabolism.[4]

Carbohydrates

Glucose partially participates in the regulation of memory and learning formation processes, probably via the cholinergic system.[27] Inadequate blood glucose regulation has shown reduced memorization; for example, moderate hypoglycemia induces general cognitive dysfunctions.[28]

Individuals with diabetes mellitus are described to have decreased memory, attention, and other cognitive domains, compared with their healthy counterparts, wherein raised insulin levels possibly play a part in this correlation.[29] Insulin is partly attributed to a neuroprotective action along with a participation in neuronal growth and survival, as well as a suggested regulative role in the gene expression involved in long-term memory.[30] In fact, in cognitively healthy nondiabetic individuals it was observed that fasting glucose levels in the upper threshold of the normal range are linked with greater impairment in the hippocampus and amygdala.[31]

A linkage between brain glucose dysregulation and the pathogenesis of AD has been revealed. A considerable glucose concentration was found in brain regions more susceptible to aggregation of hyperphosphorylated tau and Aβ, even in the period before the beginning of the disease, which in turn exacerbates their severity.[32] Moreover, this dysregulation has led to brain impairment, involving neuronal dysfunction in insulin signaling and endoplasmic reticulum, which occurs similarly in peripheral tissues in type 2 diabetes.[30,33] Bringing these statements to the progression of AD, **Fig. 3** illustrates the possible role of glucose metabolism in AD.

Proteins and amino acids

Amino acids (AAs) and their derivatives are necessary for the adequate functioning of the central nervous system (CNS). Insufficient provision of dietary protein leads to brain disturbances, such as alteration in the cerebral monoaminergic function that might influence psychosocial behavior and pathologies influenced by neurotransmitters.[34] Seemingly, 2 brain structures are more susceptible to this deficiency: the hippocampus and the cortex.[35] Large neutral AAs, particularly tryptophan, the main substrate involved in the synthesis of serotonin and catecholamines,[36] execute a modulatory role in sleep and behavioral processes. Low concentrations of tryptophan may precede mood and cognitive impairments. Some experimental data suggest a

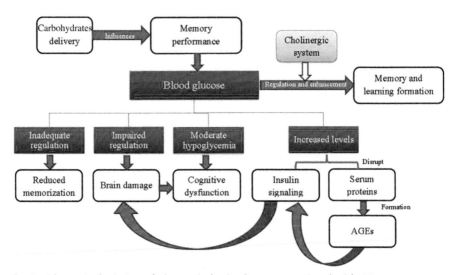

Fig. 3. Schematic depiction of glucose in brain changes associated with AD.

protective role of serotonin against the Aβ accumulation in the hippocampus by increasing its levels through dietary tryptophan supply.[37] Glutamatergic neurons are recognized for their participation in learning and memory,[38] then affected in AD, in which the synaptic levels of glutamate, an excitatory neurotransmitter, may be influenced by the Aβ aggregation.[39]

Acetyl-L-carnitine (ALC), derived from L-carnitine, may stimulate the production and delivery of acetylcholine. In nonhuman studies, ALC was found to increase brain synaptic function, thus improving memory and learning capacity in aging conditions.[40] For example, ALC was able to improve spatial learning and long-term memory performance, raise levels and modulates the activity of neurotrophins, as well as diminish homocysteine levels, tau hyperphosphorylation, and Aβ accumulation in rats.[41,42] N-acetylcysteine (NAC), derivative of cysteine, is the precursor of the most important endogenous antioxidant, glutathione.[43] In animal models, the antioxidant activity of NAC concedes its beneficial effect by preventing oxidative processes.[44,45] **Fig. 4** summarizes some associations between AAs and AD.

Lipids and fatty acids
Polyunsaturated fatty acids (PUFAs) may exert neuroprotective mechanisms against inflammation and oxidative stress in the CNS. DHA has revealed a capacity to mitigate

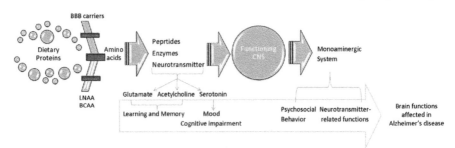

Fig. 4. Schematic depiction of AAs in brain changes associated with AD. BCAA, branched-chain amino acids; LNAA, large neutral amino acids.

Aβ secretion in animal models and cultured cells through the inhibition of Aβ42–induced neurotoxicity, and enhance microglial phagocytosis of Aβ42, promoting brain cell survival and protecting them from apoptosis induced by the amyloidosis.[46,47] In vivo and in vitro studies have suggested an antioxidant activity of n–3 PUFAs, despite that they are known for being prone to oxidation; given the reduced production of reactive oxygen species and lipid peroxidation metabolites after n–3 supplementation.[48]

Several studies propose the indirect influence of other lipids in the pathogenesis of AD. Albeit cholesterol has a significant function in neurotransmission and synaptogenesis in brain cell membranes, high levels have been involved in the Aβ formation in neuronal tissues, and may be linked to AD through vascular dementia, a risk for developing this disease.[49,50] In contrast, in elderly individuals without dementia, high total and high low-density lipoprotein cholesterol have been associated with better memory and cognitive performance.[51]

On the other hand, triglycerides have been correlated with diminished transport of leptin across the BBB. This hormone has an effect on hippocampus and is thought to positively influence memory and learning processes; leptin also increases the transport of ghrelin and insulin, which may concede positive effects on cognition, even in AD.[50] Also, in cognitively healthy individuals it was observed that high levels of triglycerides during adult years might antecede the development of the neuropathology 2 decades later[52] (**Fig. 5**).

Micronutrients

The metabolism of macronutrients is in strict relationship with the ideal amount and proportion of micronutrients, basically vitamins and minerals. A number of these micronutrients deserve special attention in brain functioning and the neuropathology of AD, which are summarized in **Table 1**.

Other Dietary Substances and Alzheimer Disease

Besides the conventional nutrients, the anti-inflammatory and/or antioxidant role of different substances present in foods has gained special attention. Herein, we highlight substances related to the control of the intestinal environment

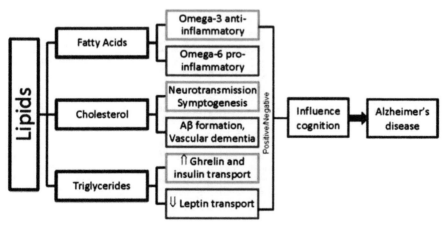

Fig. 5. Schematic depiction of lipids in brain changes associated with AD. ⇑, increase; ⇓, decrease.

Table 1
Related role of micronutrients on brain metabolism, mental functions, and the neuropathology occurring in AD

Micronutrients	Brain Metabolism	Hypothesized Roles	
		Mental Functions	Neuropathology AD
Vitamin A (retinoic acids [RAs])[53-55]	Dopaminergic cognitive function, signaling, synaptic plasticity, gene regulation, neurogenesis modulation, neuronal differentiation, and regeneration	RA supplementation improved learning and memory; enhanced cognitive decline.[b] RAs bind to retinoic acid receptors in brain areas involved in cognitive processes.[a]	Serum levels decreased in patients with AD. Deficiency enhanced Aβ deposition.[b] RAs synthesis is reduced in brain areas containing high amounts of Aβ peptides.[b] Prevented the aggregation of Aβ and tau phosphorylation.[b]
Vitamin B1 (Thiamine)[56,57]	Cofactor in glucose metabolism and pentose phosphate pathway, vital for the synthesis of some neurotransmitters, and GSH. Neuromodulation of the acetylcholine (ACh).	Deficiency produces a cholinergic deficit and induces excess glutamate release. Positive correlation of B1 deficiency with learning and memory impairment.	Serum levels decreased in AD. Long-term deficiency might promote the formation of Aβ plaques and NFT.[b]
Vitamin C (ascorbic acid)[58-60]	Cofactor in the synthesis of catecholamines. Neural maturation and neuromodulation of the activity of ACh, glutamate, GABA, dopamine and the catecholamines.	Long-term supplementation at 2 different dosages, found in the lowest dose that the anxiolytic effects were more typical, while memory improvement seemed to be confined to the highest dose.[b] Deficiency produce reduced spatial cognition in perinatal phase.[b]	Therapeutic action against the oxidative-induced damage. Moderate deficiency, mostly during initial stages of disease, has a significant effect in accelerating amyloid pathogenesis, which may be modulated by oxidative stress pathways.[b]
Vitamin D (1,25 [OH]2 D3)[61-63]	Modulation of brain development. Neurotransmission and neuroprotection via the nerve growth factor.	Regulation of sleep.	Serum levels decreased in older population. Amyloid phagocytosis and clearance. May ameliorate some calcium deleterious effects of Aβ.
Vitamin E (α-tocopherol)[64,65]	Antioxidant and free radical scavenger. Protects PUFA within biological membranes and in plasma lipoproteins.	Ancillary participation in activation and suppression of enzymatic reactions that may influence cognitive processes.[b] Influence memory, cognition, and emotional functions.	Deficiency with a simultaneous augmentation in the indexes of oxidative/nitrosative damage are found in patients with AD or MCI.

Nutrient			
Vitamin K (menaquinone-4 [MK-4])[66]	Production of sphingolipids.	Correlation in the sphingolipids metabolism changes with age-related cognitive decline, AD.	Associated to neuroprotection against oxidative stress and inflammation.
Vitamin B6[24,67-69] Vitamin B9 (folic acid)[24,68-70] Vitamin B12[24,68-71]	These 3 vitamins participate in the 1-C metabolism, which is responsible for the synthesis of neurotransmitters and nucleic acids.	From 1-C metabolism, reductions in SAM and consequent increases in HCY have consequences in the neurotransmitter synthesis, synthesis of phospholipids in the cell membrane, formation of the myelin sheath, control of Aβ, Tau phosphorylation, neurotoxicity, vasotoxicity, and risk of arterial and brain diseases.	Impaired homocysteine metabolism and deregulation methylation reactions contribute to the accumulation of phosphorylated tau and APP in the brain. Reduced SAM modifies the expression of genes responsible for APP metabolism, which increases Aβ peptide synthesis and accumulation. HCY and SAM metabolism are, therefore, related to onset of AD.
Calcium (Ca)[63]	Regulation of synaptic transmission, depolarization.	Regulation of learning processes and the formation and consolidation of memory. Aggregation of Aβ in AD induces an increase in the resting level of Ca, causing a deregulation of Ca signaling, which possibly influences cognition by interfering with the rhythm rheostat that controls the sleep/wake cycle, affecting memory formation by a rapid erasure of memories acquired during the wake period before they can be consolidated during sleep.	Ca dyshomeostasis in the aging process. Dysfunction of Ca signaling pathways in the brain is associated with AD.
Magnesium (Mg)[24,72-74]	Synthesis of nucleic acids and proteins. Potential of action conduction and neurotransmitter release. Protection of synaptic plasticity.	Deficiency triggers neuropsychiatric disturbances. Brain Mg has an inhibitory function on N-methyl-D-aspartate (NMDA) receptor regulating its excitability, which rises at an Mg-deficient state, this receptor participates in learning and memory. Supplementation improved hippocampal frequency potentiation and learning and memory functions.[b] Mg is able to protect the brain against the pathogenic effect of iron overload.	Low levels in patients with AD. Magnesium levels are decreased in various areas of AD brain. Deficiency may have a role in the pathogenesis of AD in the reduction of tau hyperphosphorylation, and modulative role of the amyloid-β protein precursor (AβPP). Regulation of oxidative stress and the release of calcitonin gene-related peptide and substance P, an inflammatory neuropeptide increased by Mg deficiency.

(continued on next page)

Table 1
(continued)

| | | Hypothesized Roles | |
Micronutrients	Brain Metabolism	Mental Functions	Neuropathology AD
Manganese (Mn)[75,76]	Synaptic neurotransmission in glutamatergic neurons. Part of Mn metalloproteins, that is, glutamine synthetase, Mn superoxide dismutase Mn-SOD.	Dietary deficiency may trigger neurologic dysfunctions. Higher levels are neurotoxic because it induces oxidative activity.	Mn-SOD offers neuroprotection to an oxidative stress. Aβ deposition may decrease its activity leading to mitochondrial dysfunction.[b]
Selenium (Se)[24,77,78]	Component of selenoproteins. Modulator of brain functions through the antioxidant and anti-inflammatory effects of Se-containing glutathione peroxidase, methionine-sulfoxide-reductase and thioredoxin reductases.	Selenoproteins play an important role in normal brain function. Deficiency leads to negative outcomes in cognitive function. Low ingestion may increase anxiety, depression, and tiredness that eventually can improve after Se supplementation.	Selenoprotein P offers neuroprotection to brain cells against the amyloid-β-induced oxidative damage inhibiting neuronal apoptosis.
Copper[24,79]	Cofactor in brain enzymatic activities.	High levels are linked to reduced neuropsychological performance and medial temporal lobe atrophy.	Aβ has a high affinity, and is able to reduce, Cu2+, Zn2+, and Fe3+, producing ROS, increasing Aβ toxicity
Iron[24,80]	Participates in a number of enzymes that mediate the synthesis of neurotransmitters.	Deficiency represents a risk for permanent cognitive deficits and behavioral affections.	With neuronal damaged occurs due to oxidative stress, bound intracellular zinc can be released into the cytosol, collaborating with further ROS production.
Zinc[24,81-84]	Fastened to metalloproteins in neurons and glial cells. Found in synaptic vesicles of some glutamatergic areas associated with episodic memory, behavior, and emotional expression. Important role in gene regulation, structural stabilization of proteins, enzymatic activity, and neurotransmission.	Influences cognition as a neuronal messenger and modulator of synaptic transmission and plasticity. Deficiency causes alterations in behavior and cognitive functioning[b] and permanent disruptions of learning and memory.[b]	Free zinc in the cytosol induces Aβ aggregation, and it can also directly bind to tau protein, facilitating the formation of neurofibrillary tangles. Magnesium also has a crucial role in AD pathogenesis.

Abbreviations: AD, Alzheimer disease; GABA, gamma aminobutyric acid; GSH, glutathione; HCY, homocysteine; MCI, mild cognitive impairment; Mn-SOD, manganese superoxide dismutase; NFT, neurofibrillary tangle; PUFA, polyunsaturated fatty acids; ROS, reactive oxygen species; SAM, S-adenosyl-L-methionine.
[a] Evidence in vivo, in vitro.
[b] Evidence in animal models.

and inflammation that can potentially contribute to AD prevention and/or attenuation.

Prebiotic, probiotic, and symbiotic substances

Having in mind the inflammatory hypothesis, it is plausible to assume that probiotics, prebiotics, or symbiotic substances could be important to prevent, postpone, or minimize some of the manifestations of AD. Several nonhuman studies, in vitro or with animals, have pointed evidence of the relationship between gut and brain disorders in AD.[6,20] However, only 1 small clinical study with humans was found in the literature up to now. Akbari and colleagues[1] investigated the effects of probiotics in subjects with AD. The intake of *Lactobacillus* and *Bifidobacterium* for 12 weeks improved the mental status (evaluated by the Mini-Mental State Examination), oxidative stress, insulin resistance, and serum triglycerides, when compared with a control group.[1]

Polyphenols

Polyphenols are ubiquitous molecules among different foods, mainly fruits and vegetables.[85] Their metabolites have activity on numerous brain processes, such as (1) interaction with neuronal/glial signaling pathways, scavenging radicals, chelating metals, upregulating the antioxidant enzymes and proteins related to synapses plasticity and neuronal repair; (2) improvement of the cerebral blood flow; (3) inhibition of pathologic processes in specific regions of the brain; and (4) interaction with neuronal signaling pathways involved in cell survival and programmed cell death, increasing synaptic plasticity and memory.[85] Epigenetic studies, most of them performed in vitro or in nonhuman models, have shown benefits in the prevention of AD.[86–88] **Table 2** shows some examples of these actions.

Finally, a few studies have shown that polyphenol supplementation may be effective in improving intestinal microbiota.[89]

ISOLATED NUTRIENTS OR DIETARY PATTERNS?

Most published interventions in AD use nutrient supplementations. In a systematic review with meta-analyses performed by our group, we gathered clinical trials using different supplementation protocols, single or combined nutrients, in patients diagnosed with AD at any stage. The results exhibited some slight, or sometimes no significant effects on different Alzheimer-related outcomes. The importance of nutrients was explicit; nonetheless, the lack of significant effectiveness suggested that single nutrient supplementation may represent a weak approach considering the complex interaction of nutrients, on the chronic and progressive damage generated by this disease; we tried to depict this complexity in **Fig. 6**.[90,91]

Different nutrients act synergistically, as dietary patterns, to influence the risk or protection of several chronic diseases, including AD. Therefore, it is consistent to think that the studies of dietary patterns can provide more concrete information regarding the development or prevention of AD. In **Box 3**, we present a summary of the most studied dietary patterns in this context.[92–99]

NUTRITION IN THE MANAGEMENT OF THE PATIENT WITH ALZHEIMER DISEASE

Once the disease is installed, one of the main concerns in its management is the body weight loss,[100–102] due to different factors. Some of these factors can be cognitive, behavioral, and motor disorders; medial and temporal lobe atrophy; and olfactory and taste disorders. Furthermore, the side effects of medication, social factors, and different comorbidities are secondary factors. All these factors are associated with

Table 2
Some epigenetic actions of food-derived polyphenols, obtained from in vitro studies

Molecules	Food Sources	Epigenetic Actions
Catechin, epicatechin (EC), epicatechin 3-gallate (ECG), epigallocatechin (EGC) and (−)-epigallocatechin-3-gallate (EGCG); bioflavonoids, such as quercetin, fisetin, myricetin, apigenin; and curcumin	Green tea, red wine, and chocolate (EC, ECG, EGC, EGCG); onions, leeks, and broccoli (quercetin); strawberries, apples, persimmons, onions, and cucumbers (fisetin); different vegetables, fruits, nuts, berries, tea, red wine (myricetin); parsley (Apigenin); spice turmeric (curcumin)	Inhibition of DNA methyltransferase (DNMT)-mediated DNA methylation in a concentration-dependent manner; therefore, they are able to demethylate and reactivate genes silenced by methylation.
EGCG	Green tea	Inhibition of DNA methylation, by forming hydrogen bonds between different residues in the active site of DNMT. ECGG contributes to histone posttranslational modifications by inhibiting histone methyltransferases.
Polyphenols	Garlic and cinnamon	Inhibition of histone deacetylases.
Resveratrol	Peanuts, mulberries, cranberries, and mostly in the skin of grapes	Inhibition of DNMT activity. Activation of SIRT1, a member of nicotinamide adenine dinucleotide (NAD+)-dependent deacetylases family. Activation of SIRT1 prevents β-amyloid–induced microglial death.
Curcumin	Spice turmeric	Reduction of Aβ level in vivo and in vitro. Potent inhibitor of histone acetyltransferases. Inhibition of DNMT1 activity.
Genistein	Soy and soy products	Regulation of gene transcription by affecting epigenetic modifications. Inhibition of DNMT1, DNMT3a and 3b, reactivating genes previously silenced by methylation.
Anthocyanins	Blueberry, raspberry, black rice, and black soybean	Reduction of age-associated oxidative stress. Inhibition of Aβ aggregation into oligomers. Inhibition of tau filament formation.

Abbreviation: EGCG, epigallocatechin-3-gallate.
 Data from Refs.[8,24,85–88]

forgetfulness of eating, refusal to eat, increases of energy expenditure, and loss of appetite.[89]

The different stages of AD present different features related to nutritional status, which demands different feeding strategies. In **Table 3**, we describe some possibilities in this regard.

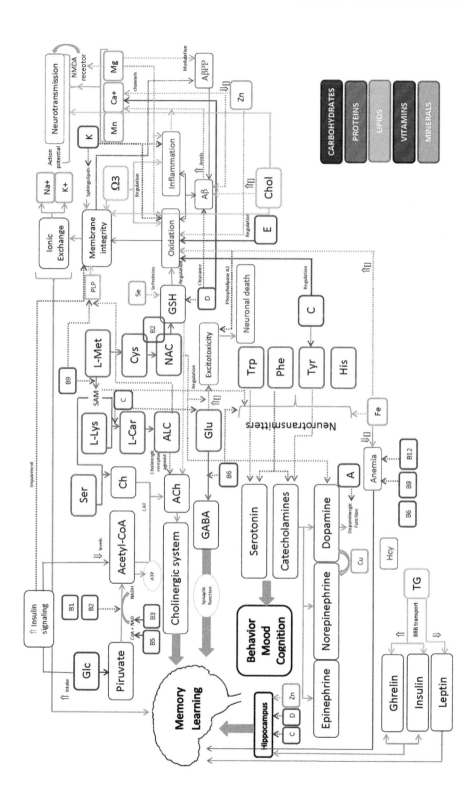

Box 3
Dietary patterns related to the development of AD

Patterns associated with the prevention or attenuation of the disease

Mediterranean diet (MeDi)
- Higher adherence to this pattern may provide some benefit to reduce the risk of cognitive impairment, cognitive decline, and dementia in cognitively healthy people and a decreased progression from mild cognitive impairment (MCI) to AD.
- Important source of nutrients such as monounsaturated fatty acids (MUFAs), polyunsaturated fatty acids (PUFAs), micronutrients, and antioxidants derived from the consumption of nuts, fruits, vegetables, legumes, cereals, and fish, with a moderate alcohol ingestion and fair intake of meat and dairy products, which confers considerable benefits acting on the aforesaid pathologic processes involved in AD.

Dietary Approaches to Stop Hypertension (DASH)
- This style has been proposed to offer neurocognitive improvements; however, there is no direct evidence examining a possible correlation between this diet and AD.

Mediterranean-DASH diet intervention for neurodegenerative delay (MIND)
- Based on the observed beneficial properties of MeDi and DASH for the brain performance, combination of both led to this modified hybrid style.
- MIND score considers 10 food groups deemed beneficial for brain health (green leafy vegetables, other vegetables, nuts, berries, beans, whole grains, seafood, poultry, olive oil, and wine) and 5 unhealthy components (red meats, butter and stick margarine, cheese, pastries and sweets, and fried/fast food).
- Higher score had a positive statistically significant association with slower rate of cognitive decline, predominantly at the level of episodic and semantic memory, as well as perceptual speed.

Fish-based diet
- Epidemiologic findings demonstrated a significant association between higher fish consumption and the low risk of developing AD.
- Additional analysis has detected a positive correlation between the intake of n-3 PUFAs and the low risk of MCI, but not for AD, dementia, or cognitive decline.
- The rapid rise in AD prevalence in Japan, which was among the lower rates, coincided with the nutritional transition when Western dietary styles were introduced to their traditional patterns of consumption typically based on rice and fish, but scanty ingestion of meat, dairy, sugar, with a low-to-moderate energy content.
- From these observations it was hypothesized that there is a possible association of these nutritional changes and the favoring in the occurrence of this disease.

Low-copper diet
- It was demonstrated a positive correlation with high levels of serum copper and poor neuropsychological performance as well as medial temporal lobe atrophy in people with AD.
- Given the assumption that copper participates in the pathogenesis of AD and its main supply comes primarily from food, a low-copper diet was postulated as a possible strategy to contribute to its risk reduction.
- Main sources of copper: animal liver, oysters, seafood, sunflower and sesame seeds, cocoa, cashew, pumpkin, sun-dried tomatoes, and dried herbs.

◀───

Fig. 6. Schematic depiction of the impact of brain nutrient interactions network on some brain functions affected in AD. ⇑[], increase concentration/levels; ⇓[], decrease concentration/levels; A, vitamin A; Acetyl-CoA, Acetyl coenzyme A; ACh, acetylcholine; ALC, acetyl-L-carnitine; Aβ, amyloid-β; AβPP, amyloid-β protein precursor; B, vitamin-B complex; C, vitamin C; Car, carnitine; CAT, choline acetyltransferase; Ch, choline; Chol, cholesterol; Cu, copper; Cys, cysteine; D, vitamin D; E, vitamin E; GABA, gamma aminobutyric acid; Glc, glucose; Glu, glutamate; GSH, glutathione; His, histidine; K, vitamin K; K+, potassium; Lys, lysine; Met, methionine; Mg, magnesium; Mn, manganese; Na+, sodium; NAC, N-acetyl-cysteine; NMDA, N-methyl-D-aspartate receptor; Phe, phenylalanine; PLP, phospholipids; SAM, S-adenosyl-L-methionine; Se, selenium; Ser, serine; TG, triglycerides; Trp, tryptophan; Tyr, tyrosine; Zn, zinc; Ω3, FA omega-3.

Patterns associated with the increased risk of the disease

High-carbohydrate diet
- A low fat and high intake of processed carbohydrates instantly increases levels of postprandial blood glucose; this condition disrupts serum proteins, favoring the formation of advanced glycation end-products (AGEs).
- AGEs are highly induced by the consumption of fructose, commonly used by the food industry.
- AGEs alter lipid homeostasis in the brain and permanent augmented insulin/insulinlike growth factor signaling, affecting the normal function and integrity of neuronal membrane, including glucose transporters and the APP, promoting brain cellular damage, followed by the later behavioral and cognitive changes. These biochemical activities have been observed in ApoE4 carriers that can be worsened when exposed to high-carbohydrate diets.

Data from Refs.[92–99]

Table 3
Possibilities to improve feeding, according to the stage of the disease

Stage of the Disease	Aspects Associated with Food Intake	Possibilities of Strategies to Minimize the Problem
Initial stage	Loss of taste sensibility and loss of the thirst threshold.	The use of herbs and spices can improve the pleasure of eating. The person can benefit if he or she can take part in food preparation, even with small tasks. It is important to stimulate water intake. The use of a food diary can help as a cognitive training tool (for instance, a notebook in which the patient could take notes of the meals, including some memories that the type of food could bring to them). Involvement of the patient in interaction groups (family, friend, or community centers) can help the patient to avoid reductions in food intake.
Intermediary stage	It is common to forget meals; that is, the patient eats, but forget almost immediately. Dysphagia occurs more frequently.	Fractionation of the meals throughout the day can be a good option to deal with forgetfulness. Although difficult, it is very important to maintain having meals together with the family, in an attempt to minimize or delay the forgetfulness. It is important to be aware of the need for thickeners, and to pay attention to the consistency of the meals. It seems to be helpful to use flavored water with mint, peel of lemon or orange, or cinnamon, among others.
Advanced stage and palliative care	This stage of the disease is characterized by apathy, and total cognitive loss. Feeding is associated with a high risk of bronchoaspiration and asphyxia. The patient generally is unable to feed by him/herself. It is common to forget the function of cutlery, and when the food is inside the mouth, he or she does not know what to do next.	A good strategy is to eat together with the patient, simulating to him or her the mouth movements. The risk of dysphagia in this stage is very high, which demands special attention during eating. In the terminal stage, it is necessary to consider a diet with a gummy consistency, liquids with thickening. It is important to consider the use of nutritional supplements, such as hypercaloric. In this stage, many times it is necessary to decide about tube feeding.

SUMMARY AND PERSPECTIVES

Nutrients participate in the formation, physiologic and anatomic development, and maintenance of brain health. Several nutrients have been studied in the pursuit of the mechanism triggered by the pathology of AD. The findings suggest a modulator and protective effect of nutrients against dementia. Nevertheless, more research is necessary to draw definite conclusions. Understanding this role is a key determinant to search for adequate nutritional interventions and identify the gaps in research in this area and thus conduct new investigations.

Finally, it is important to highlight the multifactorial origin of AD development and progression. Nutrition, despite its importance, can be considered only one path in this complex network of factors.

REFERENCES

1. Akbari E, Asemi Z, Daneshvar Kakhaki R, et al. Effect of probiotic supplementation on cognitive function and metabolic status in Alzheimer's disease: a randomized, double-blind and controlled trial. Front Aging Neurosci 2016;8:256.
2. National Academies of Sciences, Engineering and Medicine, Leshner AI, Landis S, Stroud C, et al, editors. Preventing cognitive decline and dementia. Washington, DC: National Academies Press; 2017.
3. He Z, Guo JL, McBride JD, et al. Amyloid-β plaques enhance Alzheimer's brain tau-seeded pathologies by facilitating neuritic plaque tau aggregation. Nat Med 2018;24(1):29–38.
4. Mancuso C, Santangelo R. Alzheimer's disease and gut microbiota modifications: the long way between preclinical studies and clinical evidence. Pharmacol Res 2018;129:329–36.
5. Akiyama H, Barger S, Barnum S, et al. Inflammation and Alzheimer's disease. Neurobiol Aging 2000;21(3):383–421.
6. Cattaneo A, Cattane N, Galluzzi S, et al. Association of brain amyloidosis with pro-inflammatory gut bacterial taxa and peripheral inflammation markers in cognitively impaired elderly. Neurobiol Aging 2017;49:60–8.
7. Sadleir KR, Kandalepas PC, Buggia-Prévot V, et al. Presynaptic dystrophic neurites surrounding amyloid plaques are sites of microtubule disruption, BACE1 elevation, and increased Aβ generation in Alzheimer's disease. Acta Neuropathol 2016;132(2):235–56.
8. Rubio-Perez JM, Morillas-Ruiz JM. A review: inflammatory process in Alzheimer's disease, role of cytokines. ScientificWorldJournal 2012;2012:1–15.
9. Franceschi C, Bonafè M, Valensin S, et al. Inflamm-aging. An evolutionary perspective on immunosenescence. Ann N Y Acad Sci 2000;908:244–54.
10. Cacquevel M, Lebeurrier N, Chéenne S, et al. Cytokines in neuroinflammation and Alzheimer's disease. Curr Drug Targets 2004;5(6):529–34.
11. Franceschi C, Campisi J. Chronic inflammation (inflammaging) and its potential contribution to age-associated diseases. J Gerontol A Biol Sci Med Sci 2014; 69(Suppl 1):S4–9.
12. Streit WJ, Xue QS. Alzheimer's disease, neuroprotection, and CNS immunosenescence. Front Pharmacol 2012;3:138.
13. Alkasir R, Li J, Li X, et al. Human gut microbiota: the links with dementia development. Protein Cell 2017;8(2):90–102.
14. García-Peña C, Álvarez-Cisneros T, Quiroz-Baez R, et al. Microbiota and aging. A review and commentary. Arch Med Res 2017;48(8):681–9.

15. Zhao Y, Lukiw WJ. Microbiome-generated amyloid and potential impact on amyloidogenesis in Alzheimer's disease (AD). J Nat Sci 2015;1(7):e138.
16. Pistollato F, Sumalla Cano S, Elio I, et al. Role of gut microbiota and nutrients in amyloid formation and pathogenesis of Alzheimer disease. Nutr Rev 2016; 74(10):624–34.
17. Friedland RP. Mechanisms of molecular mimicry involving the microbiota in neurodegeneration. J Alzheimers Dis 2015;45(2):349–62.
18. Caricilli AM, Saad MJA. The role of gut microbiota on insulin resistance. Nutrients 2013;5(3):829–51.
19. Cani PD, Delzenne NM. The role of the gut microbiota in energy metabolism and metabolic disease. Curr Pharm Des 2009;15(13):1546–58.
20. Harach T, Marungruang N, Duthilleul N, et al. Reduction of Abeta amyloid pathology in APPPS1 transgenic mice in the absence of gut microbiota. Sci Rep 2017;7:41802.
21. Bischof GN, Park DC. Obesity and aging: consequences for cognition, brain structure, and brain function. Psychosom Med 2015;77(6):697–709.
22. Dye L, Boyle NB, Champ C, et al. The relationship between obesity and cognitive health and decline. Proc Nutr Soc 2017;76(4):443–54.
23. Fotenos AF, Snyder AZ, Girton LE, et al. Normative estimates of cross-sectional and longitudinal brain volume decline in aging and AD. Neurology 2005;64(6):1032–9.
24. Sezgin Z, Dincer Y. Alzheimer's disease and epigenetic diet. Neurochem Int 2014;78:105–16.
25. Chouliaras L, Rutten BPF, Kenis G, et al. Epigenetic regulation in the pathophysiology of Alzheimer's disease. Prog Neurobiol 2010;90(4):498–510.
26. Sarris J, Logan AC, Akbaraly TN, et al. Nutritional medicine as mainstream in psychiatry. Lancet Psychiatry 2015;2(3):271–4.
27. Benton D, Owens S, Parker PY. Blood glucose influences memory in young adults and attention. Neuropsychologia 1994;32(5):595–607.
28. Warren RE, Frier BM. Hypoglycaemia and cognitive function. Diabetes Obes Metab 2005;7:493–503.
29. Kodl CT, Seaquist ER. Cognitive dysfunction and diabetes mellitus. Endocr Rev 2008;29(4):494–511.
30. Vieira MNN, Lima-Filho RAS, De Felice FG. Connecting Alzheimer's disease to diabetes: underlying mechanisms and potential therapeutic targets. Neuropharmacology 2018;136(Pt B):160–71.
31. Cherbuin N, Sachdev P, Anstey KJ. Higher normal fasting plasma glucose is associated with hippocampal atrophy: The PATH Study. Neurology 2012;79: 1019–26.
32. An Y, Varma VR, Varma S, et al. Evidence for brain glucose dysregulation in Alzheimer's disease. Alzheimers Dement 2018;14(3):318–29.
33. Wijesekara N, Gonçalves da Silva RA, De Felice FG, et al. Impaired peripheral glucose homeostasis and Alzheimer's disease. Neuropharmacology 2018; 136(Pt B):172–81.
34. Kar BR, Rao SL, Chandramouli BA. Cognitive development in children with chronic protein energy malnutrition. Behav Brain Funct 2008;4(1):31.
35. Georgieff MK. Nutrition and the developing brain: nutrient priorities and measurement. Am J Clin Nutr 2007;85(2):614–20.
36. Fernstrom JD, Fernstrom MH. Tyrosine, phenylalanine, and catecholamine synthesis and function in the brain. J Nutr 2007;137(6 Suppl 1):1539S–47S [discussion: 1548S].

37. Noristani HN, Verkhratsky A, Rodríguez JJ. High tryptophan diet reduces CA1 intraneuronal β-amyloid in the triple transgenic mouse model of Alzheimer's disease. Aging Cell 2012;11(5):810–22.
38. Greenamyre JT, Young AB. Excitatory amino acids and Alzheimer's disease. Neurobiol Aging 1989;10(5):593–602.
39. Revett TJ, Baker GB, Jhamandas J, et al. Glutamate system, amyloid β peptides and tau protein: functional interrelationships and relevance to Alzheimer disease pathology. J Psychiatry Neurosci 2013;38(1):6–23.
40. Kobayashi S, Iwamoto M, Kon K, et al. Acetyl-l-carnitine improves aged brain function. Geriatr Gerontol Int 2010;10(SUPPL. 1):99–106.
41. Yin Y-Y, Liu H, Cong X-B, et al. Acetyl-L-carnitine attenuates okadaic acid induced tau hyperphosphorylation and spatial memory impairment in rats. J Alzheimers Dis 2010;19(2):735–46.
42. Zhou P, Chen Z, Zhao N, et al. Acetyl-L-carnitine attenuates homocysteine-induced Alzheimer-like histopathological and behavioral abnormalities. Rejuvenation Res 2011;14(6):669–79.
43. Zhao Y, Zhao B. Oxidative stress and the pathogenesis of Alzheimer's disease. Oxid Med Cell Longev 2013;2013:1–10.
44. Fu A-L, Dong Z-H, Sun M-J. Protective effect of N-acetyl-l-cysteine on amyloid β-peptide-induced learning and memory deficits in mice. Brain Res 2006; 1109(1):201–6.
45. Robinson RAS, Joshi G, Huang Q, et al. Proteomic analysis of brain proteins in APP/PS-1 human double mutant knock-in mice with increasing amyloid β-peptide deposition: insights into the effects of in vivo treatment with N-acetylcysteine as a potential therapeutic intervention in mild cognitive. Proteomics 2012;11(21):4243–56.
46. Cunnane SC, Plourde M, Pifferi F, et al. Fish, docosahexaenoic acid and Alzheimer's disease. Prog Lipid Res 2009;48(5):239–56.
47. Hjorth E, Zhu M, Toro VC, et al. Omega-3 fatty acids enhance phagocytosis of Alzheimer's disease-related amyloid-β42 by human microglia and decrease inflammatory markers. J Alzheimers Dis 2013;35(4):697–713.
48. Richard D, Kefi K, Barbe U, et al. Polyunsaturated fatty acids as antioxidants. Pharmacol Res 2008;57(6):451–5.
49. Di Paolo G, Kim T-W. Linking lipids to Alzheimer's disease: cholesterol and beyond. Nat Rev Neurosci 2011;12(5):284–96.
50. Morley JE. Banks WA. Lipids and cognition. J Alzheimers Dis 2010;20(3): 737–47.
51. West R, Beeri MS, Schmeidler J, et al. Better memory functioning associated with higher total and low-density lipoprotein cholesterol levels in very elderly subjects without the apolipoprotein e4 allele. Am J Geriatr Psychiatry 2008; 16(9):781–5.
52. Nägga K, Gustavsson A-M, Stomrud E, et al. Increased midlife triglycerides predict brain β-amyloid and tau pathology 20 years later. Neurology 2018;90(1): e73–81.
53. Olson CR, Mello CV. Significance of vitamin A to brain function, behavior and learning. Mol Nutr Food Res 2010;54(4):489–95.
54. Krezel W, Kastner P, Chambon P. Differential expression of retinoid receptors in the adult mouse central nervous system. Neuroscience 1999;89(4):1291–300.
55. Ono K, Yamada M. Vitamin A and Alzheimer's disease. Geriatr Gerontol Int 2012; 12(2):180–8.

56. Gibson GE, Hirsch JA, Fonzetti P, et al. Vitamin B1 (thiamine) and dementia. Ann N Y Acad Sci 2016;1:21–30.
57. Karuppagounder SS, Xu H, Shi Q, et al. Thiamine deficiency induces oxidative stress and exacerbates the plaque pathology in Alzheimer's mouse model. Neurobiol Aging 2009;30(10):1587–600.
58. Hughes RN, Hancock NJ, Thompson RM. Anxiolysis and recognition memory enhancement with long-term supplemental ascorbic acid (vitamin C) in normal rats: possible dose dependency and sex differences. Ann Neurosci Psychol 2015;2(2):1–9.
59. Harrison FE, Bowman GL, Polidori MC. Ascorbic acid and the brain: rationale for the use against cognitive decline. Nutrients 2014;6(4):1752–81.
60. Dixit S, Bernardo A, Walker JM, et al. Vitamin C deficiency in the brain impairs cognition, increases amyloid accumulation and deposition, and oxidative stress in APP/PSEN1 and normally aging mice. ACS Chem Neurosci 2015;6(4): 570–81.
61. Kesby JP, Eyles DW, Burne THJ, et al. The effects of vitamin D on brain development and adult brain function. Mol Cell Endocrinol 2011;347(1–2):121–7.
62. Schlogl M, Holick MF. Vitamin D and neurocognitive function. Clin Interv Aging 2014;9:559–68.
63. Berridge MJ. Calcium regulation of neural rhythms, memory and Alzheimer's disease. J Physiol 2014;592(Pt 2):281–93.
64. Mangialasche F, Xu W, Kivipelto M, et al. Tocopherols and tocotrienols plasma levels are associated with cognitive impairment. Neurobiol Aging 2012;33: 2282–90.
65. Morris MC, Evans DA, Tangney CC, et al. Relation of the tocopherol forms to incident Alzheimer disease and to cognitive change. Am J Clin Nutr 2005;81: 508–14.
66. Ferland G. Vitamin K, an emerging nutrient in brain function. Biofactors 2012; 38(2):151–7.
67. Kennedy DO, Haskell CF. Vitamins and cognition: what is the evidence? Drugs 2011;71(15):1957–71.
68. Flicker L, Martins RN, Thomas J, et al. B-vitamins reduce plasma levels of beta amyloid. Neurobiol Aging 2008;29(2):303–5.
69. Selhub J, Troen A, Rosenberg IH. B vitamins and the aging brain. Nutr Rev 2010;68(Suppl 2):S112–8.
70. Black MM. Effects of vitamin B 12 and folate deficiency on brain development in children. Food Nutr Bull 2008;29(2_suppl1):S126–31.
71. Rafiee S, Asadollahi K, Riazi G, et al. Vitamin B12 inhibits tau fibrillization via binding to cysteine residues of tau. ACS Chem Neurosci 2017;8(12):2676–82.
72. Veronese N, Zurlo A, Solmi M, et al. Magnesium status in Alzheimer's disease: a systematic review. Am J Alzheimers Dis Other Demen 2015;31(3):208–13.
73. Xu ZP, Li L, Bao J, et al. Magnesium protects cognitive functions and synaptic plasticity in streptozotocin-induced sporadic Alzheimer's model. PLoS One 2014;9(9):1–11.
74. Yu J, Sun M, Chen Z, et al. Magnesium modulates amyloid-β protein precursor trafficking and processing. J Alzheimers Dis 2010;20(4):1091–106.
75. Takeda A. Manganese action in brain function. Brain Res Brain Res Rev 2003; 41:79–87.
76. Thomas H, Rupniak R, Joy KA, et al. Oxidative neuropathology and putative chemical entities for Alzheimer's disease: neuroprotective effects of salen-manganese catalytic anti-oxidants. Neurotox Res 2000;2(2):167–78.

77. Schweizer U, Bräuer AU, Köhrle J, et al. Selenium and brain function: a poorly recognized liaison. Brain Res Brain Res Rev 2004;45(3):164–78.

78. Rayman M, Thompson A, Warren-perry M, et al. Impact of selenium on mood and quality of life: a randomized, controlled trial. Biol Psychiatry 2006;59: 147–54.

79. Squitti R, Lupoi D, Pasqualetti P, et al. Elevation of serum copper levels in Alzheimer's disease. Neurology 2002;59(8):1153–61.

80. Rouault TA, Cooperman S. Brain iron metabolism. Semin Pediatr Neurol 2006; 13(3):142–8.

81. Sensi SL, Paoletti P, Koh J-Y, et al. The neurophysiology and pathology of brain zinc. J Neurosci 2011;31(45):16076–85.

82. Huang X, Cuajungco MP, Atwood CS, et al. Alzheimer's disease, beta-amyloid protein and zinc. J Nutr 2000;130(5S Suppl):1488S–92S.

83. Adlard PA, Parncutt J, Lal V, et al. Metal chaperones prevent zinc-mediated cognitive decline. Neurobiol Dis 2015;81:196–202.

84. Frederickson CJ, Koh J-Y, Bush AI. The neurobiology of zinc in health and disease. Nat Rev Neurosci 2005;6(6):449–62.

85. Williams RJ, Spencer JPE. Flavonoids, cognition, and dementia: actions, mechanisms, and potential therapeutic utility for Alzheimer disease. Free Radic Biol Med 2012;52(1):35–45.

86. Sahu BD, Kalvala AK, Koneru M, et al. Ameliorative effect of fisetin on cisplatin-induced nephrotoxicity in rats via modulation of NF-κB activation and antioxidant defence. PLoS One 2014;9(9):e105070.

87. Basli A, Soulet S, Chaher N, et al. Wine polyphenols: potential agents in neuroprotection. Oxid Med Cell Longev 2012;2012:805762.

88. Ross JA, Kasum CM. Dietary flavonoids: bioavailability, metabolic effects, and safety. Annu Rev Nutr 2002;22:19–34.

89. Dueñas M, Muñoz-González I, Cueva C, et al. A survey of modulation of gut microbiota by dietary polyphenols. Biomed Res Int 2015;2015:1–15.

90. Muñoz Fernández SS, Ivanauskas T, Lima Ribeiro SM. Nutritional strategies in the management of Alzheimer disease: systematic review with network meta-analysis. J Am Med Dir Assoc 2017;18(10):897.e13-30.

91. Cao L, Tan L, Wang H, et al. Dietary patterns and risk of dementia: a systematic review and meta-analysis of cohort studies. Mol Neurobiol 2016;53:6144–54.

92. Singh B, Parsaik AK, Mielke MM, et al. Association of Mediterranean diet with mild cognitive impairment and Alzheimer's disease: a systematic review and meta-analysis. J Alzheimers Dis 2014;39(2):271–82.

93. Petersson SD, Philippou E. Mediterranean diet, cognitive function, and dementia: a systematic review of the evidence. Adv Nutr 2016;(7):889–904.

94. Gu Y, Scarmeas N. Dietary patterns in Alzheimer's disease and cognitive aging. Curr Alzheimer Res 2011;8:510–9.

95. Morris MC, Tangney CC, Wang Y, et al. MIND diet associated with reduced incidence of Alzheimer's disease. Alzheimers Dement 2015;11(9):1007–14.

96. Zeng L-F, Cao Y, Liang W-X, et al. An exploration of the role of a fish-oriented diet in cognitive decline: a systematic review of the literature. Oncotarget 2017;8(24):39877–95.

97. Squitti R, Siotto M, Polimanti R. Low-copper diet as a preventive strategy for Alzheimer's disease. Neurobiol Aging 2014;35(SUPPL.2):S40–50.

98. Seneff S, Wainwright G, Mascitelli L. Nutrition and Alzheimer's disease: the detrimental role of a high carbohydrate diet. Eur J Intern Med 2011;22(2):134–40.

99. Perrone L, Grant WB. Observational and ecological studies of dietary advanced glycation end products in national diets and Alzheimer's disease incidence and prevalence. J Alzheimers Dis 2015;45(3):965–79.
100. Gillette-Guyonnet S, Nourhashemi F, Andrieu S, et al. Weight loss in Alzheimer disease. Am J Clin Nutr 2000;71(2):637S–42S.
101. Droogsma E, van Asselt D, De Deyn PP. Weight loss and undernutrition in community-dwelling patients with Alzheimer's dementia: from population-based studies to clinical management. Z Gerontol Geriatr 2015;48(4):318–24.
102. Saragat B, Buffa R, Mereu E, et al. Nutritional and psycho-functional status in elderly patients with Alzheimer's disease. J Nutr Health Aging 2012;16(3):231–6.

UNITED STATES POSTAL SERVICE ®

Statement of Ownership, Management, and Circulation (All Periodicals Publications Except Requester Publications)

1. Publication Title	2. Publication Number		3. Filing Date
CLINICS IN GERIATRIC MEDICINE	000 – 704		9/18/2018

4. Issue Frequency	5. Number of Issues Published Annually	6. Annual Subscription Price
FEB, MAY, AUG, NOV	4	$278.00

7. Complete Mailing Address of Known Office of Publication (Not printer) (Street, city, county, state, and ZIP+4®)

ELSEVIER INC.
230 Park Avenue, Suite 800
New York, NY 10169

Contact Person
STEPHEN R. BUSHING
Telephone (Include area code)
215-239-3688

8. Complete Mailing Address of Headquarters or General Business Office of Publisher (Not printer)

ELSEVIER INC.
230 Park Avenue, Suite 800
New York, NY 10169

9. Full Names and Complete Mailing Addresses of Publisher, Editor, and Managing Editor (Do not leave blank)

Publisher (Name and complete mailing address)

TAYLOR E. BALL, ELSEVIER INC.
1600 JOHN F KENNEDY BLVD. SUITE 1800
PHILADELPHIA, PA 19103-2899

Editor (Name and complete mailing address)

JESSICA MCCOOL, ELSEVIER INC.
1600 JOHN F KENNEDY BLVD. SUITE 1800
PHILADELPHIA, PA 19103-2899

Managing Editor (Name and complete mailing address)

PATRICK MANLEY, ELSEVIER INC.
1600 JOHN F KENNEDY BLVD. SUITE 1800
PHILADELPHIA, PA 19103-2899

10. Owner (Do not leave blank. If the publication is owned by a corporation, give the name and address of the corporation immediately followed by the names and addresses of all stockholders owning or holding 1 percent or more of the total amount of stock. If not owned by a corporation, give the names and addresses of the individual owners. If owned by a partnership or other unincorporated firm, give its name and address as well as those of each individual owner. If the publication is published by a nonprofit organization, give its name and address.)

Full Name	Complete Mailing Address
WHOLLY OWNED SUBSIDIARY OF REED/ELSEVIER US HOLDINGS	1600 JOHN F KENNEDY BLVD. SUITE 1800 PHILADELPHIA, PA 19103-2899

11. Known Bondholders, Mortgagees, and Other Security Holders Owning or Holding 1 Percent or More of Total Amount of Bonds, Mortgages, or Other Securities. If none, check box ► ☐ None

Full Name	Complete Mailing Address
N/A	

12. Tax Status (For completion by nonprofit organizations authorized to mail at nonprofit rates) (Check one)
The purpose, function, and nonprofit status of this organization and the exempt status for federal income tax purposes:
☒ Has Not Changed During Preceding 12 Months
☐ Has Changed During Preceding 12 Months (Publisher must submit explanation of change with this statement)

PS Form 3526, July 2014 [Page 1 of 4 (see instructions page 4)] PSN: 7530-01-000-9931   PRIVACY NOTICE: See our privacy policy on www.usps.com.

---

13. Publication Title			14. Issue Date for Circulation Data Below
CLINICS IN GERIATRIC MEDICINE			MAY 2018

15. Extent and Nature of Circulation			Average No. Copies Each Issue During Preceding 12 Months	No. Copies of Single Issue Published Nearest to Filing Date
a. Total Number of Copies (Net press run)			127	204
b. Paid Circulation (By Mail and Outside the Mail)	(1)	Mailed Outside-County Paid Subscriptions Stated on PS Form 3541 (Include paid distribution above nominal rate, advertiser's proof copies, and exchange copies)	60	86
	(2)	Mailed In-County Paid Subscriptions Stated on PS Form 3541 (Include paid distribution above nominal rate, advertiser's proof copies, and exchange copies)	0	0
	(3)	Paid Distribution Outside the Mails Including Sales Through Dealers and Carriers, Street Vendors, Counter Sales, and Other Paid Distribution Outside USPS®	30	44
	(4)	Paid Distribution by Other Classes of Mail Through the USPS (e.g., First-Class Mail®)	0	0
c. Total Paid Distribution (Sum of 15b (1), (2), (3), and (4))		►	90	130
d. Free or Nominal Rate Distribution (By Mail and Outside the Mail)	(1)	Free or Nominal Rate Outside-County Copies included on PS Form 3541	29	61
	(2)	Free or Nominal Rate In-County Copies Included on PS Form 3541	0	0
	(3)	Free or Nominal Rate Copies Mailed at Other Classes Through the USPS (e.g. First-Class Mail)	0	0
	(4)	Free or Nominal Rate Distribution Outside the Mail (Carriers or other means)	0	0
e. Total Free or Nominal Rate Distribution (Sum of 15d (1), (2), (3) and (4))		►	29	61
f. Total Distribution (Sum of 15c and 15e)		►	119	191
g. Copies not Distributed (See Instructions to Publishers #4 (page #3))		►	8	13
h. Total (Sum of 15f and g)		►	127	204
i. Percent Paid (15c divided by 15f times 100)		►	75.63%	68.06%

* If you are claiming electronic copies, go to line 16 on page 3. If you are not claiming electronic copies, skip to line 17 on page 3.

16. Electronic Copy Circulation		Average No. Copies Each Issue During Preceding 12 Months	No. Copies of Single Issue Published Nearest to Filing Date
a. Paid Electronic Copies	►	0	0
b. Total Paid Print Copies (Line 15c) + Paid Electronic Copies (Line 16a)	►	90	130
c. Total Print Distribution (Line 15f) + Paid Electronic Copies (Line 16a)	►	119	191
d. Percent Paid (Both Print & Electronic Copies) (16b divided by 16c × 100)	►	75.63%	68.06%

☒ I certify that 50% of all my distributed copies (electronic and print) are paid above a nominal price.

17. Publication of Statement of Ownership

☒ If the publication is a general publication, publication of this statement is required. Will be printed ☐ Publication not required
in the NOVEMBER 2018 issue of this publication.

18. Signature and Title of Editor, Publisher, Business Manager, or Owner   Date

STEPHEN R. BUSHING - INVENTORY DISTRIBUTION CONTROL MANAGER   *Stephen R. Bushing*   9/18/2018

I certify that all information furnished on this form is true and complete. I understand that anyone who furnishes false or misleading information on this form or who omits material or information requested on the form may be subject to criminal sanctions (including fines and imprisonment) and/or civil sanctions (including civil penalties).

PS Form 3526, July 2014 (Page 3 of 4)   PRIVACY NOTICE: See our privacy policy on www.usps.com

Moving?

Make sure your subscription moves with you!

To notify us of your new address, find your **Clinics Account Number** (located on your mailing label above your name), and contact customer service at:

Email: journalscustomerservice-usa@elsevier.com

800-654-2452 (subscribers in the U.S. & Canada)
314-447-8871 (subscribers outside of the U.S. & Canada)

Fax number: **314-447-8029**

Elsevier Health Sciences Division
Subscription Customer Service
3251 Riverport Lane
Maryland Heights, MO 63043

*To ensure uninterrupted delivery of your subscription, please notify us at least 4 weeks in advance of move.

Printed and bound by CPI Group (UK) Ltd, Croydon, CR0 4YY

07/10/2024

01040503-0017